MR Imaging of the Fetus

R. Rajeswaran

MR Imaging of the Fetus

Springer

R. Rajeswaran
Department of Radiology
Sri Ramachandra Institute of Higher Education and Research
Chennai, Tamil Nadu, India

ISBN 978-981-16-9208-6 ISBN 978-981-16-9209-3 (eBook)
https://doi.org/10.1007/978-981-16-9209-3

This Springer imprint is published by the registered company Springer Nature Singapore Pte Ltd.
The registered company address is: 152 Beach Road, #21-01/04 Gateway East, Singapore 189721, Singapore

Dedicated to
My Parents and family members
Who gave me a world to live.
My Teachers
Who showed me how to live in the world.
My patients
Who made my life and world meaningful!

Foreword

I consider it a great privilege to preview the book, "MR imaging of the Fetus." Ultrasound is the primary mode of imaging the fetus. MRI serves as an excellent secondary imaging tool for problem-solving. MRI may confirm or refute ultrasound findings, detect additional findings and sort out differential diagnosis. Ultrasound imaging is often suboptimal due to maternal habitus, fetal position, or oligohydramnios. MRI under these circumstances is indeed a boon. The application of newer MR techniques is opening exciting vistas in fetal imaging.

Dr. Rajeswaran R. is a radiologist with over 20 years of fetal MR imaging experience. He has published several scientific papers dealing with various aspects of fetal MRI. This textbook is the culmination of his rich experience as well as his yen to share the knowledge that he has acquired. The book is well structured into *16* chapters dealing with safety, indications, contraindications, and technique moving on to system-wise applications. The normal fetal MR anatomy has been described in every chapter followed by the abnormalities of that organ system. The text has been constructed in an easy-to-read numbered points format. The book is sumptuously illustrated from the author's vast archives to include a wide range of anomalies. Top-quality images and elaborate annotation aid in effortless interpretation. Wherever necessary the capabilities of MRI vis-à-vis ultrasound have been highlighted. Judicious and appropriate use of fetal MRI is, in itself, a skill that has to be developed and this textbook will go a long way in addressing the same.

I am sure that this book will be a handy resource on the desk of all specialists with an interest in prenatal imaging and diagnosis. I wish Dr. Rajeswaran R. all the very best in all his endeavors.

Srinivasa Ultrasound Scanning Centre
Bangalore, India

B. S. Ramamurthy

Preface

This book presents the anatomy and MRI features of the normal fetus at different gestational ages and describes the anomalies of each system in a systematic way. It also addresses the MRI techniques of fetal examination as the MRI technology is showing rapid advancements. It features a treasure of MR images illustrating several clinical conditions. Sonographic images, schematic diagrams, and post-natal images are supplemented for easy learning. It also addresses the differential diagnoses and prognostic indicators of the various fetal anomalies.

This book will help the residents and consultants involved in fetal care to understand the fetal anomalies and in patient counseling.

Chennai, India R. Rajeswaran

Acknowledgment

I thank **GOD** for showering His blessings, without which this work would have been impossible.

My sincere thanks to the Management of my institution, Sri Ramachandra Institute of Higher Education and Research, Chennai, India.

Special thanks to Prof. Anupama Chandrasekaran, Dr. B.S. Ramamurthy, and Dr. R. Rajkali, who served as my companions in Fetal Imaging and for lending a hand to make this book as complete as possible. I am grateful to my colleagues, gynecologists, neonatologists, pathologists of our institution, and also to the Consultants of Mediscan systems for collaborating in this journey.

I am also grateful to the MR technologists who showed enormous patience to obtain good-quality images. Thanks to the pregnant mothers and their families without whom this would not have been possible.

Finally, my thanks to everyone, whom I could not mention individually but are in my heart as a source of motivation and inspiration.

Contents

1 **Introduction and Indications for Fetal MRI** 1
1.1 Safety of Fetal MRI 1
1.1.1 Static Magnetic Fields 1
1.1.2 Radiofrequency (RF) Fields 1
1.1.3 Time-Varying Magnetic Fields 2
1.2 Contrast Agents During Pregnancy 2
1.3 Indications for Fetal MR Examination 2
1.3.1 Confirmation of Inconclusive Sonographic Findings 2
1.3.2 To Obtain Additional Information/Detect Associated Anomalies or Confirm that the Anomaly Is Isolated 2
1.3.3 Fetus with High Risk for Anomalies Though Sonography Is Normal . . . 3
1.3.4 Technical Difficulty While Performing US 4
1.3.5 Placental Conditions 8
1.4 Timing of MRI Scan 8
1.5 Contraindications 8
References 8

2 **Fetal MR Examination Technique** 11
2.1 The Basic Sequences for Fetal Imaging 11
2.2 Fetal Imaging at 18–20 Weeks 14
2.3 Fetal Volumetry 14
2.4 Dynamic Imaging 14
2.5 Artifacts While Imaging the Fetus 15
2.6 Imaging at 3 Tesla MRI 19
2.7 MR Spectroscopy 20
2.8 Diffusion Tensor Imaging (DTI) 20
2.9 Postmortem Magnetic Resonance Imaging 20
References 20

3 **Embryology and Normal Appearance of Fetal Central Nervous System** 23
3.1 Normal Development of the CNS 23
3.1.1 Induction 23
3.1.2 Dorsal Induction 23
3.1.3 Ventral Induction 23
3.1.4 Proliferation, Migration, and Organization 24
3.2 The Normal Fetal Brain on MRI 25
3.3 The Normal Fetal Spine on MRI 31
References 32

4 **Midline Brain Anomalies I: Anomalies of Septum Pellucidum and Corpus Callosum** 33
4.1 Anomalies of Septum Pellucidum 33

4.1.1 Absent Septum Pellucidum 33
4.1.2 Septo-Optic Dysplasia (SOD) 34
4.1.3 Narrow CSP 35
4.1.4 Enlarged CSP 35
4.1.5 Cyst of Cavum Septi Pellucidi 37
4.1.6 Cavum Vergae and Cavum Vergae Cyst 39
4.1.7 Cavum Veli Interpositi (CVI) and Cyst 40
4.2 Corpus Callosal Abnormalities (CCA) 40
4.2.1 Hypoplastic CC 40
4.2.2 Dysplastic CC 42
4.2.3 Hypoplastic and Dysplastic CC 42
4.2.4 Complete Agenesis 42
4.2.5 Mega Corpus Callosum (MCC) 42
4.2.6 CCA with Interhemispheric Cyst 42
4.2.7 CCA with Pericallosal Lipoma 44
4.2.8 Association 44
References 47

5 Midline Brain Anomalies II: Holoprosencephaly 49
5.1 Embryology 49
5.2 Aprosencephaly, Atelencephaly 49
5.3 Holoprosencephaly (HPE) 49
5.3.1 Alobar HPE 50
5.3.2 Semilobar HPE 51
5.3.3 Lobar HPE 53
5.3.4 Middle Interhemispheric Variant (MIH) 54
5.3.5 Septo Optic Dysplaia 54
5.3.6 Minimal HPE 54
5.3.7 Microform HPE 54
References 54

6 Neural Tube Defects 57
6.1 Cranial Neuropore Defects 57
6.1.1 Anencephaly 57
6.1.2 Encephalocele 58
6.2 Cranial and Caudal Neuropore Defects 59
6.2.1 Craniorachischisis Totalis 59
6.3 Caudal Neuropore Defects 59
6.3.1 Myeloschisis 59
6.3.2 Myelomeningocele (Syn—Spina Bifida Cystica) 61
6.3.3 Hemimyelomeningocele and Hemimyelocele 62
6.3.4 Chiari Malformation 62
6.3.5 Lipomyelomeningoceles, Lipomeningocele and Lipomyelocele 64
6.3.6 Meningocele 64
6.3.7 Myelocystocele 65
6.3.8 Caudal Regression Syndrome (CRS) 67
6.3.9 Dorsal Dermal Sinus Tract (DDS) 67
6.3.10 Diastematomyelia 67
6.3.11 Lipoma 68
6.3.12 Tethered Cord/Tight Filum Terminale Syndrome 69
6.4 Scoliosis 69
6.5 Sacrococcygeal Teratoma (SCT) 70
References 71

7 Ventriculomegaly 73
7.1 Ventriculomegaly 73
7.2 Aqueductal Stenosis 74
7.3 Ventriculomegaly Due to Infection 75
7.4 Approach to Mild and Moderate Ventriculomegaly 76
7.5 Unilateral Ventriculomegaly 78
References 78

8 Posterior Fossa Anomalies 81
8.1 Embryology 81
8.2 The MR Imaging Checklist While Examining the Posterior Fossa 81
8.3 Cystic Malformations 82
8.3.1 Mega Cisterna Magna 82
8.3.2 Blake's Pouch Cyst (BPC) 84
8.3.3 Vermian Hypoplasia 85
8.3.4 Dandy–Walker Malformation 85
8.3.5 Posterior Fossa Arachnoid Cyst 86
8.4 Hypoplasia 86
8.4.1 Global Cerebellar Hypoplasia 86
8.4.2 Unilateral Cerebellar Hypoplasia 86
8.4.3 Ponto-Cerebellar Hypoplasia 88
8.4.4 Vermian Agenesis 88
8.5 Dysgenesis 90
8.5.1 Rhombencephalosynapsis 90
8.5.2 Joubert Syndrome and Molar Tooth Sign Related Disorders 90
8.5.3 Kinked/z-Shaped Brainstem 92
8.5.4 Cerebellar Cortical Dysplasia 92
8.5.5 Ponto Tegmental Cap Dysplasia 92
8.6 Chiari Malformations 92
References 93

9 Abnormalities of Proliferation, Neuronal Migration, and Cortical Organization 95
9.1 Embryology 95
9.2 Group I: Abnormal Cell Proliferation or Apoptosis 99
9.2.1 Microcephaly 99
9.2.2 Megalencephaly 100
9.2.3 Abnormal Proliferation: Abnormal Cell Type—Tuberous Sclerosis 101
9.3 Group II: Abnormal Neuronal Migration 102
9.3.1 Diffuse Neuronal Migration Arrest: Classical Lissencephaly (Type I) 103
9.3.2 Neuronal Overmigration: Cobblestone Lissencephaly (Type 2) 103
9.3.3 Focal Neuronal Migration Arrest: Heterotopia 103
9.4 Group III: Abnormal Post Migrational Development (Organization) 104
9.4.1 Polymicrogyria (PMG) 105
9.4.2 Schizencephaly 105
9.4.3 Cortical Dysplasia 106
9.5 Group IV: Inborn Errors of Metabolism 107
References 107

10 Intracranial Cysts, Tumors, and Masses . . . 109
10.1 Intracranial Cysts . . . 109
10.1.1 Arachnoid Cyst . . . 109
10.1.2 Porencephalic Cyst . . . 109
10.1.3 Choroid Plexus Cyst . . . 111
10.1.4 Periventricular Pseudocysts . . . 111
10.2 Vascular Abnormalities . . . 111
10.2.1 Vein of Galen Malformation . . . 111
10.2.2 Dural Sinus Malformation (DSM) . . . 112
10.3 Tumors . . . 113
10.3.1 Teratoma . . . 113
10.3.2 Lipoma . . . 113
References . . . 114

11 Intracranial Hemorrhage, Destructive Pathologies, and Infection . . . 115
11.1 Intracranial Hemorrhage . . . 115
11.2 Encephalomalacia . . . 115
11.3 In Utero Infections . . . 116
11.3.1 Cytomegalovirus . . . 117
11.3.2 Toxoplasmosis . . . 118
11.3.3 Rubella . . . 119
11.3.4 Human Parvovirus B19 . . . 119
11.3.5 Zika Virus (ZIKV) . . . 120
References . . . 120

12 Fetal Face and Neck Anomalies . . . 121
12.1 Cleft Lip and Palate . . . 121
12.2 Fetal Goiter . . . 122
12.3 Cystic Hygroma . . . 123
12.4 Cervical Teratoma . . . 126
12.5 Abnormal Orbits . . . 126
12.6 Micrognathia–Retrognathia . . . 126
References . . . 128

13 Fetal Thoracic Anomalies . . . 129
13.1 Bronchopulmonary Anomalies . . . 130
13.1.1 Pulmonary Underdevelopment . . . 130
13.1.2 Congenital Pulmonary Airway Malformations (CPAM) . . . 130
13.1.3 Bronchopulmonary Sequestration (BPS) . . . 132
13.1.4 Congenital Lobar Overinflation (CLO) . . . 132
13.1.5 Bronchogenic Cyst . . . 134
13.1.6 Bronchial Atresia . . . 135
13.2 Diaphragmatic Anomalies . . . 135
13.2.1 Congenital Diaphragmatic Hernia (CDH) . . . 135
13.2.2 Congenital Diaphragmatic Eventration (CDE) . . . 136
13.3 Mediastinal Cysts and Masses . . . 137
13.4 Pleural Effusion . . . 137
13.5 Fetal Cardiovascular System . . . 137
References . . . 140

14 Fetal Gastrointestinal and Abdominal Wall Anomalies . . . 141
14.1 Esophageal Atresia . . . 143
14.2 Duodenal Atresia . . . 144
14.3 Jejunal/Ileal Atresia . . . 144
14.4 Colonic Atresia . . . 144

14.5 Anal Atresia 145
14.6 Cloaca 145
14.7 Choledochal Cyst 146
14.8 Hepatic Tumors and Hemochromatosis 147
14.8.1 Congenital Hepatic Hemangioma 147
14.8.2 Mesenchymal Hepatic Hamartoma 147
14.8.3 Hepatoblastoma 147
14.8.4 Neonatal Hemochromatosis 147
14.9 Omphalocele 147
14.10 Heterotaxy 147
14.11 Fetal Ascites 148
References 150

15 Fetal Genito Urinary System Anomalies and Miscellaneous Conditions 153
15.1 Genito Urinary System Anomalies 153
15.1.1 Unilateral Renal Agenesis 154
15.1.2 Ectopic Kidney 154
15.1.3 Fusion Abnormality of Kidneys 154
15.1.4 Multicystic Dysplastic Kidney 154
15.1.5 Obstructive Uropathy 155
15.1.6 Mesoblastic Nephroma 157
15.1.7 Adrenal Neuroblastoma 157
15.1.8 Ovarian Cyst 158
15.2 Musculoskeletal System 160
15.3 Miscellaneous Fetal Conditions 161
15.3.1 Fetal Growth Restriction (FGR) 161
15.3.2 Hydrops Fetalis 161
15.3.3 Twin–Twin Transfusion Syndrome (TTTS) 161
15.3.4 Single Umbilical Artery 162
References 164

16 Placental Diseases, Ectopic Pregnancy, and Other Obstetric Applications 167
References 179

Abbreviations

ADC	Apparent diffusion coefficient
CC	Corpus callosum
CDH	Congenital diaphragmatic hernia
CMV	Cytomegalovirus
CNS	Central Nervous System
CSF	Cerebrospinal fluid
CSP	Cavum Septum pellucidum
DSM	Dural sinus malformation
DTI	Diffusion tensor imaging
DWI	Diffusion-weighted imaging
EPI	Echo planar imaging
EXIT procedure	Ex Utero Intrapartum Treatment
FGR	Fetal growth restriction
FIESTA	Fast Imaging Employing Steady State Acquisition
FISP	Fast imaging with steady precession
FLASH	Fast Low Angle Shot
FOV	Field of view
FSE	Fast spin-echo
FSPGR	Fast Spoiled Gradient Echo
GRASS	Gradient- refocused or recalled acquisition in the steady state
GRE	Gradient Recalled Echo
HASTE	Half Fourier Acquisition Single Shot Turbo Spine Echo
HPE	Holoprosencephaly
LSCS	Lower Segment Cesarean Section
MR/MRI	Magnetic Resonance Imaging
NTD	Neural tube defect
RARE	Rapid acquisition with relaxation enhancement
RF	Radiofrequency
ROI	Region of Interest
SAR	Specific Absorption Ratio
SNR	Signal to Noise Ratio
SOD	Septo-optic dysplasia
SSFSE	Single-shot Fast spin-echo
TORCH	Toxoplasmosis, Other [Varicella-Zoster, syphilis], Rubella, Cytomegalovirus, Herpes
T1w	T1-weighted
T2w	T2-weighted
US/USG	Ultrasonography
WI	Weighted images

1 Introduction and Indications for Fetal MRI

Sonography (USG) is the primary modality in imaging fetuses as it is widely available, accurate, inexpensive, and allows real-time examination of the fetus. It is also widely used in imaging pregnant patients with pelvic and abdominal pathologies. However, USG is operator dependent and suffers from limitations like inability to image a large field of view (FOV), limited contrast resolution, inability to differentiate hemorrhage from fluids, poor acoustic window in advanced pregnancy, and obesity. MRI is the preferred alternative modality for fetal imaging when there are limitations on sonography and when the findings are inconclusive [1].

MR imaging during pregnancy was first described by Smith et al. in 1983 [2]. In the early studies, maternal sedation by administering benzodiazepine or fetal paralysis by directly injecting pancuronium was employed to suppress fetal motion. Subsequently, fetal MR imaging has been revolutionized with the advent of ultra-fast sequences, high channel coils, and better scanners [3–5]. Presently sedation techniques are infrequently used.

MRI is also being increasingly used in pelvic and abdominal pathologies associated with pregnancy and in placental abnormalities [6]. With advancing pregnancy and posteriorly located pathologies like posterior placenta previa, MRI has a definite role when US may not be able to clearly delineate the abnormalities. MRI is useful in uterine pathologies like red degeneration because of its ability to characterize the various stages of hemorrhage. MRI is complementary to US in the diagnosis of placenta accreta, unusual ectopic pregnancies, and abruptio placenta because of its ability to image a large FOV, detect hemorrhage, and produce high image contrast.

1.1 Safety of Fetal MRI

Several reports in literature indicate that fetal MRI is safe during pregnancy [3, 5]. MRI scanners up to 3 Tesla and below are being routinely used for fetal examinations and there had been no adverse effect reported so far. As per the American College of Radiology (ACR) guidance document published in 2015, MRI can be performed at any stage of pregnancy if risk-benefit ratio to the patient warrants that the study is performed. Written informed consent needs to be taken from all patients. Potential harmful effects due to MR examination are mainly due to the following causes [7]:

1.1.1 Static Magnetic Fields

This refers to the constant fields due to the main magnet, which do not change in strength or direction over time. To ensure safety, it is important that a full metal-related questionnaire is completed with the pregnant women. This will ensure that they do not inadvertently carry any metallic objects into the scanning room. Similarly, the history of metallic implants needs to be elicited as they can cause heating effects or localized artifacts.

Pregnant MRI workers exposed to the static magnetic field have not shown any significant adverse effects [8]. Several MRI examinations have been performed during the first trimester for maternal reasons and there had been no adverse effects reported so far [9, 10].

1.1.2 Radiofrequency (RF) Fields

The potential harmful effect associated with RF waves is heating effect. Each pulse sequence has a specified Specific Absorption ratio (SAR) being mentioned by the scanner manufacturer [7]. The fetus is sensitive to elevated temperature during organogenesis, the Central Nervous System being more vulnerable. In human fetuses a temperature rise of 2 °C for 24 h or more can result in craniofacial and neural tube defects. It has been recommended to keep the maternal body temperature below 37.5 °C to prevent adverse effects in the fetus. This will ensure that the fetal temperature is 38 °C or less. (The normal fetal body temperature is 0.5 °C higher than that of the maternal body temperature.)

R. Rajeswaran, *MR Imaging of the Fetus*, https://doi.org/10.1007/978-981-16-9209-3_1

1.1.3 Time-Varying Magnetic Fields

This refers to the high volume of noise generated by the gradient coils when they receive electrical pulses. These electric pulses make the coils vibrate and produce a loud noise. The potential harmful effects due to the pulsed electromagnetic gradient fields are - biological effects, acoustic noise damage and rarely peripheral nerve stimulation, muscle stimulation, and cardiac fibrillation. The biological effect of time-varying electromagnetic fields has been reviewed and no measurable adverse effects have so far been recorded. Similarly, there had been no significant adverse effects relating to anxiety levels/stress levels/intelligence quotient/reaction time, memory disturbances, nerve stimulation, and teratogenicity [11]. MR examination can generate noise of 80–100 db depending upon the type of sequence and this may be partially attenuated by the maternal tissues and amniotic fluid. As occupational prolonged exposure of noise greater than 99 dB during pregnancy are associated with hearing loss, decreased birth weight, and shortened gestation, it is recommended to keep the effective noise levels for the fetus below 65 db [12, 13]. Louder sequences may be used with reduced acquisition time or after the application of noise reduction software [7].

1.2 Contrast Agents During Pregnancy

It is better to avoid MRI contrast agents in pregnant women. Gadolinium is a pregnancy class C drug, i.e., the safety has not been fully established. Gadolinium can cross the placenta into the fetal circulation and is excreted by the fetal kidneys into the amniotic fluid. It is then swallowed by the fetus, and due to this cycle, can remain in the circulation for a long period. The adverse effects of gadolinium on the developing fetus are unknown and hence is not recommended [14, 15]. Gadolinium injection should be limited to conditions where the benefits will outweigh the potential risks. The potential risks include stillbirth, inflammatory/infiltrative conditions of the skin and they are very rare [16]. However, gadolinium can be administered to mothers if the situation warrants, and breastfeeding need not be interrupted after gadolinium administration.

1.3 Indications for Fetal MR Examination

The indications for fetal MR examination depend to a large extent on the local availability of quality Sonography centers. MRI referrals from dedicated Sonography centers may be infrequent.

The important indications are discussed in the following section [17]. Detailed discussion on the indications regarding a particular organ or system can be found in the concerned chapters.

1.3.1 Confirmation of Inconclusive Sonographic Findings

Corpus callosal anomalies—MRI is useful to confirm the diagnosis of agenesis of corpus callosum, to identify hypoplastic/dysplastic corpus callosum (Fig. 1.1) [18] and the associated lipoma.

Posterior fossa anomalies—MR is complementary to US in the diagnosis of cerebellar anomalies and is extremely useful to diagnose conditions like Joubert syndrome. The excellent sagittal depiction helps in the diagnosis of ponto-cerebellar hypoplasia, ponto-tegmental cap dysplasia, Blake's pouch cyst, and kinked brainstem [19–21].

MR is also useful to identify *migrational abnormalities, lissencephaly, and cortical dysplasia* (Fig. 1.2). The sulcation at various gestational ages is also better visualized by MRI [22].

Sometimes in *septal agenesis*, the fornix may falsely appear as septum on US and MRI is useful to clarify this by virtue of its coronal imaging [23].

1.3.2 To Obtain Additional Information/Detect Associated Anomalies or Confirm that the Anomaly Is Isolated

Ventriculomegaly- Isolated mild and moderate ventriculomegaly carry a good prognosis and MRI is useful to demonstrate additional anomalies like heterotopia, cortical malformation, encephalomalacia (Fig. 1.3) which may not be obvious on US [24].

In anomalies of *corpus callosum, cavum septum pellucidum*, etc., MRI is useful to demonstrate additional sonographically occult anomalies.

Intracranial hemorrhage—Fetal intracranial hemorrhage is sometimes misdiagnosed as a mass lesion on US. Besides US is not sensitive to subarachnoid and intraventricular extension of the hemorrhage. MRI is useful to identify the size, stage of hemorrhage, intraventricular/subarachnoid/intraparenchymal extensions (Fig. 1.4), and the ischemic component when present [25].

In *fetal masses and cysts*, MRI is useful to characterize the lesion and to demonstrate the mass effect/infiltration of adjacent structures.

Face and Neck—MRI is useful in demonstration of facial clefts [26, 27], retrognathism (Fig. 1.5), neck masses, and the airway compromise.

In *Congenital diaphragmatic hernia/eventration and other thoracic anomalies* MRI is useful to obtain fetal lung volume which is more accurate than US. The volume of the herniated liver can also be calculated (Fig. 1.6a, b) [28]. This information is important for counseling the couple and for the management of the fetus. MRI is also useful to demon-

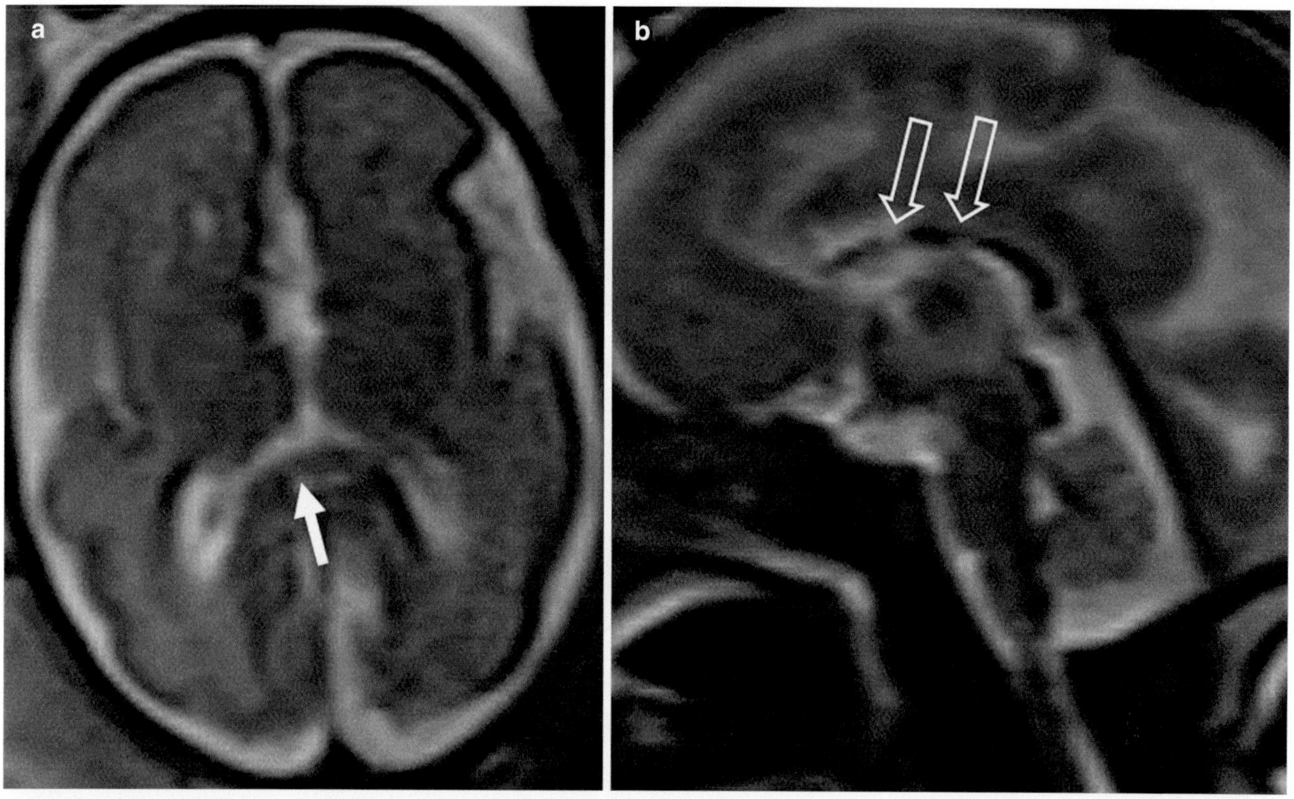

Fig. 1.1 Axial T2W image (**a**) of a 29-week fetus showing the absence of genu of CC, cavum septum pellucidum and the presence of splenium (arrow). Sagittal T2W image (**b**) showing diffuse thinning and irregularity of CC (open arrows) and the absence of genu suggesting hypoplasia with dysplasia. There was a suspicion of dysplastic corpus callosum on sonography. CC-corpus callosum

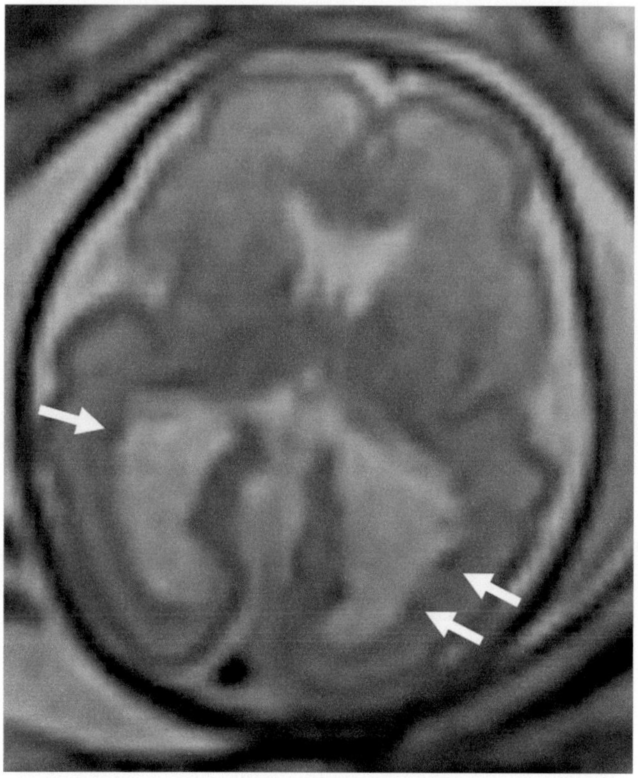

Fig. 1.2 Axial T2W image of a fetus shows ventriculomegaly with associated bilateral periventricular nodular heterotopia

strate the position and dimensions of the great vessels though it is so far not indicated for cardiac anomalies.

Genitourinary system—MR is useful to identify ectopic kidneys (Fig. 1.7). On DWI fetal kidney appears hyperintense and is easily demonstrable. In complex cloacal abnormalities and complicated ovarian cysts, MR is complementary to US.

Abdomen—Liver appears hyperintense on T1WI (Fig. 1.6b) and is better delineated by MRI in CDH, heterotaxy and heptomegaly. MR is useful in conditions like congenital hemochromatosis, intraabdominal sequestration, neuroblastoma, and complex abdominal masses [29].

1.3.3 Fetus with High Risk for Anomalies Though Sonography Is Normal

'Familial Genetic disorders—In fetuses having family history of congenital anomalies like Joubert syndrome and metabolic disorders, MRI is complementary to US to exclude anomalies (Fig. 1.8a, b).

Feto-maternal infection—In mothers diagnosed to have infections like CMV, toxoplasmosis, MRI is an additional tool besides amniocentesis to exclude malformations (Fig. 1.9a, b, c).

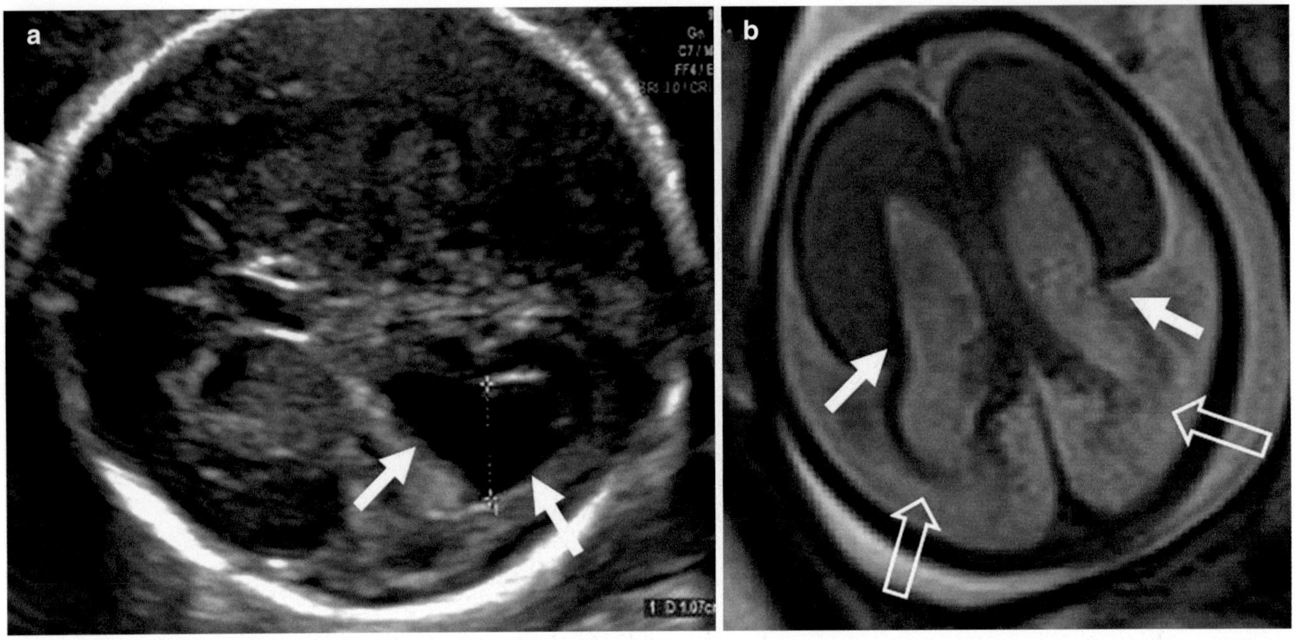

Fig. 1.3 Sonographic image of a 26-week fetus (**a**) shows ventriculomegaly (arrows). Axial MR image (**b**) shows ventriculomegaly with associated encephalomalacia (open arrows) of bilateral parieto occipital lobes

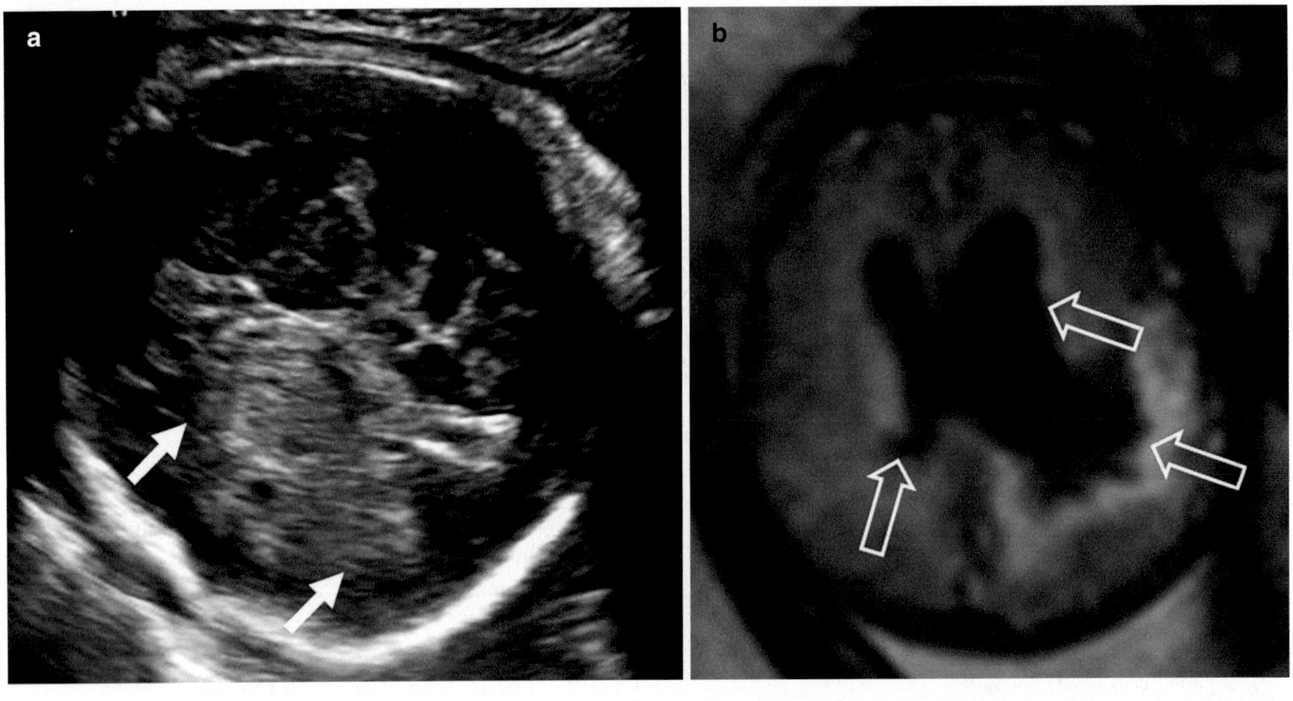

Fig. 1.4 Sonographic image of a 34-week fetus (**a**) shows an echogenic "mass" (arrows) in the left cerebral hemisphere. Axial T2W image (**b**) shows germinal matrix hemorrhage with intraventricular and intraparenchymal extension (open arrows)

In fetuses with *Twin-to-Twin transfusion Syndrome and co-twin demise,* MRI is useful to demonstrate acute/chronic ischemic changes (Fig. 1.10a, b).

Previous syndromic baby, previous stillbirths, recent maternal trauma—when the couple are anxious about the ongoing pregnancy MRI helps in reassuring them.

1.3.4 Technical Difficulty While Performing US

Factors such as maternal obesity, thickened/scarred maternal anterior abdominal wall, and oligohydramnios may hinder satisfactory US imaging of the fetus. MR imaging is not

Fig. 1.5 Sagittal T2W images of a 34-week fetus showing severe retrognathism (arrow). The airway is severely narrowed (open arrows). The fetus was delivered by EXIT procedure and tracheostomy was performed subsequently

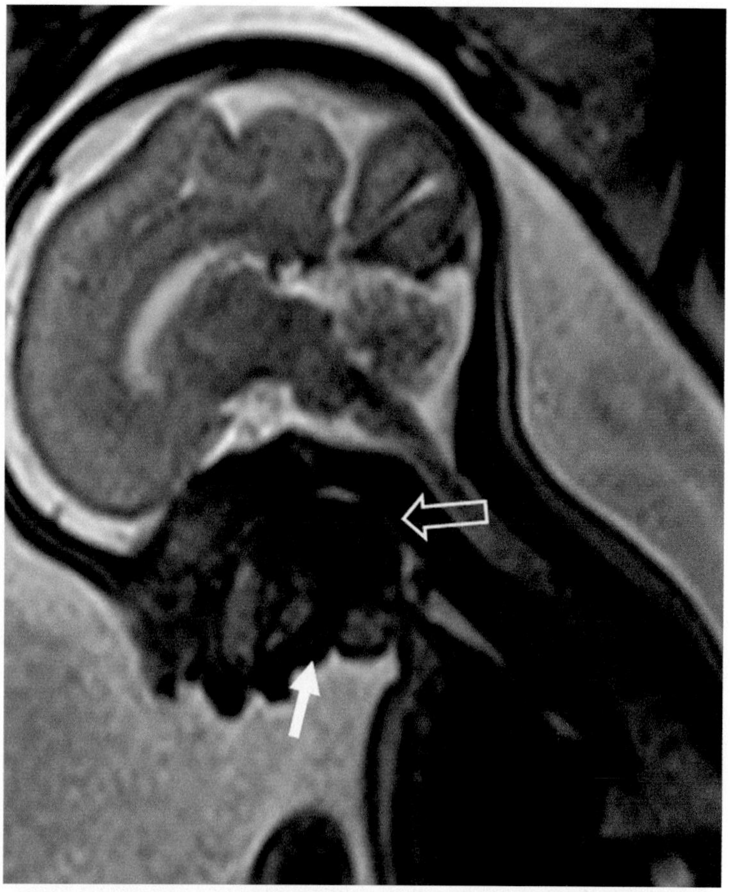

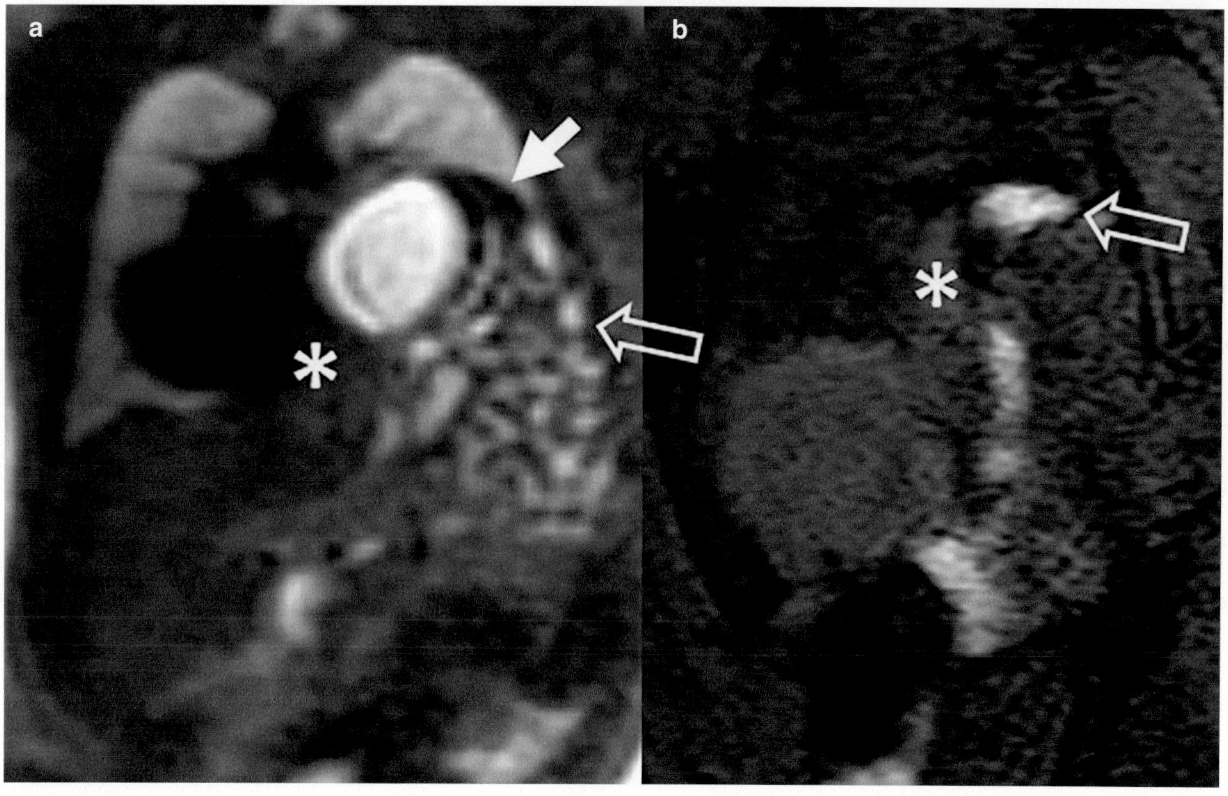

Fig. 1.6 Coronal T2 (**a**), Coronal T1W (**b**) Images, showing eventration of left hemidiaphragm. The left hemidiaphragm is seen as a thin dark band (arrow). The stomach, left lobe of liver (asterisk), small bowel, large bowel (open arrows) are seen at the level of thorax. The left lobe of liver, large bowel appear hyperintense on T1W images

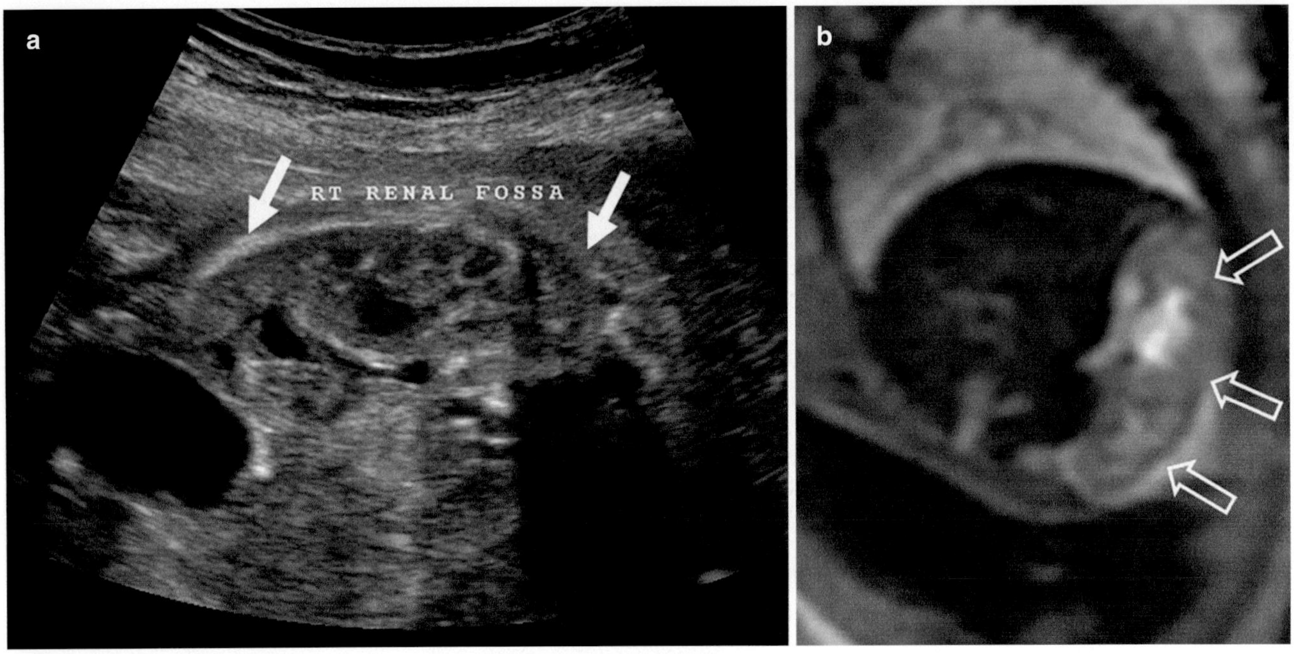

Fig. 1.7 Sonographic (**a**) image shows an "enlarged kidney" in the right renal fossa (arrow). Sagittal T2w MR image (**b**) shows crossed fused ectopia of the left kidney (open arrows)

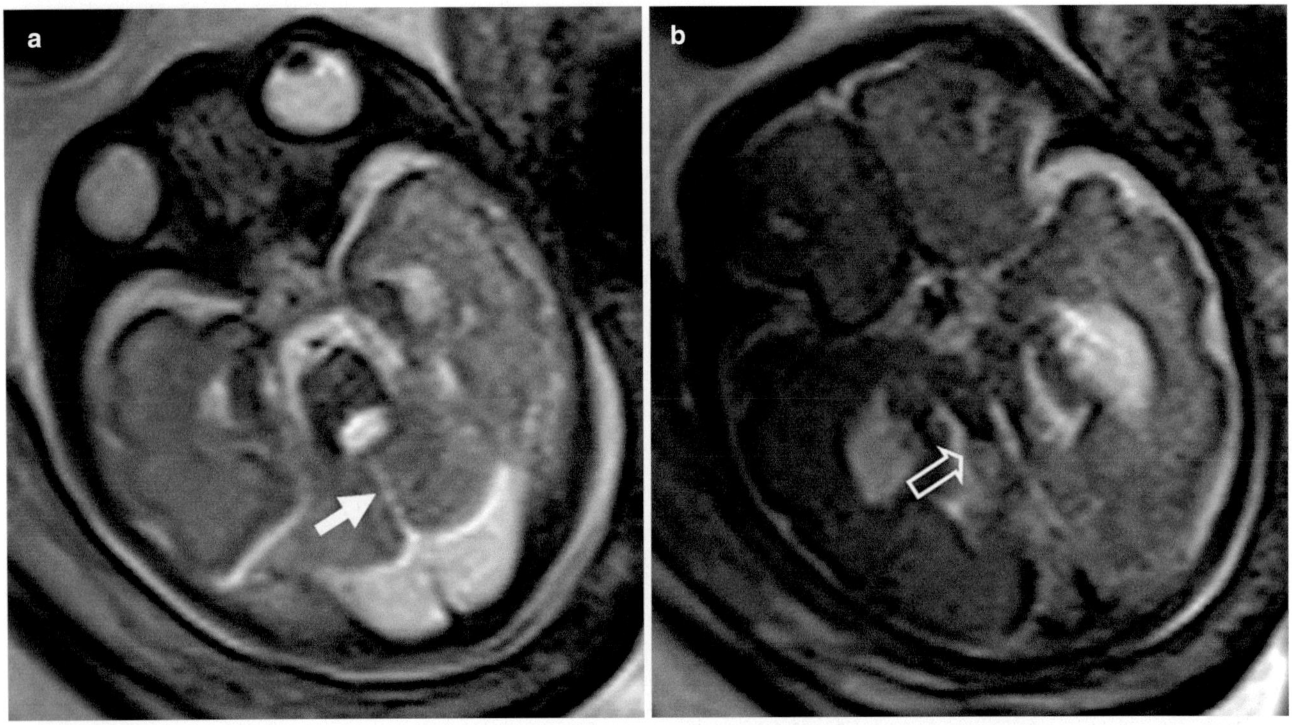

Fig. 1.8 The previous child had Joubert syndrome and the ongoing pregnancy was referred for fetal MRI. Axial (**a**, **b**) images of the 30-week fetus show absence of the vermis (arrow). Bilateral superior cerebellar peduncles are elongated (open arrows) giving a molar tooth appearance to midbrain suggesting Joubert syndrome

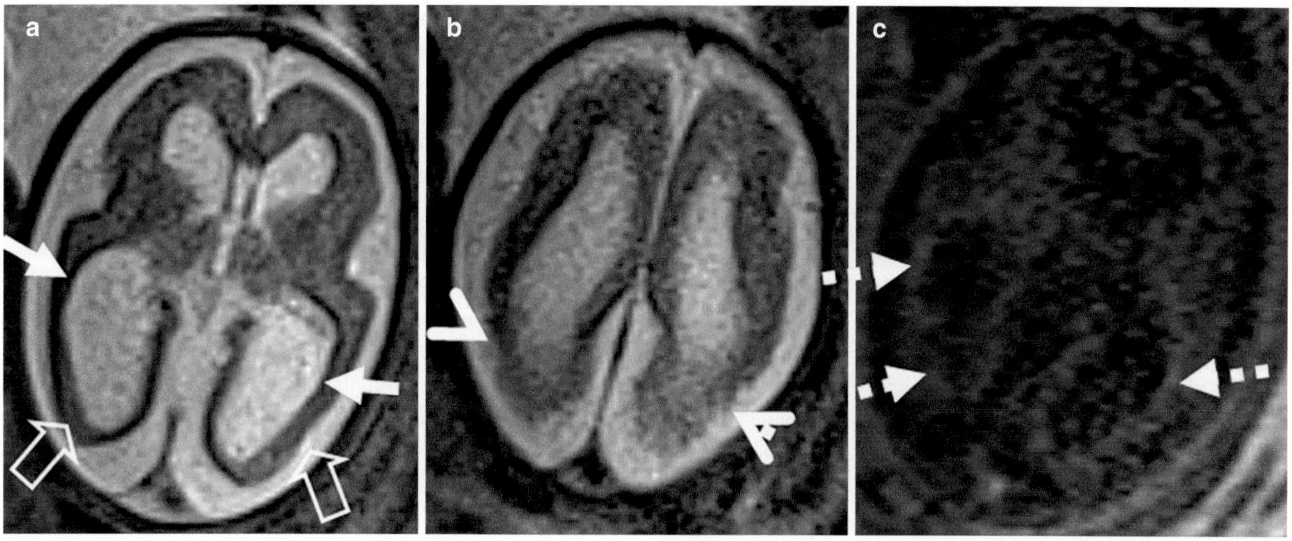

Fig. 1.9 Axial (**a**, **b**) T2W images of a 31-week CMV infected fetus show ventriculomegaly, diffuse cerebral cortical thinning with generalized reduced sulcation and polymicrogyria (arrowheads). Axial (**c**) T1W image shows numerous small periventricular hyperintense foci (broken arrows) suggesting calcifications

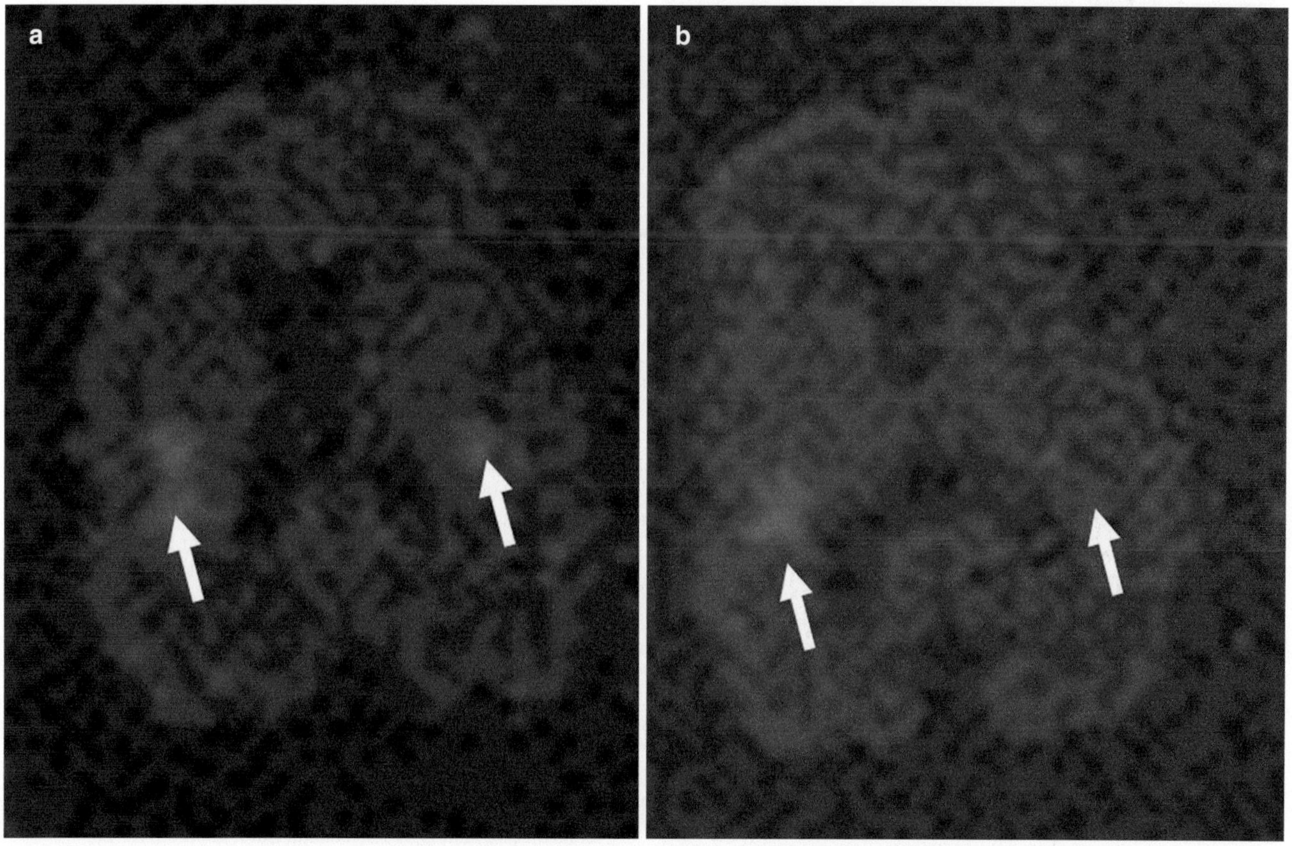

Fig. 1.10 Axial diffusion-weighted images (**a**, **b**) showing acute infarcts in bilateral parietal region in the surviving twin following co-twin demise

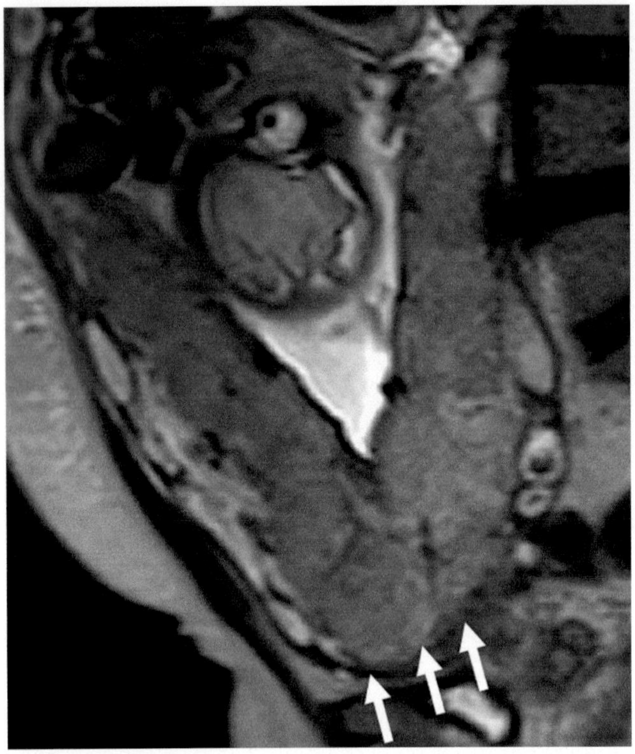

Fig. 1.11 Sagittal T2 image of a 36-year-old woman with history of previous Cesarean section, shows placenta previa with loss of interface and focal bulge (arrows) and heterogenous placenta. Elective Cesarean section confirmed the diagnosis of placenta acreta and obstetric hysterectomy was performed

affected by these factors and hence is preferred to overcome these shortcomings.

1.3.5 Placental Conditions

MR is useful in the assessment of placenta acreta (Fig. 1.11), placental tumors, placental ischemia associated with fetal growth retardation (FGR). In chronic maternal illnesses like SLE and antiphospholipid Antibody syndrome, MRI is useful in the placental evaluation to diagnose infarcts, edema, and intervillous thrombosis [30].

1.4 Timing of MRI Scan

MRI scan may be performed as soon as the anomaly is detected on sonography, 19–24 weeks is preferable. Legal termination of pregnancy varies in different countries and is generally between 20 and 24 weeks. MRI scan at the appropriate time will help the couple to make a decision on further continuation of pregnancy [31].

A third trimester MRI scan is useful to demonstrate cortical malformations and migrational disorders. MR examination may also be needed prior to some EXIT procedures (e.g., fetus with neck mass) [32]. Similarly, MRI is indicated toward term if there is a suspicion that the immediate postnatal period will be stormy and unstable and postnatal MRI evaluation may not be possible.

1.5 Contraindications

Contraindications to MR examination include the presence of a Pacemaker, patient in labor, or an unstable patient. Claustrophobia can be managed by appropriate counseling or feet first examination or patient sedation.

References

1. Levine D, Barnes PD, Edelman RR. Obstetric MR imaging. Radiology. 1999;211:609–17.
2. Smith F, Adam A, Phillips W. NMR imaging in pregnancy. Lancet. 1983;1:61–2.
3. Levine D. Ultrasound versus magnetic resonance imaging in fetal evaluation. Top Magn Reson Imaging. 2001;12:25–38.
4. Quinn TM, Hubbard AM, Adzick NS. Prenatal magnetic resonance imaging enhances fetal diagnosis. J Paediatr Surg. 1998;33:553–8.
5. Rajeswaran R, Chandrasekharan A, Joseph S, Venkata Sai PM, Dev B, Reddy S. Ultrasound versus MRI in the diagnosis of fetal head and trunk anomalies. J Matern-Fetal Neonatal Med. 2009;22(2):115–23.
6. Nagenthran G, Rangasami R, Chandrasekharan A, et al. Role of magnetic resonance imaging in pregnancy-associated obstetric and gynecological complications. Egypt J Radiol Nucl Med. 2019;50:98. https://doi.org/10.1186/s43055-019-0112-x.
7. Story L, Rutherford M. Advances and applications in fetal magnetic resonance imaging. Obstet Gynaecol. 2015;17:189–99.
8. Kanal E, Gillen J, Evans JA, Savitz DA, Shellock FG. Survey of reproductive health among female MR workers. Radiology. 1993;187:395–9.
9. Arai Y, Nabe K, Ikeda H, Honjo S, Wada Y, Hamamoto Y, et al. A case of lymphocytic panhypophysitis (LPH) during pregnancy. Endocrine. 2007;32:117–21.
10. Patenaude Y, Pugash D, Lim K, Morin L, Lim K, Bly S, et al. The use of magnetic resonance imaging in the obstetric patient. J Obstet Gynaecol Can. 2014;36:349–63.
11. De Wilde JP, Rivers AW, Price DL. A review of the current use of magnetic resonance imaging in pregnancy and safety implications for the fetus. Prog Biophys Mol Biol. 2005;87:335–53.
12. American Academy of Pediatrics. Committee on Environmental Health. Noise: a hazard for the fetus and newborn. Pediatrics. 1997;100:724–7.
13. Darcy AE, Hancock LE, Ware EJ. A descriptive study of noise in the neonatal intensive care unit: ambient levels and perceptions of contributing factors. Adv Neonatal Care. 2008;8:S16–26.
14. Gupta R, Bajaj SK, Kumar N, et al. Magnetic resonance imaging - a troubleshooter in obstetric emergencies: a pictorial review. Indian J Radiol Imaging. 2016;26:44–51.
15. Shellock FG, Kanal E. Safety of magnetic resonance imaging contrast agents. J Magn Reson Imaging. 1999;10:477–84.
16. Ray JG, Vermeulen MJ, Bharatha A, Montanera WJ, Park AL. Association between MRI exposure during pregnancy and fetal and childhood outcomes. JAMA. 2016;316:952–61.

17. Prayer D, Brugger PC, Asenbaum U. Indications for fetal MRI. In: Prayer D, editor. Fetal MRI. Medical radiology. Berlin: Springer; 2010. https://doi.org/10.1007/174_2010_24.
18. Manor C, Rangasami R, Suresh I, Suresh S. Magnetic resonance imaging findings in fetal corpus callosal developmental abnormalities: a pictorial essay. J Pediatr Neurosci. 2020;15:352–7.
19. Mahalingam HV, Rangasami R, Seshadri S, Suresh I. Imaging spectrum of posterior fossa anomalies on foetal magnetic resonance imaging with an algorithmic approach to diagnosis. Pol J Radiol. 2021;86:e183–94. https://doi.org/10.5114/pjr.2021.105014.
20. Lerman-Sagie T, Prayer D, Stöcklein S, Malinger G. Fetal cerebellar disorders. Handb Clin Neurol. 2018;155:3–23.
21. Shekdar K. Posterior fossa malformations. Semin Ultrasound CT MR. 2011;32(3):228–41.
22. Azoulay R, Fallet-Bianco C, Garel C, Grabar S, Kalifa G, Adamsbaum C. MRI of the olfactory bulbs and sulci in human fetuses. Pediatr Radiol. 2006;36(2):97–107.
23. Usman N, Rangasami R, Ramachandran R. 'Pseudo-septum' appearance in septal agenesis on fetal MRI. J Fetal Med. 2021; https://doi.org/10.1007/s40556-021-00300-y.
24. Mailath-Pokorny M, Tauscher V, Krampl-Bettelheim E, Prayer D, Messerschmidt A, Brugger PC. P05.14: fetal cerebral ventriculomegaly: prenatal diagnosis, chromosomal abnormalities and associated anomalies in 146 fetuses. Ultrasound Obstet Gynecol. 2009;34:196.
25. Prayer D, Brugger PC. Investigation of normal organ development with fetal MRI. Eur Radiol. 2007;17(10):2458–71.
26. Robson CD, Barnewolt CE. MR imaging of fetal head and neck anomalies. Neuroimaging Clin N Am. 2004;14(2):273–91.
27. Mirsky DM, Shekdar KV, Bilaniuk LT. Fetal MRI: head and neck. Magn Reson Imaging Clin N Am. 2012;20(3):605–18.
28. Cannie M, Jani J, Chaffiotte C, Vaast P, Deruelle P, Houfflin-Debarge V, Dymarkowski S, Deprest J. Quantification of intrathoracic liver herniation by magnetic resonance imaging and prediction of postnatal survival in fetuses with congenital diaphragmatic hernia. Ultrasound Obstet Gynecol. 2008;32(5):627–32.
29. Manganaro L, Antonelli A, Bernardo S, Capozza F, Petrillo R, Satta S, Vinci V, Saldari M, Maccioni F, Ballesio L, Catalano C. Highlights on MRI of the fetal body. Radiol Med. 2018;123(4):271–85.
30. Meroni PL, di Simone N, Testoni C, D'Asta M, Acaia B, Caruso A. Antiphospholipid antibodies as cause of pregnancy loss. Lupus. 2004;13(9):649–52.
31. Ramdass S, Adam S, Lockhat Z, Masenge A, Suleman FE. Foetal magnetic resonance imaging: a necessity or adjunct? A modality comparison of *in-utero* ultrasound and ultrafast foetal magnetic resonance imaging. SA J Radiol. 2021;25(1):2010. https://doi.org/10.4102/sajr.v25i1.2010.
32. Walz PC, Schroeder JW Jr. Prenatal diagnosis of obstructive head and neck masses and perifnatal airway management: the ex-utero intrapartum treatment procedure. Otolaryngol Clin N Am. 2015;48(1):191–207.

2 Fetal MR Examination Technique

The fetal MR examination can be challenging because of fetal movements, small size of the fetal organs, dynamic changes in the fast-growing fetus, and maternal factors like habitus and breathing movements. These can be overcome by appropriate patient–coil positioning, using higher channel coils, applying parallel imaging, more signal averaging (NEX), and phase oversampling methods [1, 2]. Prior patient counseling and encouraging her to take shallow breaths can reduce the motion artifacts arising from the mother.

Either a torso or cardiac phased array surface coil is used for fetal imaging. The scan, which may last for 30–45 min, is done with the mother in supine. In case the mother is not able to lie supine as may happen in the third trimester, due to back pain or respiratory difficulty, then the MR examination can be performed in the left lateral decubitus position. The feet-first examination helps to avoid claustrophobia. Ultrafast MRI sequences are employed to limit the effects of fetal motion [3–5]. These sequences generate images at the rate of 1 image in less than a second. Maternal fasting 3 h before the MR examination also helps in reducing fetal motion.

It is important to follow patient safety protocol by using a standard questionnaire to exclude metallic objects and contraindicating factors. The mother needs to be explained about the procedure in detail and an informed consent has to be taken. It is better to know the indication for fetal MRI and the US findings prior to the study. This will facilitate optimal MR imaging and use of optional sequences appropriately. For example, GRE sequence may be needed to assess calcifications/hemorrhage in a case of suspected fetal intracranial infection/hemorrhage.

Initially, localizer images with respect to the maternal lower abdomen are obtained in three orthogonal planes using a 6-mm HASTE/SSFSE sequence, with a 1-mm interslice gap, and large field of view (FOV) (Fig. 2.1a, b). The localizer is useful in identifying the position of the fetus and its sidedness. The localizer is also useful to verify that that maximal signal intensity is obtained from the region that needs to be scanned. It is important to reposition the coil after the localizer scan, if required, to obtain maximum Signal-to-Noise Ratio (SNR).

From this localizer set, HASTE T2 weighted images are then obtained in axial, coronal, and sagittal planes with respect to the fetal head or trunk (Fig. 2.1c, d). Multiple acquisitions may be necessary to obtain optimal images. We routinely acquire at least three sets of images in each plane as information lost in any image due to artifacts may be compensated from the other set of images. A FOV of 24–30 cm and slice thickness of 3–4 mm is recommended. Images can be acquired during maternal free breathing or using respiratory triggering. The parameters used in our institution for fetal imaging are given in Table 2.1.

Some machines have interactive scanning techniques that allow adjustment of scanning parameters, such as section orientation and angle, in "real-time" [6]. The technologist can thus correct the angle/orientation of prescribed forthcoming images in case the fetus moves in the middle of the scan. Using this technique, true axial, coronal, and sagittal images can be obtained more rapidly.

2.1 The Basic Sequences for Fetal Imaging

1. T2/T2* weighted imaging using Half-Fourier Single-shot Turbo spin-Echo (HASTE/SSFSE), true fast imaging with steady-state free precession (trueFISP/FIESTA), respectively.
2. T1 weighted imaging using Fast Spoiled Gradient Echo (FSPGR/Turbo FLASH).
3. Gradient/Echo planar Imaging Gradient (EPI GRE).
4. Diffusion-weighted imaging (DWI) with b value of 0 and 700.

Half-Fourier acquired single-shot turbo spin-echo (HASTE) or single-shot, fast spin-echo (SS-FSE) This is the basic and most widely used sequence used to study the

R. Rajeswaran, *MR Imaging of the Fetus*, https://doi.org/10.1007/978-981-16-9209-3_2

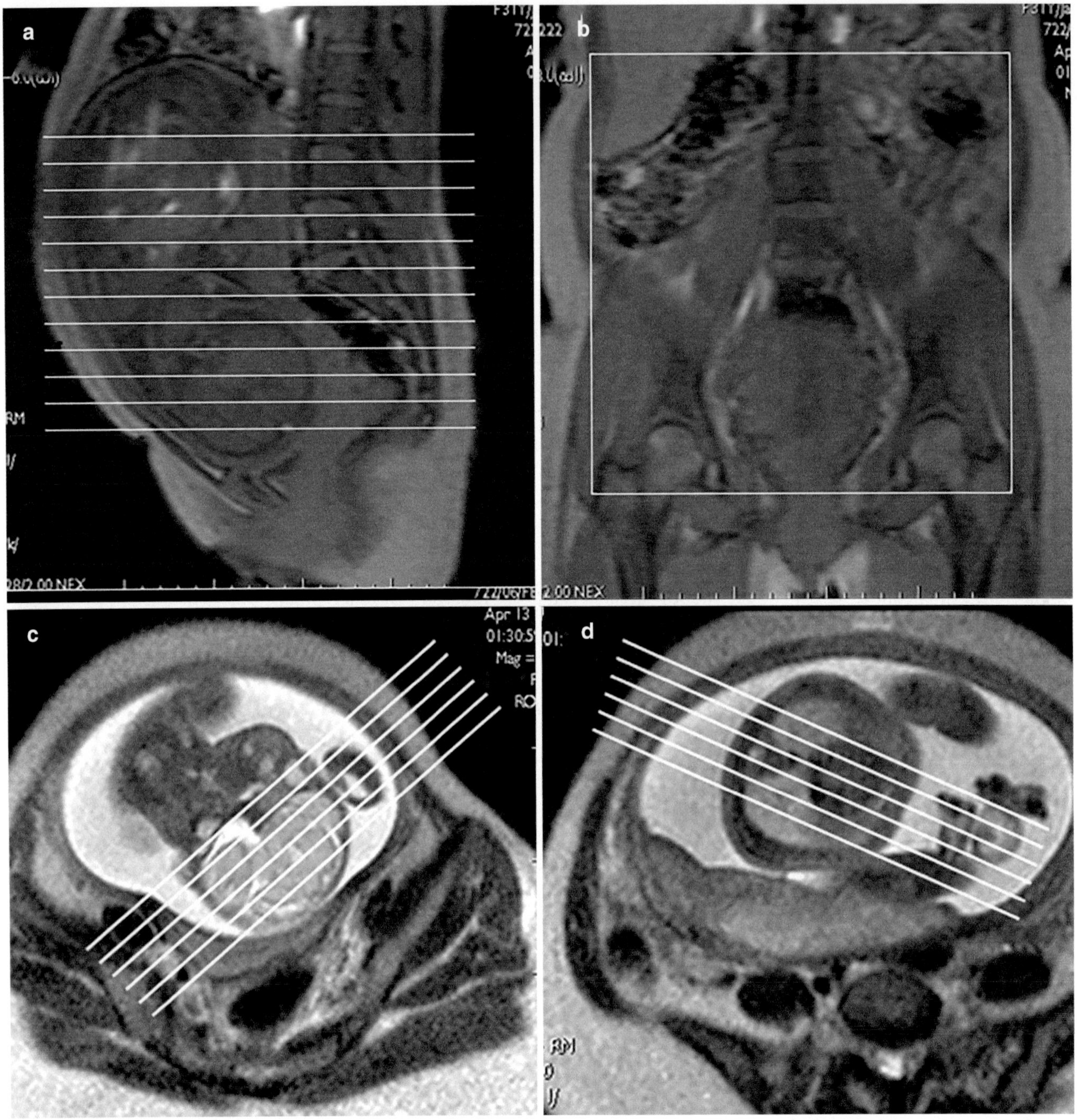

Fig. 2.1 Initial localizer images (**a**, **b**) with respect to the maternal lower abdomen. Axial sections of the fetal brain (**c**) and sagittal (**d**) sections of the fetal thorax are planned from the HASTE images obtained from this localizer set

fetal anatomy, anomalies, and pathologies (Fig. 2.2a, b, c). This sequence produces the best contrast resolution and is not affected by mild fetal movements [7–10]. The visualization of various fetal organs, their anomalies, placenta, and umbilical cord are better using this ultrafast sequence. Similarly, the pathologies like ventricular dilatation, vascular malformation, mass lesions, destructive lesions, infective lesions, and migrational disorders are well demonstrated using the HASTE sequence [8, 9]. However, the depiction of calcification and hemorrhage are suboptimally depicted [11].

True fast imaging with steady-state free precession (true FISP/2D FIESTA)

This is a gradient-based ultrafast sequence with a high signal-to-noise ratio that can produce images at the rate of one slice per sec. This sequence is an alternative to HASTE

Table 2.1 Parameters in the routine sequences used for fetal MR imaging

Imaging parameters	T2 HASTE	T1 TURBO FLASH	DWI	GRE
TR (milliseconds)	1000	100	4500	600
TE (milliseconds)	90	4.7	101	26
Flip angle	–	70 degrees	–	20 degrees
FOV (cm)	24–28 cm	24–28 cm	28–32 cm	26–30 cm
Matrix	256 × 205	256 × 160	192 × 192	256 × 135
Slice thickness	3–4 mm	4–5 mm	4–5	4–5 mm
Intersection gap	0.2 mm	0.5 mm	0.5 mm	0.5 mm
No. of excitations	1	1	NA	1

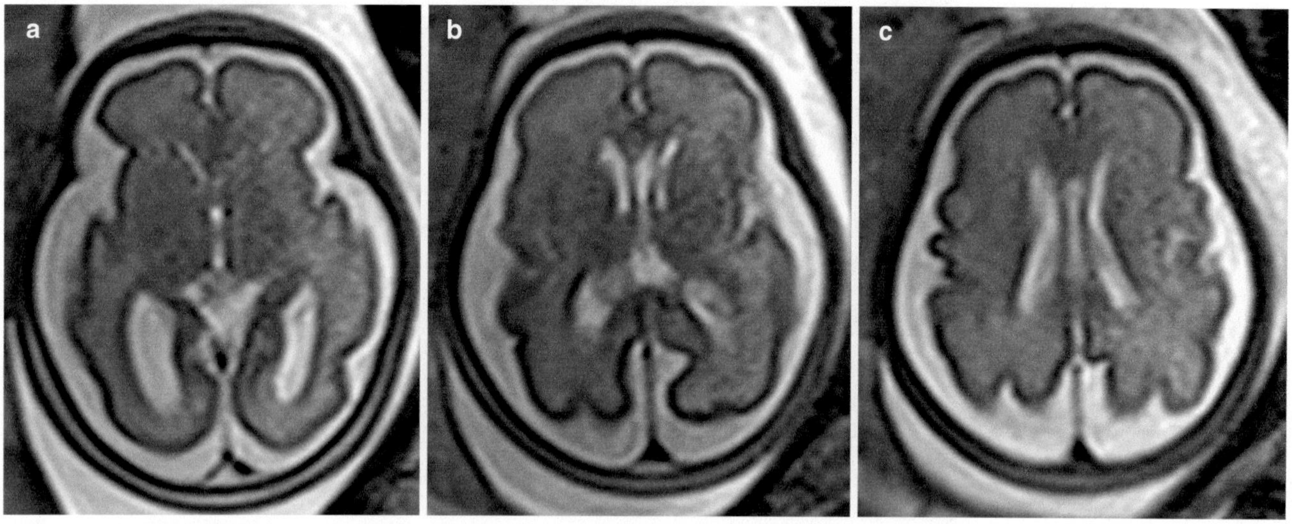

Fig. 2.2 Axial sections of the fetal brain (**a**, **b**, **c**) obtained using HASTE sequence

and produces T2* images. The advantages are better depiction of myelination and low specific radiofrequency absorption rate (SAR). This sequence is also useful in the depiction of spine (Fig. 2.3a), heart (Fig. 2.3b), bony parts (Fig. 2.3c), and great vessels. However, true FISP is rarely used in fetal imaging because of its sensitivity to field heterogeneity that leads to banding artifacts (Fig. 2.3a) [12, 13].

T1 weighted imaging using Fast Spoiled Gradient Echo (FSPGR/Turbo FLASH)

T1 weighted fetal images are poorer in quality than T2, with less contrast resolution, and are prone to motion artifacts [14]. Hence, it is recommended that T1 weighted images be obtained with maternal breath-hold in 1 or 2 orthogonal planes. T1 weighted images are useful for confirming the presence of hemorrhage, fat, and early calcification which may appear hyperintense [15]. While imaging the fetal neck and trunk, T1 weighted images are also useful in the identification of thyroid, meconium, and liver (in Congenital Diaphragmatic hernia) (Fig. 2.4a, b). The recently developed Snapshot inversion recovery sequence (SNAPIR) offers better image contrast and T1 weighted imaging.

Gradient (GRE)/Echo Planar Imaging Gradient (EPI GRE) sequences are useful to confirm hemorrhage and calcifications (Fig. 2.5a, b) [11]. Gradient sequence imaging takes around 1.5 min and is prone to motion artifacts. This can be overcome by using the ultrafast Echo Planar Imaging Gradient sequence.

Diffusion-weighted imaging (DWI) with b values of 0 and 700

Diffusion-weighted images (b700) are useful to identify subacute hemorrhage (Fig. 2.6) and acute ischemia, both appearing hyperintense. These images may show motion artifacts, because of the relatively long scan time. Acute infarcts occurring after co-twin demise can be demonstrated by DWI (Fig. 2.7).

Diffusion-weighted images (with b0 value) are like T2* images. Hemorrhage and calcifications [11] appear hypointense on this sequence (Fig. 2.8).

Thick-slab MR fetography is an optional sequence. Like MR myelography it is a heavily T2-weighted sequence that is employed to scan the entire fetus, preferably in the coronal

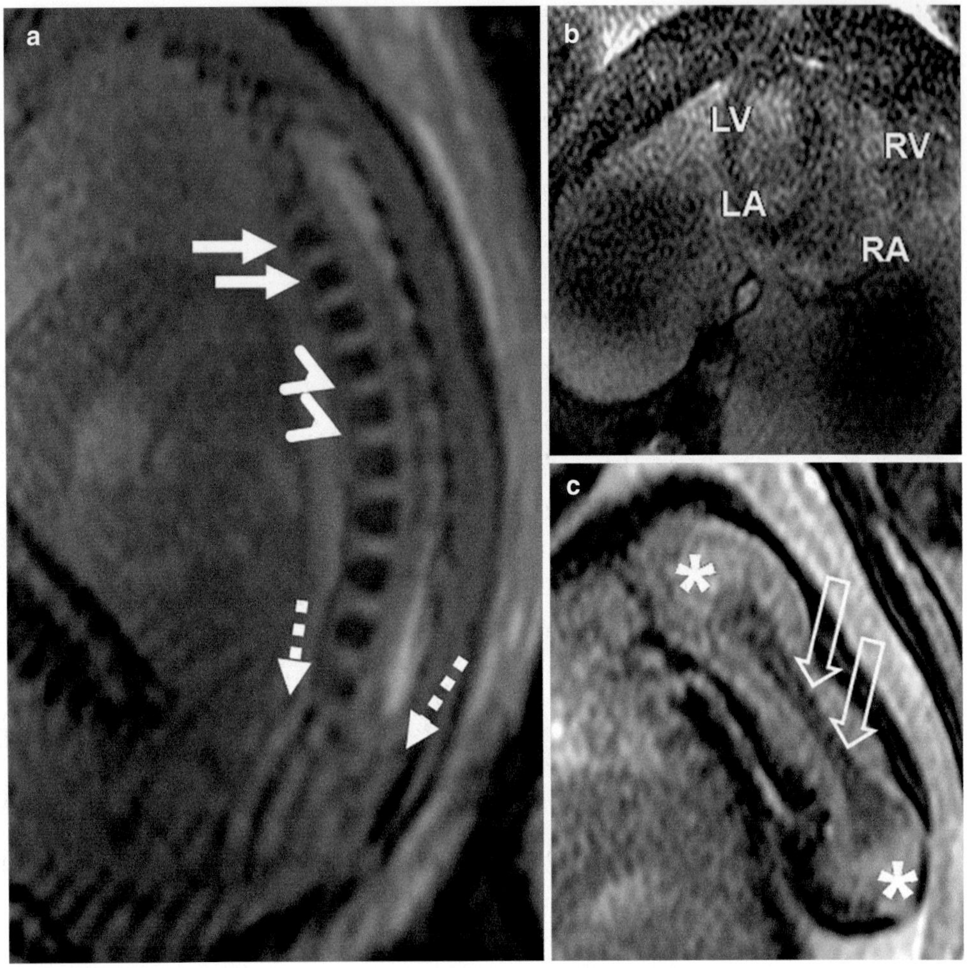

Fig. 2.3 Sagittal section of a 32-week fetal spine (**a**), axial section of fetal heart (**b**) and coronal section (**c**) of fetal arm obtained using true FISP sequence; (**a**) the vertebral bodies (arrows) and discs (arrowheads) are well demonstrated. Banding artifacts are seen in the pelvic region (broken arrows); (**b**) the chambers of heart are seen; (**c**) humeral shaft (open arrows) and epiphyseal cartilage (asterisk) are well seen

and sagittal planes. This sequence provides an overview of the fetus, fetal spine (Fig. 2.9), distended bowel loops, dilated urinary tracts, and cystic lesions.

The MR Sequences used for fetal imaging are summarized in Table 2.1.

2.2 Fetal Imaging at 18–20 Weeks

In some countries, medical termination of pregnancy is allowed till 20 weeks. In these circumstances, there are referrals from clinicians to perform fetal MR examination at 18–20 weeks after US examination to confirm certain anomalies and to decide on the future course. The various limitations can be overcome by meticulously planning the MR examination [2]. Proper coil placement at the region of interest and higher channel coil increase the signal-to-noise ratio. Using parallel imaging can reduce the scan time, increase the image resolution, and cause reduction in specific absorption rate. The aliasing arising due to the use of short FOV can be overcome by oversampling and/or changing the phase encoding and frequency encoding directions [1]. However, the fetal medicine physician needs to be cautious as certain anomalies (like microcephaly, ventriculomegaly, infections) are better diagnosed in the late II trimester or III trimester. Higher density coils and advanced scanner technology will in future improve the quality of fetal MRI scans during this gestational period.

2.3 Fetal Volumetry

MRI-based calculations of volumes and weight are now available [16, 17]. They are commonly used to calculate brain and lung volumes. Fetal weight has also been estimated by MRI to study FGR.

2.4 Dynamic Imaging

Steady-state free precession cine sequences can be utilized to assess fetal limb motion, swallowing, diaphragmatic movements, and cardiac motion [18–20].

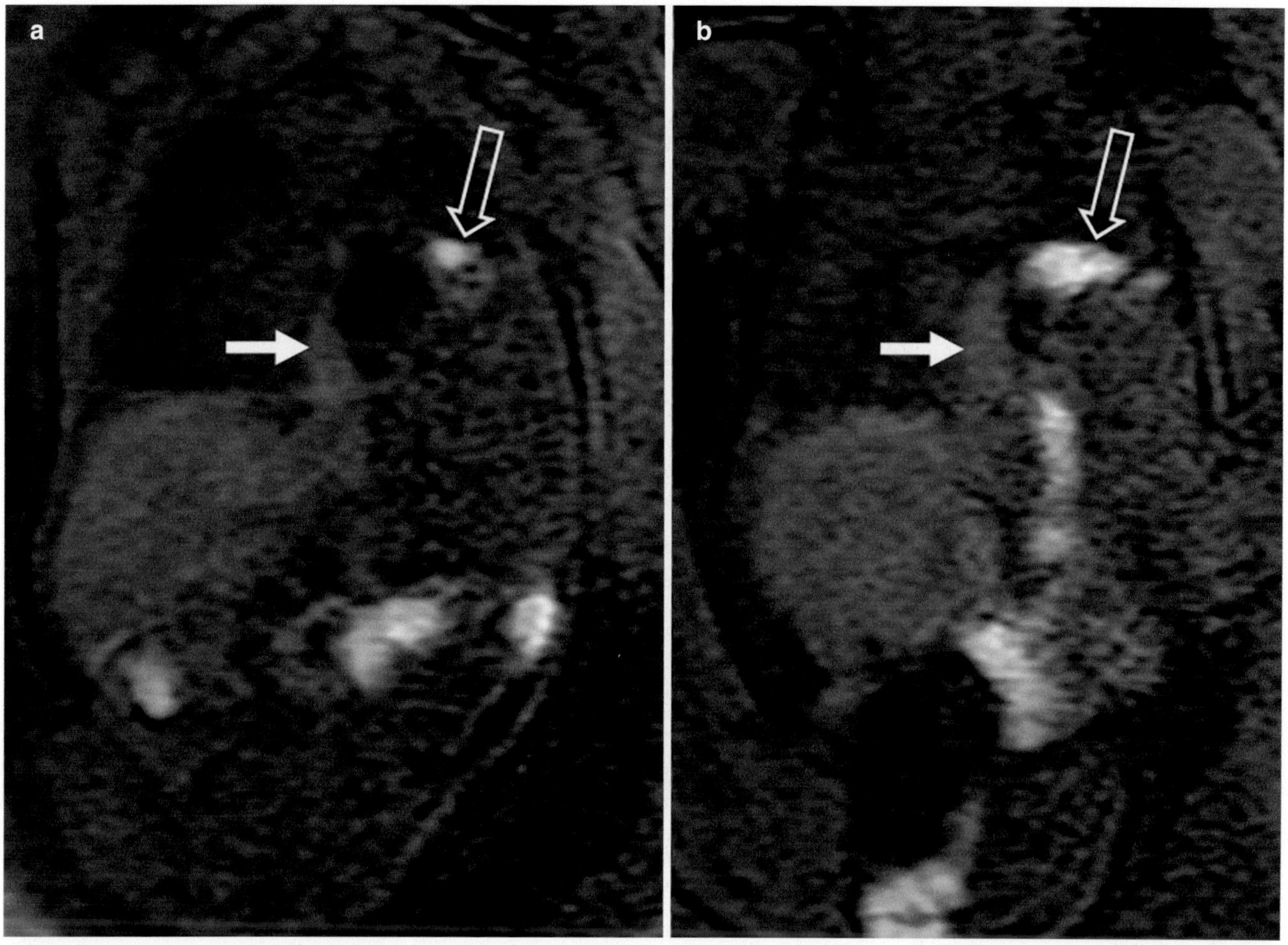

Fig. 2.4 T1-weighted coronal sections (**a**, **b**) of a fetus with congenital diaphragmatic hernia. The hyperintense left lobe of liver (arrows) and large intestine (open arrows) are seen in the left thoracic cavity

2.5 Artifacts While Imaging the Fetus [21–23]

1. *Motion Artifacts*—can occur due to fetal movements, maternal breathing (Fig. 2.10) and to a lesser extent due to maternal bowel peristalsis and arterial pulsations. However, HASTE images are acquired at less than 1 s per image and inherently produce diagnostic quality images despite motion.
2. *Bulk motion*: Movement of the entire object while scanning results in blurring of the entire image, with ghost images in the phase encoding direction. The mother can be advised to keep still and/or to perform shallow breathing.
3. *Fluid Motion*: This artifact occurs when there is movement of fluid while it is being scanned. This results in the fluid appearing as a signal void. It results when spins excited by a slice-selective radiofrequency pulse change position before their signal is recorded (Fig. 2.11). Since fetal imaging is performed with single-shot sequences, mild fetal movement will result in artifacts in a few slices. If there is continuous movement of the fetus, it results in artifacts in several slices and the sequence needs to be repeated.
4. *Non-visualization of a structure/Repeat visualization of a structure*: If the fetus moves during the sequence, it is possible that a structure may not be visualized if the structure moves out of the imaging plane. Conversely, a structure may be seen more than once if there is movement of that structure in plane with the imaging (Fig. 2.12).
5. *Aliasing or wrap-around artifact*: This artifact occurs when a short FOV is selected and anatomic structures that are outside the FOV appear to "wrap around" into the opposite side of image. This artifact can be eliminated by increasing the FOV to include the anatomic structures or by using "Phase oversampling." One pitfall of increasing the FOV is that the spatial resolution gets reduced.
6. *Susceptibility artifact*: This artifact occurs when there are inhomogeneities in the main magnetic field resulting in localized distortions of the geometry or distortions in

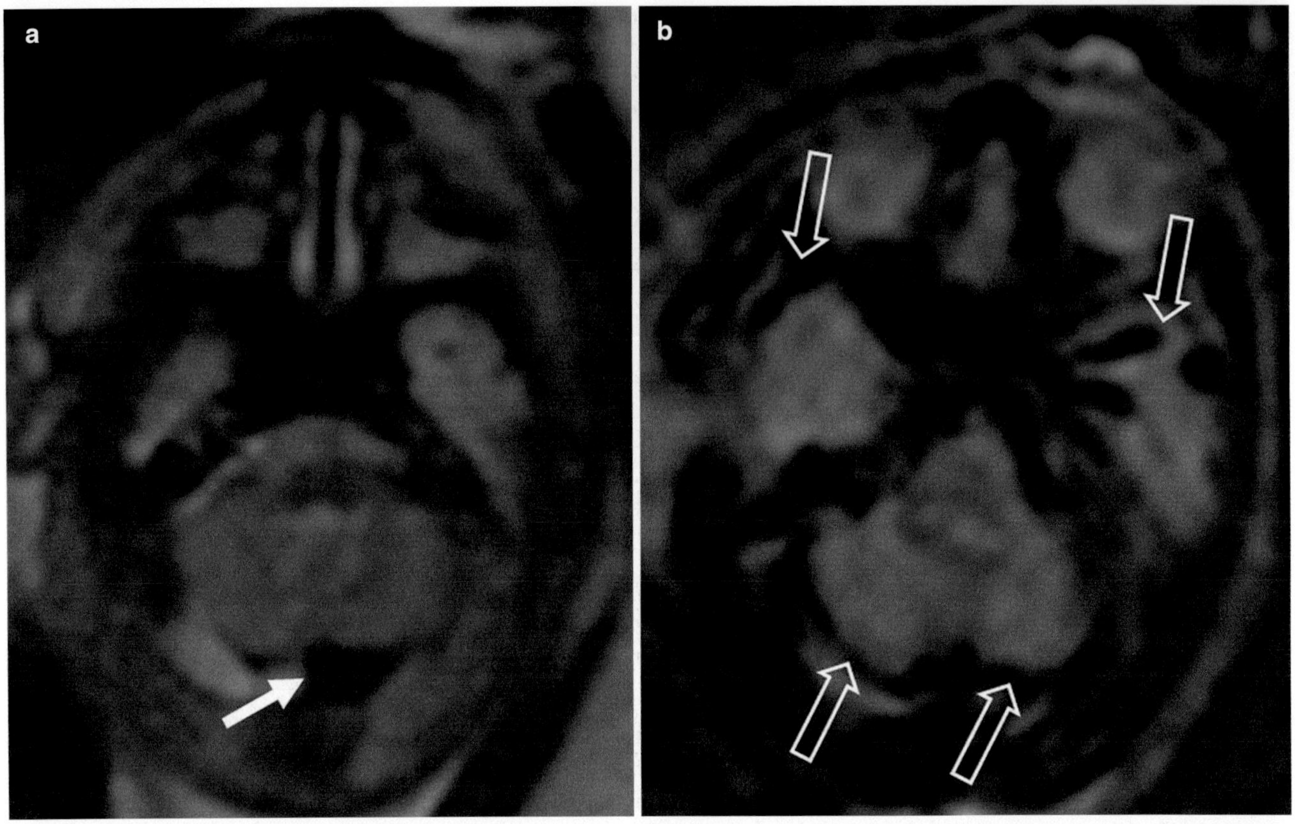

Fig. 2.5 T2-weighted axial image of a 34-week fetus using HASTE sequence (**a**) showing subarachnoid hemorrhage (arrows) in the basal cisterns. GRE axial image (**b**) confirms the subarachnoid hemorrhage (open arrows) and demonstrates the hemorrhage better

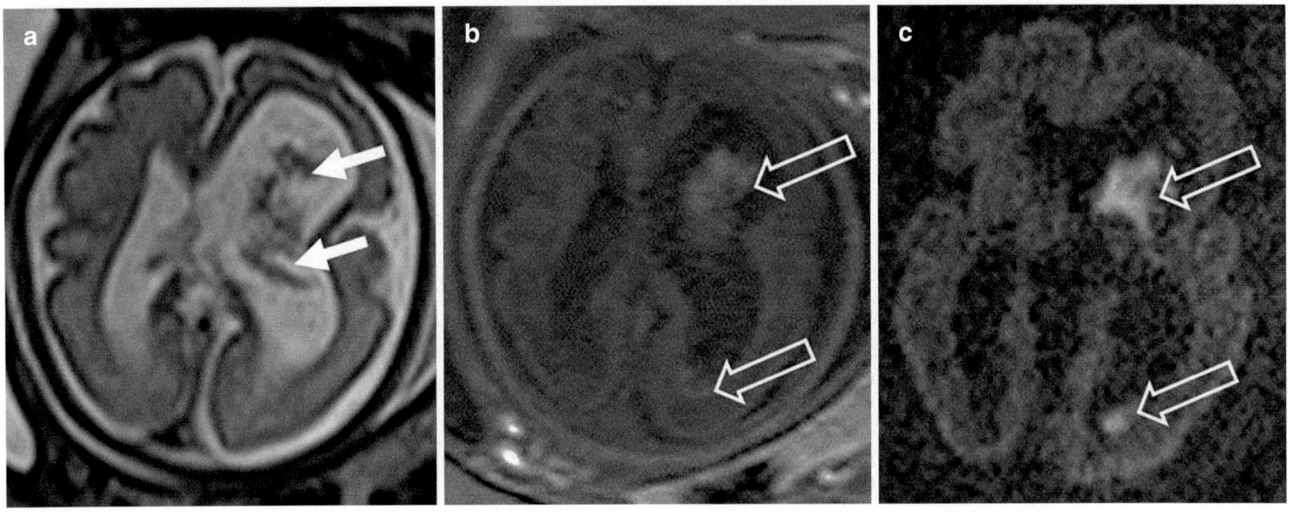

Fig. 2.6 T2-weighted axial image of a fetus using HASTE sequence (**a**) showing intraventricular hemorrhage (arrows). T1 weighted (**b**) and Diffusion-weighted (**c**) axial images confirm the subacute stage of the hemorrhage (open arrows) as it is seen as a hyperintense lesion

the intensity of the image. Susceptibility artifact is rare with HASTE sequence but is common with trueFISP sequence. This artifact can be reduced by performing shimming to improve the magnetic field homogeneity, reducing the TE, and increasing the readout bandwidth.

7. *Partial volume artifact*: This artifact occurs when two different tissues happen to be within a slice and the resultant image is an average of the two tissues. It can be eliminated by obtaining thinner sections or comprehending with the images obtained from other orthogonal planes.

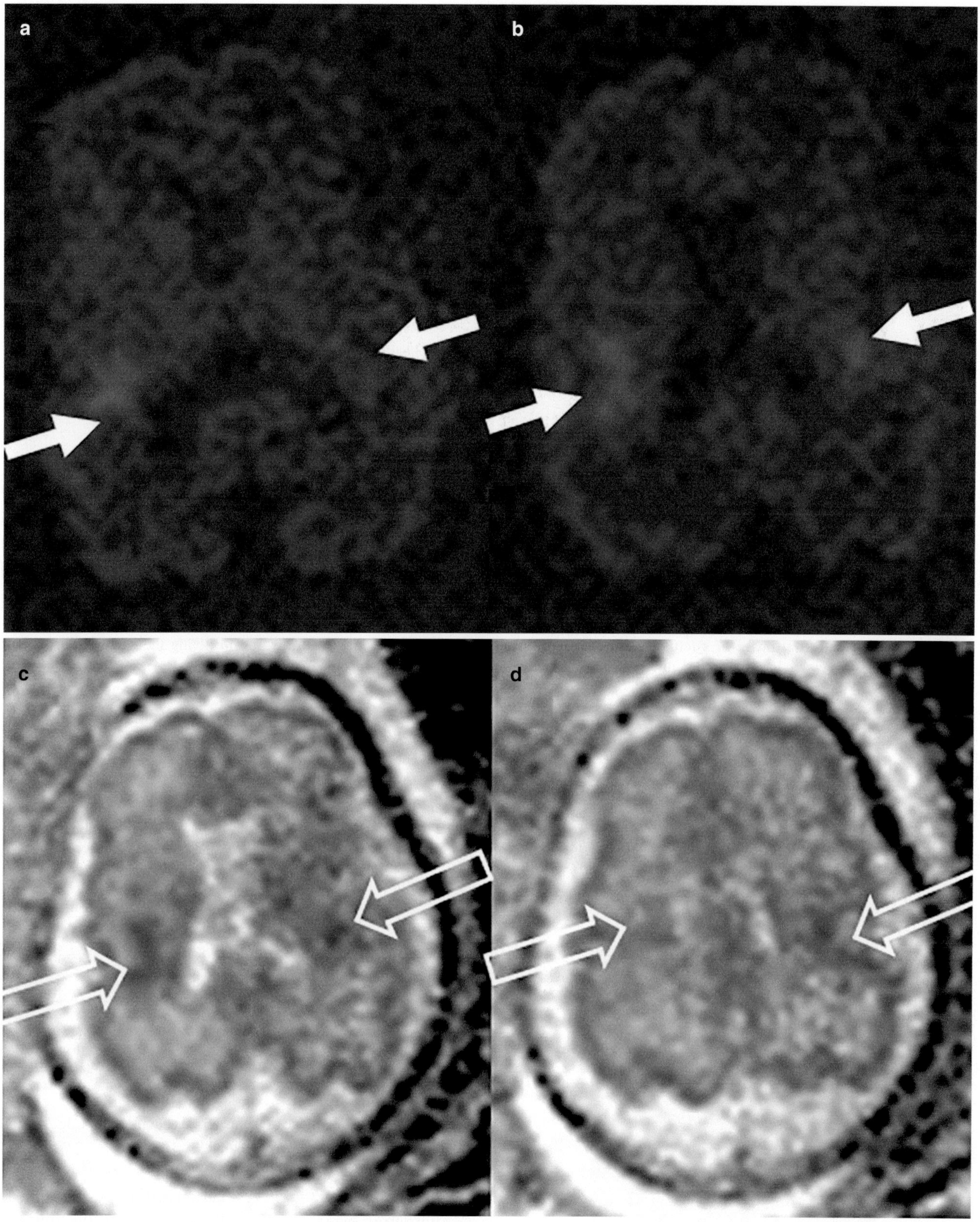

Fig. 2.7 Diffusion-weighted axial images (**a**, **b**) of a surviving twin showing acute infarcts (arrows) following cotwin demise. ADC images (**c**, **d**) showing restricted diffusion in these lesions (open arrows)

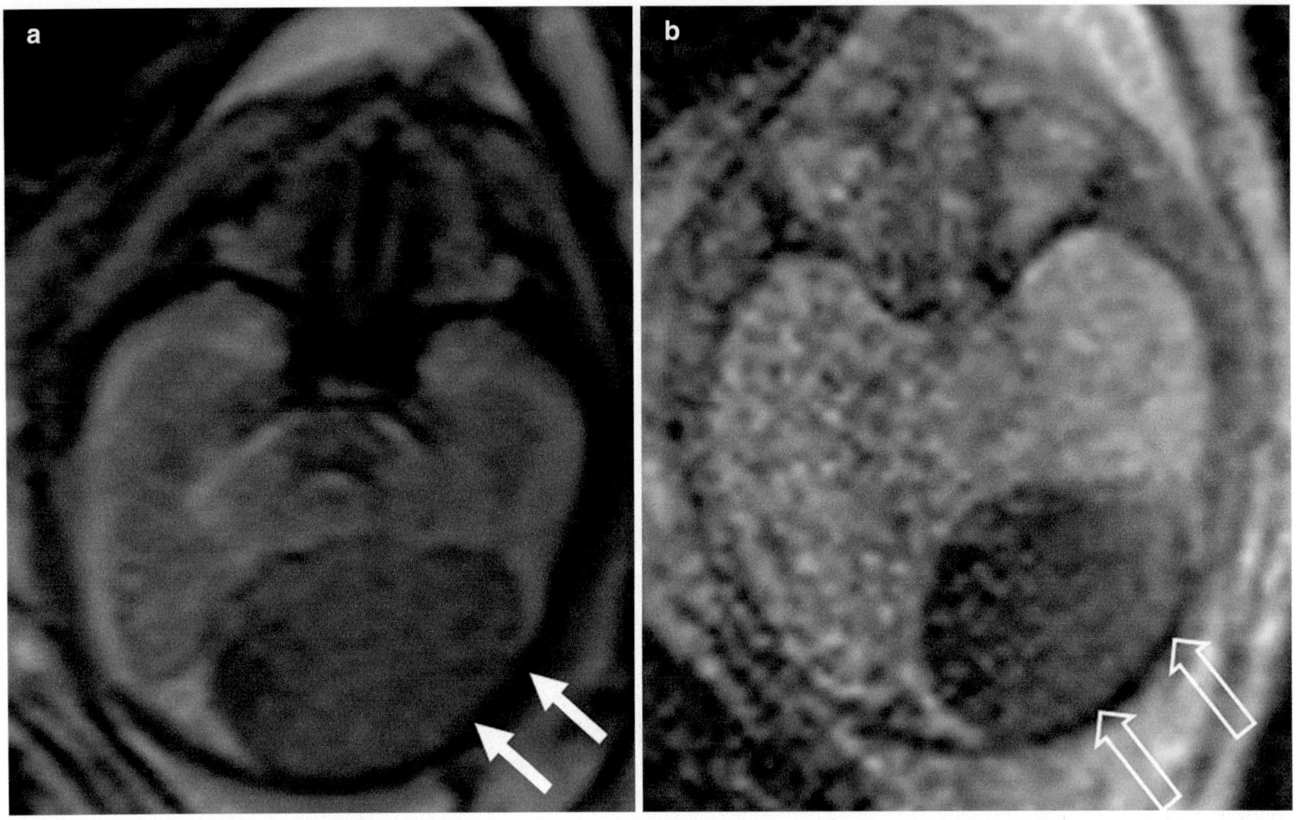

Fig. 2.8 T2 weighted axial image of a fetus using HASTE sequence (**a**) shows dural sinus malformation involving the left transverse sinus (arrows). Diffusion-weighted axial image with b0 value (**b**) shows hypointensity within the lesion (open arrows)

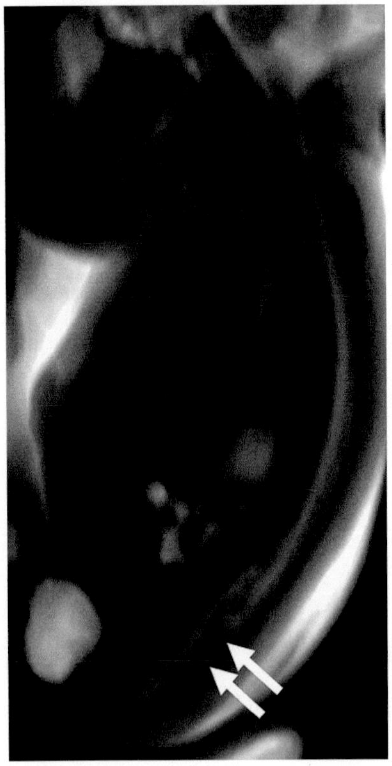

Fig. 2.9 Thick-slab MR fetography demonstrating low ending tethered cord in a case of diastematomyelia (arrows)

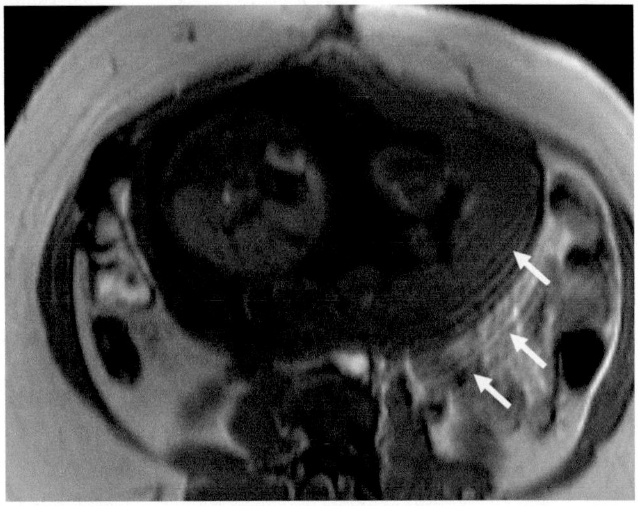

Fig. 2.10 Axial T1W image of the maternal abdomen showing "motion artifact" (arrows) due to maternal breathing

8. *Gibbs ringing artifact* (Truncation artifact)—It is seen as alternating bright and dark lines parallel to the sides of an object and they fade with distance. This artifact can be reduced by increasing the matrix size or by using filters. However, increasing the matrix size will increase the scan time and the use of filter will reduce image resolution.

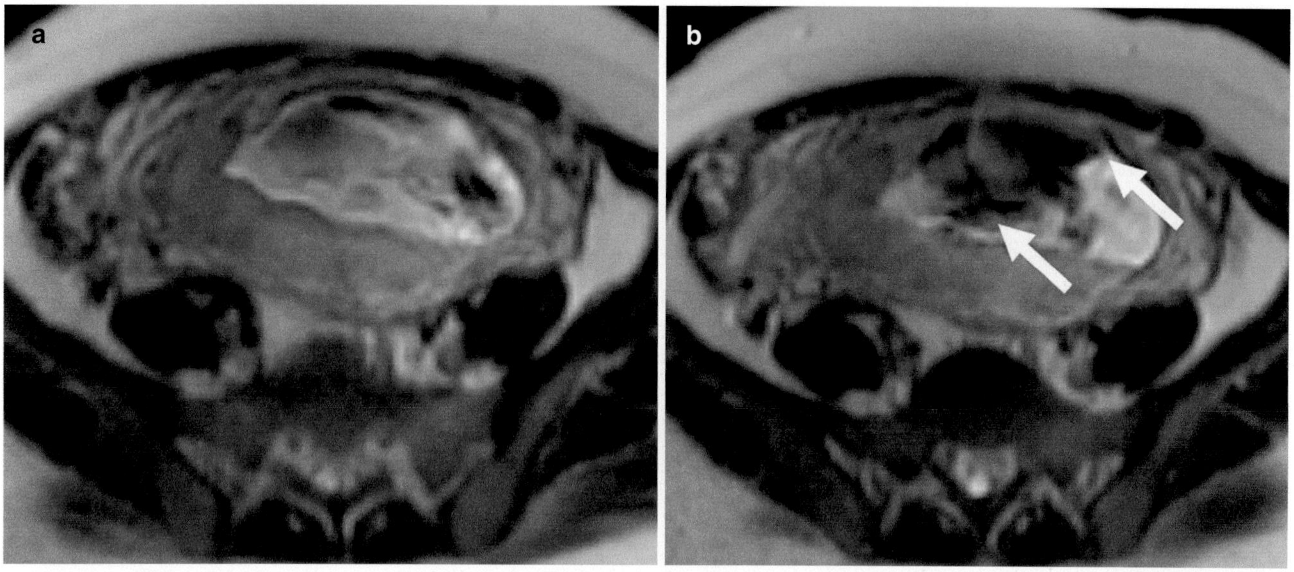

Fig. 2.11 Axial T2W images (**a**, **b**) of the maternal pelvis showing fluid motion artifact (arrows)

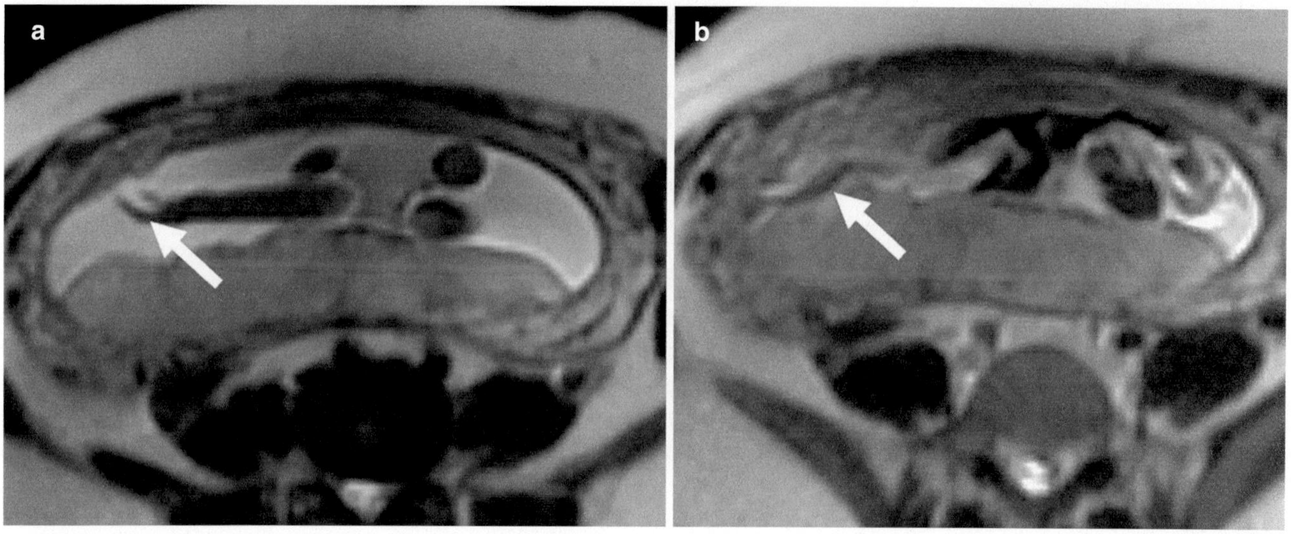

Fig. 2.12 Axial sections of the maternal Lower abdomen (**a**) and pelvis (**b**) shows the repeat of fetal hand (arrows) in the inferiorly taken images due to fetal movements

9. *Radio frequency (RF) interference*: This artifact occurs when aberrant RF signals outside the magnet are absorbed during data reception and is characterized by broad bands of lines in the phase encoding direction (Fig. 2.13) or a single area of very high signal intensity. This artifact can be eliminated by ensuring that the scanner room door is fully closed and shutting down any extraneous equipment within the scanner room. In case if it does not get eliminated, the vendor's service team may be summoned.

2.6 Imaging at 3 Tesla MRI

The advantages of imaging at 3 Tesla are high field strength, the high-density coils, and the advanced software that comes inherent with a 3 T system. This translates into a higher Signal-to-Noise Ratio (SNR) and lesser scanning time in clinical practice [24]. However, some artifacts can come up while using a 3 T system besides the increased Specific Absorption Ratio (SAR). Some authors recommend modification of the sequences to reduce the artifacts. This includes

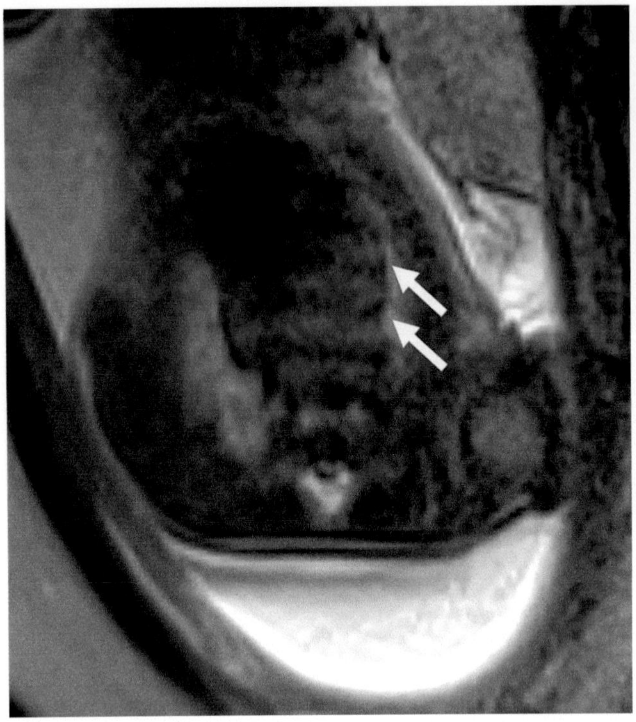

Fig. 2.13 Axial T2W Image of fetal thorax shows parallel bands due to RF interference (arrows)

mildly increasing the repetition time, decreasing the field of view while keeping the matrix values the same as 1.5 T system [24].

Radiofrequency field inhomogeneity and standing wave artifacts (dielectric resonance artifacts) can occur due to high field strength and imaging a large FOV like a pregnant woman with liquor. Some ways to decrease these artifacts include the use of dielectric pads or radiofrequency cushions, use of multichannel transmission body coils [25], and active radiofrequency shimming coupled with parallel imaging [26].

To reduce susceptibility-related artifacts, certain modifications like changing the readout direction, implementing parallel imaging, and using shorter echo are recommended [24].

2.7 MR Spectroscopy

The application of MR spectroscopy (MRS) in clinical practice is limited due to long acquisition times but progress is being made [27]. Girard et al. performed MRS after fetal sedation with oral administration of flunitrazepam to the mothers. The studies were performed using Point-resolved spectroscopy sequence (PRESS) with long and short TEs (135 and 30 ms). They used a voxel size of 20 × 15 × 15 mm and located them in the centrum semiovale. With increasing gestational age, there is an increase in *N*-acetyl aspartate, creatine and decrease in choline and myo-inositol. In FGR there may be a reduction in NAA and increase in lactate. MRS has the potential to diagnose metabolic disorders in utero [27]. MR spectroscopy can also be performed in the third trimester when the fetal head is engaged in the pelvis. The sequence may be modified to shorten acquisition times but this will also result in the reduction of SNR.

2.8 Diffusion Tensor Imaging (DTI)

Because of long acquisition time, DTI exists more as a research tool. Few studies highlight the potential of diffusion tensor imaging (DTI) to investigate fiber tracts in utero [28–31]. A customized DTI sequence lasting for less than 2 min has depicted association fibers in a recent study on 24 fetuses [32]. Association fibers are white matter tracts that connect cortical areas within the same hemisphere. DTI and tractography are potential tools that can be used in the evaluation of intrauterine white matter damage.

2.9 Postmortem Magnetic Resonance Imaging

This non-invasive procedure can provide information about the cause of intrauterine death and the associated anomalies and is an alternative for conventional autopsy. This procedure is more acceptable to some of the couples than the conventional autopsy [33]. It can provide significant information when autolysis may hamper detailed neuropathological examination. The limitations are that it cannot provide histological details, but can be overcome by obtaining additional biopsies at multiple sites [34]. MR Imaging has also been used prenatally immediately after fetal demise to ascertain the cause of intrauterine death [35]. The other limitations are the availability of fewer centers and few radiologists trained for this purpose.

References

1. Glenn OA, Barkovich AJ. Magnetic resonance imaging of the fetal brain and spine: an increasingly important tool in prenatal diagnosis, part 1. Am J Neuroradiol. 2006;27:1604–11.
2. Mohan A, Rangasami R, Chandrasekharan A, et al. Role of MRI in the diagnosis of fetal anomalies at 18–20 weeks gestational age. J South Asian Feder Obst Gynae. 2019;11(5):292–6.
3. Quinn TM, Hubbard AM, Adzick NS. Prenatal magnetic resonance imaging enhances fetal diagnosis. J Paediatr Surg. 1998;33:553–8.
4. Levine D. Ultrasound versus magnetic resonance imaging in fetal evaluation. Top Magn Reson Imaging. 2001;12:25–38.
5. Rajeswaran R, Chandrasekharan A, Joseph S, Venkata Sai PM, Dev B, Reddy S. Ultrasound versus MRI in the diagnosis of fetal head and trunk anomalies. J Matern-Fetal Neonatal Med. 2009;22(2):115–23.

6. Busse R, Carrillo A, Brittain J, et al. On-demand real-time imaging: interactive multislice acquisition applied to prostate and fetal imaging. In: Proceedings of the Tenth Scientific Meeting and Exhibition of the International Society for Magnetic Resonance in Medicine; May 18–24, 2002; Honolulu, Hawaii.
7. Levine D, Hatabu H, Gaa J, Atkinson MW, Edelman RR. Fetal anatomy revealed with fast MR sequences. AJR. 1996;167:905–8.
8. Yamashita Y, Namimoto T, Abe Y, et al. MR imaging of the fetus by a HASTE sequence. AJR. 1997;168:513–9.
9. Tsuchiya K, Katase S, Seki T, Mizutani Y, Hachiya J. Short communication: MR imaging of fetal brain abnormalities using a HASTE sequence. Br J Radiol. 1996;69:668–70.
10. Quinn TM, Hubbard AM, Adzick NS. Prenatal magnetic resonance imaging enhances fetal diagnosis. J Pediatr Surg. 1998;33:553–8.
11. Baburaj R, Rangasami R, Chandrasekharan A, Suresh I, Suresh S, Seshadri S. Utility of various ultrafast magnetic resonance sequences in the detection of fetal intracranial hemorrhage. Ann Indian Acad Neurol. 2018;21:275–9.
12. Haacke EM, Wielopolski PA, Tkach JA, Modic MT. Steady-state free precession imaging in the presence of motion: application for improved visualization of the cerebrospinal fluid. Radiology. 1990;175:545–52.
13. Van der Meulen P, Groen JP, Tinus AM, Bruntink G. Fast field echo imaging: an overview and contrast calculations. Magn Reson Imaging. 1988;6:355–68.
14. Story L, Rutherford M. Advances and applications in fetal magnetic resonance imaging. Obstet Gynaecol. 2015;17:189–99.
15. Huppi PS, Inder TE. Magnetic resonance techniques in the evaluation of the perinatal brain: recent advances and future directions. Semin Neonatol. 2001;6:195–210.
16. Baker PN, Johnson IR, Gowland PA, et al. Fetal weight estimation by echo-planar magnetic resonance imaging. Lancet. 1994;343(8898):644–5.
17. Gong QY, Roberts N, Garden AS, Whitehouse GH. Fetal and fetal brain volume estimation in the third trimester of human pregnancy using gradient echo MR imaging. Magn Reson Imaging. 1998;16(3):235–40.
18. Hayat TT, Nihat A, Martinez-Biarge M, et al. Optimization and initial experience of a multisection balanced steady-state free precession cine sequence for the assessment of fetal behavior in utero. AJNR Am J Neuroradiol. 2011;32(2):331–8.
19. Houshmand G, Hosseinzadeh K, Ozolek J. Prenatal magnetic resonance imaging (MRI) findings of a foregut duplication cyst of the tongue: value of real-time MRI evaluation of the fetal swallowing mechanism. J Ultrasound Med. 2011;30(6):843–50.
20. Roy CW, Seed M, van Amerom JFP, Al Nafisi B, Grosse-Wortmann L, Yoo S-J, Macgowan CK. Dynamic imaging of the fetal heart using metric optimized gating. Magn Reson Med. 2013;70:1598–607.
21. Levine D. Magnetic resonance imaging in prenatal diagnosis. Curr Opin Pediatr. 2001;13:572–8.
22. Levine D. MR imaging of fetal central nervous system abnormalities. Brain Cogn. 2002;50(3):432–48.
23. Levine D, Barnes PD. Edelman RR state of the art: obstetric MR imaging. Radiology. 1999;211:609–17.
24. Victoria T, Johnson AM, Edgar JC, Zarnow DM, Vossough A, Jaramillo D. Comparison between 1.5-T and 3-T MRI for fetal imaging: is there an advantage to imaging with a higher field strength? AJR Am J Roentgenol. 2016;206(1):195–201.
25. Vernickel P, Roschmann P, Findeklee C, et al. Eightchannel transmit/receive body MRI coil at 3 T. Magn Reson Med. 2007;58:381–9.
26. Ullmann P, Junge S, Wick M, et al. Experimental analysis of parallel excitation using dedicated coil setups and simultaneous RF transmission on multiple channels. Magn Reson Med. 2005;54:994–1001.
27. Girard N, Fogliarini C, Viola A, Confort-Gouny S, Fur YL, Viout P, Chapon F, Levrier O, Cozzone P. MRS of normal and impaired fetal brain development. Eur J Radiol. 2006;57(2):217–25. https://doi.org/10.1016/j.ejrad.2005.11.021.
28. Bui T, Daire JL, Chalard F, Zaccaria I, Alberti C, Elmaleh M, et al. Microstructural development of human brain assessed in utero by diffusion tensor imaging. Pediatr Radiol. 2006;36(11):1133–40.
29. Huppi PS, Murphy B, Maier SE, Zientara GP, Inder TE, Barnes PD, et al. Microstructural brain development after perinatal cerebral white matter injury assessed by diffusion tensor magnetic resonance imaging. Pediatrics. 2001;107(3):455–60.
30. Kasprian G, Brugger PC, Weber M, Krssak M, Krampl E, Herold C, et al. In utero tractography of fetal white matter development. NeuroImage. 2008;43(2):213–24. https://doi.org/10.1016/j.neuroimage.2008.07.026.
31. Partridge SC, Mukherjee P, Berman JI, Henry RG, Miller SP, Lu Y, et al. Tractography-based quantitation of diffusion tensor imaging parameters in white matter tracts of preterm newborns. J Magn Reson Imaging. 2005;22(4):467–74.
32. Mitter C, Prayer D, Brugger PC, Weber M, Kasprian G. In vivo tractography of fetal association fibers. PLoS One. 2015;10(3):e0119536. https://doi.org/10.1371/journal.pone.0119536.
33. Hellkvist A, Wikström J, Mulic-Lutvica A. Postmortem magnetic resonance imaging vs autopsy of second trimester fetuses terminated due to anomalies. Acta Obstet Gynecol Scand. 2019;98:865–76.
34. Breeze AC, Jessop FA, Set PA, et al. Minimally-invasive fetal autopsy using magnetic resonance imaging and percutaneous organ biopsies: clinical value and comparison to conventional autopsy. Ultrasound Obstet Gynecol. 2011;37:317–23.
35. Shankar H, Rajeswaran R, Bhuvana. MRI findings in a fetus with cord around the neck. Neurol India. 2017;65(5):1130–1.

Embryology and Normal Appearance of Fetal Central Nervous System

3

Advances in various subspecialities of medicine have made it possible to understand Central nervous system (CNS) development better. Congenital CNS malformations may occur due to spontaneous mutations within the embryo's genes, inherited genetic defects, or damage to the fetus caused by maternal exposure to infection, toxins, drugs, or trauma. The advent of high-resolution imaging techniques and genetic analysis have revolutionized the diagnosis of malformations and we are able to identify specific gene defects in several congenital anomalies. The CNS anomalies can be classified based on embryological development or on the organ/region involved.

3.1 Normal Development of the CNS

We shall briefly review the normal development of the CNS before discussing the various anomalies [1].

3.1.1 Induction

In the early embryo, there is formation of three cell lines—ectoderm, mesoderm, and endoderm. Soon a separate cell line develops from the ectoderm (induced) that forms the neural ectoderm. By the third week, there is formation of a thickened structure, called neural plate.

3.1.2 Dorsal Induction

Between 3 and 5 weeks of gestation, by the process called *primary neurulation*, the neural plate folds and forms a neural tube, which is present along its entire length. This primary neurulation is responsible for establishing brain and spinal cord regions up to S2. This neural tube is initially open at both ends forming the neuropores that subsequently close by a zippering process. Failure of these openings to close leads to neural tube defects. During neural tube closure, the superficial epidermal cells form the ectodermal layer of the skin. Subsequently, the neural tube separates from the superficial ectoderm by a process called dysjunction.

Secondary neurulation This process results in the formation of spinal cord caudal to S2 level. Totipotent mesodermal cells called tail bud or caudal cell mass coalesce to form neural tube which then reorganizes around a lumen and become continuous with the neural tube initially formed by primary neurulation [1, 2]. The caudal cell mass undergoes regression and differentiation to form the tip of conus medullaris, terminal ventricle, filum terminale, and most of the sacrum and coccyx.

The important abnormalities of dorsal induction are presented in Table 3.1 [3, 4].

3.1.3 Ventral Induction

This stage occurs between 5 and 10 weeks of gestation. From the cranial part of the neural tube 3 primary vesicles viz., prosencephalon, mesencephalon, and rhombencephalon differentiate and form forebrain, midbrain, and hindbrain, respectively (Fig. 3.1). Prosencephalon further differentiates to form telencephalon and diencephalon that develop into cerebrum and thalami respectively. The optic placode also develops at the same time as the forebrain and this is followed by the formation of the olfactory vesicle 1 week later. Any insult during this phase not only affects the development of brain vesicles but also the development of facial skeleton, orbits and nose. The common forebrain ventral induction malformations are (1) atelencephaly, (2) holoprosencephaly, (3) Septal agenesis/septo-optic dysplasia, (4) anomalies of the corpus callosum, (5) olfactory aplasia [5].

The rhombencephalon differentiates into metencephalon (that develops as pons and cerebellum) and myelencephalon (that develops as medulla). The caudal part of the neural tube

R. Rajeswaran, *MR Imaging of the Fetus*, https://doi.org/10.1007/978-981-16-9209-3_3

Table 3.1 Malformations of dorsal induction

Abnormality	Pathogenesis	Time of onset
Primary neurulation/neural tube abnormalities (3–4 weeks gestation)		
Craniorachischisis totalis	The brain and spinal cord are open to varying degrees	3 weeks
Anencephaly	Failure of closure of cephalic end of neural tube	4 weeks
Myeloschisis	Failure of the closure of posterior aspect of the neural tube	4 weeks
Encephalocele	Failure of the closure of anterior aspect of the neural tube leading to herniation of brain tissue	4 weeks
Myelomeningocele	Inadequate closure of the dorsal part of the neural tube resulting in herniation of neural contents	4 weeks
Chiari malformation	Descent of the brainstem and cerebellum	4 weeks
Lipomyelomeningocele	Failure of closure of posterior neural tube with lipomatous mass in the subcutaneous plane and connected to neural placode	4 weeks
Secondary neurulation/occult dysraphic states (4 weeks gestation to postpartum)		
Myelocystocele	Cystic dilatation of central canal that herniates posteriorly	4 weeks
Diastematomyelia/diplomyelia [4]	Longitudinal split in the spinal cord or its duplication	4–5 weeks
Meningocele	Protrusion of meninges through a defect in the skull or spine due to failure of closure of posterior neural tube	4–5 weeks
Dermal sinus with or without dermoid	Nondysjunction leading to sinus tract connecting skin dimple to the dural sac, conus, or central canal of spinal cord	3–5 weeks
Tethered cord/tight filum terminale syndrome	Associated with several types of spinal dysraphism, shows a low ending cord	4–5 weeks
Anterior dysraphic disturbances	Inadequate closure of the anterior part of the neural tube resulting in herniation of neural elements/meninges.	4–5 weeks
Caudal regression syndrome	Anomaly of notochord formation	4–7 weeks

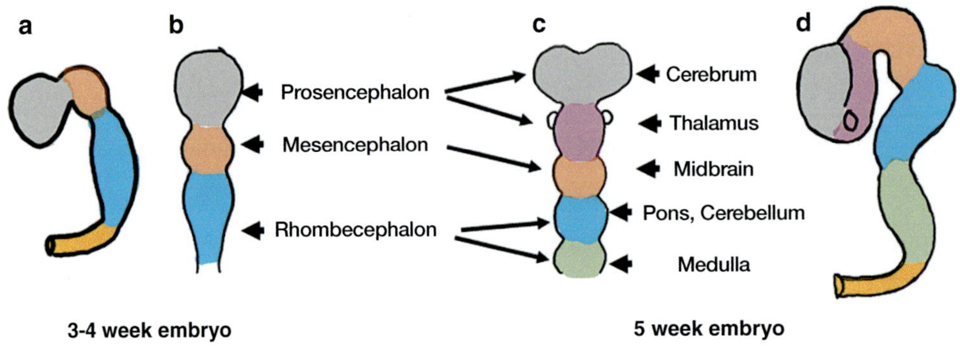

Fig. 3.1 Schematic diagram showing the development of three primary vesicles—prosencephalon, mesencephalon, and rhombencephalon (**a**, **b**) from the cranial part of the neural tube that differentiate and form forebrain, midbrain, and hindbrain, respectively (**c**, **d**)

develops to form the spinal cord. Malformations of the rhombencephalon are discussed in detail in Chap. 8.

3.1.4 Proliferation, Migration, and Organization

The dorsal cells within the neural tube migrate to form the majority of the peripheral nervous system [5]. Cell proliferation occurs within the tube and the cells later move to their correct locations. The area adjacent to the lumen of the neural tube (the future ventricles) called the germinal matrix contains neural stem cells that are precursors of the neurons, astrocytes, and oligodendrocytes. Neuronal precursor cells migrate in a radial fashion to their final locations in the six-layered cerebral cortex. Each cell line then gets organized for specific location, axonal growth, and synapse formation so that they can carry out a specific function.

Disorders of *abnormal cell proliferation* might result in too many neurons or too few neurons or abnormal neurons [6–9]. This can result in anomalies like Megalencephaly, hemimegalencephaly, microcephaly, and focal cortical dysplasia.

Abnormal neuronal migration can result in malformations like lissencephaly when there is the cessation of neuronal migration or heterotopia when there is presence of collections of neurons in abnormal locations. *Abnormal post migrational development* can result in malformations like polymicrogyria, schizencephaly, type I and type III focal cortical dysplasia.

3.2 The Normal Fetal Brain on MRI

The MRI appearance of the fetal brain needs to be correlated with the gestational age obtained from clinical history or dating scan. The supratentorial brain shows a three-layer pattern in the early II trimester gestation (Fig. 3.2), viz.—ventricular zone/germinal matrix (hypointense on T2 WI due to increased neuron density), intermediate zone (hyperintense on T2 WI due to increased water content), and cortical plate (hypointense on T2 WI) [10]. The germinal matrix neurons migrate peripherally from the ventricular wall during the II trimester, resulting in a five-layered pattern by 24–28 weeks gestation [11]. The five layers from inner to outer are the ventricular zone/germinal matrix (hypointense on T2 WI), periventricular zone (hyperintense on T2 WI), intermediate zone (hypointense on T2 WI), subplate (hyperintense on T2 WI), and cortical zone (hypointense on T2 WI). These zones are best displayed on T2-weighted images (Fig. 3.3). Subsequently, the multilayered pattern matures to acquire the typical postnatal brain appearance [11].

There is progressive appearance of sulci with increasing gestational age. The fetal brain shows a smooth surface with few shallow sulci until 23 weeks (Figs. 3.4 and 3.5) [12]. The MRI appearance of sulci lags behind those described in pathology by 2–4 weeks. The Sylvian fissure is first seen by 18 weeks on MRI, shows an obtuse angle and progresses to show acute angulation by 25 weeks (Figs. 3.4 and 3.6). The parieto occipital and calcarine sulci are visualized by 22–23 weeks, cingulate sulci by 25–26 weeks, the central sulcus by 27 weeks and convexity sulci by 27–29 weeks (Figs. 3.7, 3.8, 3.9, 3.10, 3.11 and 3.12) [13]. The subarachnoid space overlying the cerebral convexities appear mildly dilated throughout the gestation, most marked at 21–26 weeks.

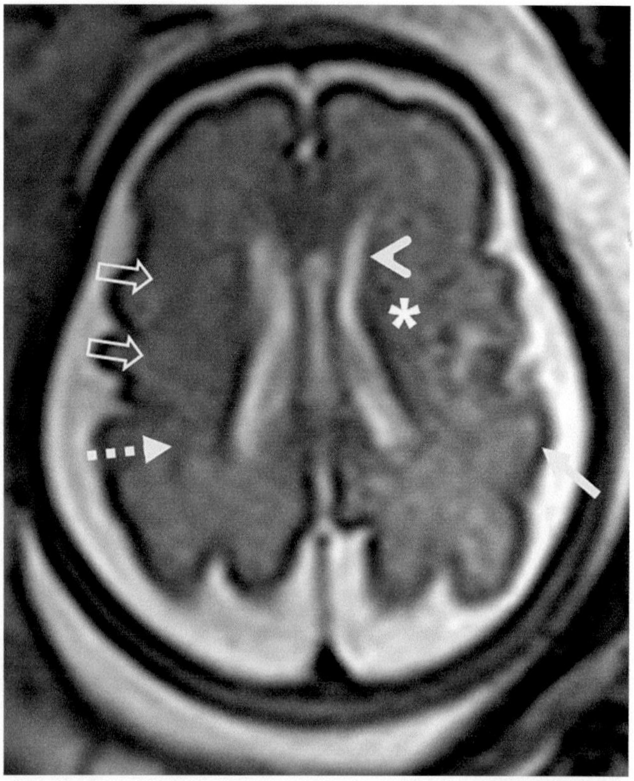

Fig. 3.3 Axial T2 image of a 29-week fetus showing five layers—the germinal matrix (arrowhead), periventricular zone (asterisk), intermediate zone (broken arrow), subplate (open arrow), and cortical zone (arrows)

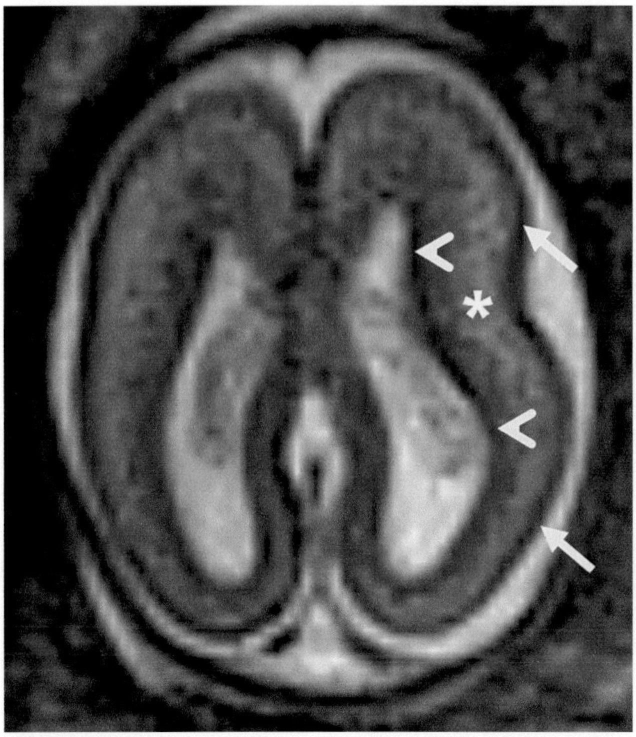

Fig. 3.2 Axial T2W image of 21-week fetus showing three layers, from inner to outer—germinal matrix (arrowhead), intermediate zone (asterisk), and cortical plate (arrows)

The corpus callosum develops between 8 and 19 weeks, beginning with the development of genu anteriorly and proceeds to form the splenium posteriorly, except for the rostrum, which is the last to develop [14, 15]. The final configuration is attained by 19–20 weeks (Fig. 3.4). The fetal ventricles also change during gestation. In early gestation, they are prominent due to the relative reduced volume of the brain parenchyma. The atrial width of normal lateral ventricles (Fig. 3.13) remains constant during 15–35 weeks (≤10 mm) and later begins to decrease.

Myelination usually occurs after birth. However certain structures in the fetus can show mild myelination and appear hyperintense on T1WI and hypointense on T2WI. At 20 weeks, some myelin is visible in the posterior brainstem. By 27 weeks, some myelination occurs in the vermis, middle cerebellar peduncles, and central basal ganglia [16, 17]. By 33–36 weeks, some myelin is also visible in the posterior limbs of the internal capsules and globus pallidus (Figs. 3.11b, c and 3.12b, c) [18].

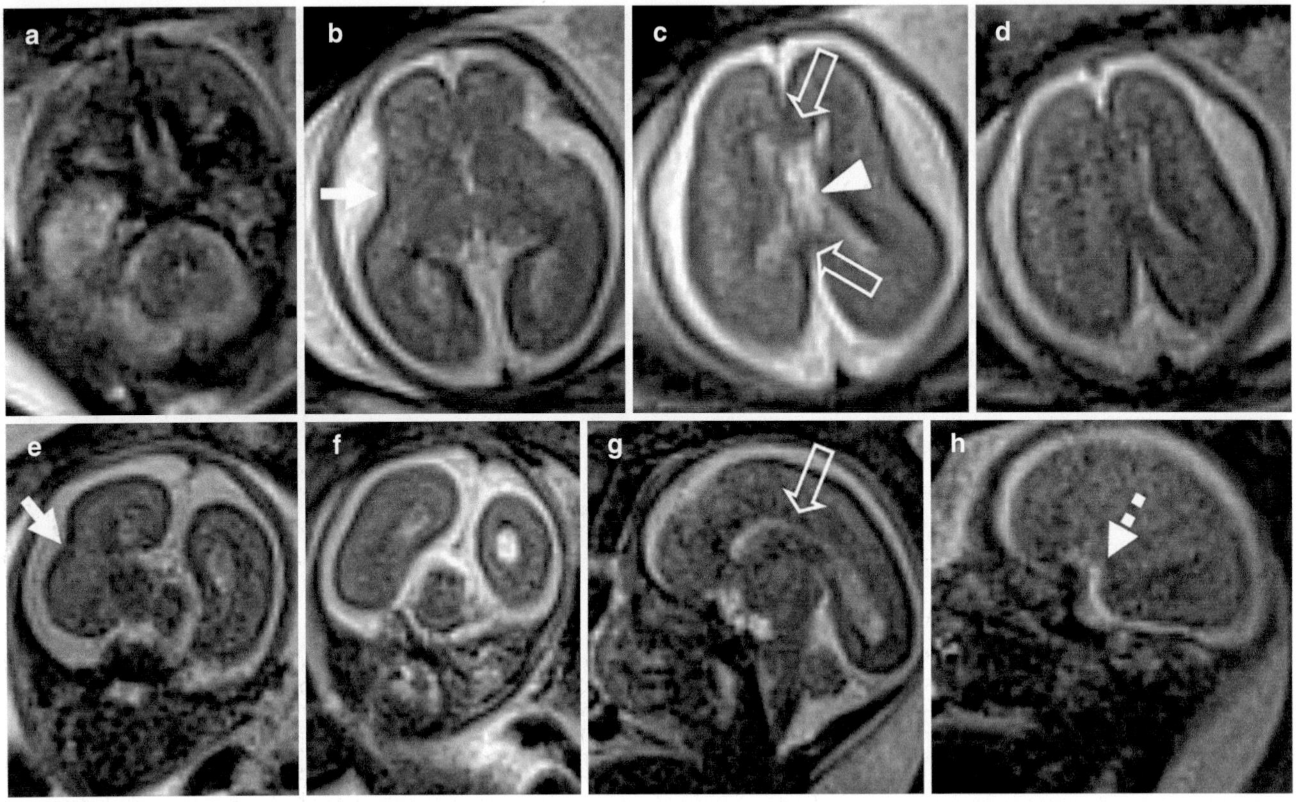

Fig. 3.4 (**a**, **b**, **c**, **d**) Axial T2W images of a 20-week fetus at the level of cerebellum, III ventricle, CSP and centrum semiovale. (**e**, **f**) coronal images at the level of sella and occipital region. (**g**, **h**) Sagittal images at the level of midline and parasagittal region. The Sylvian fissure (arrow), Cavum septum pellucidum (arrowhead), corpus callosum (open arrows) and lateral sulcus (dotted arrow) are identified

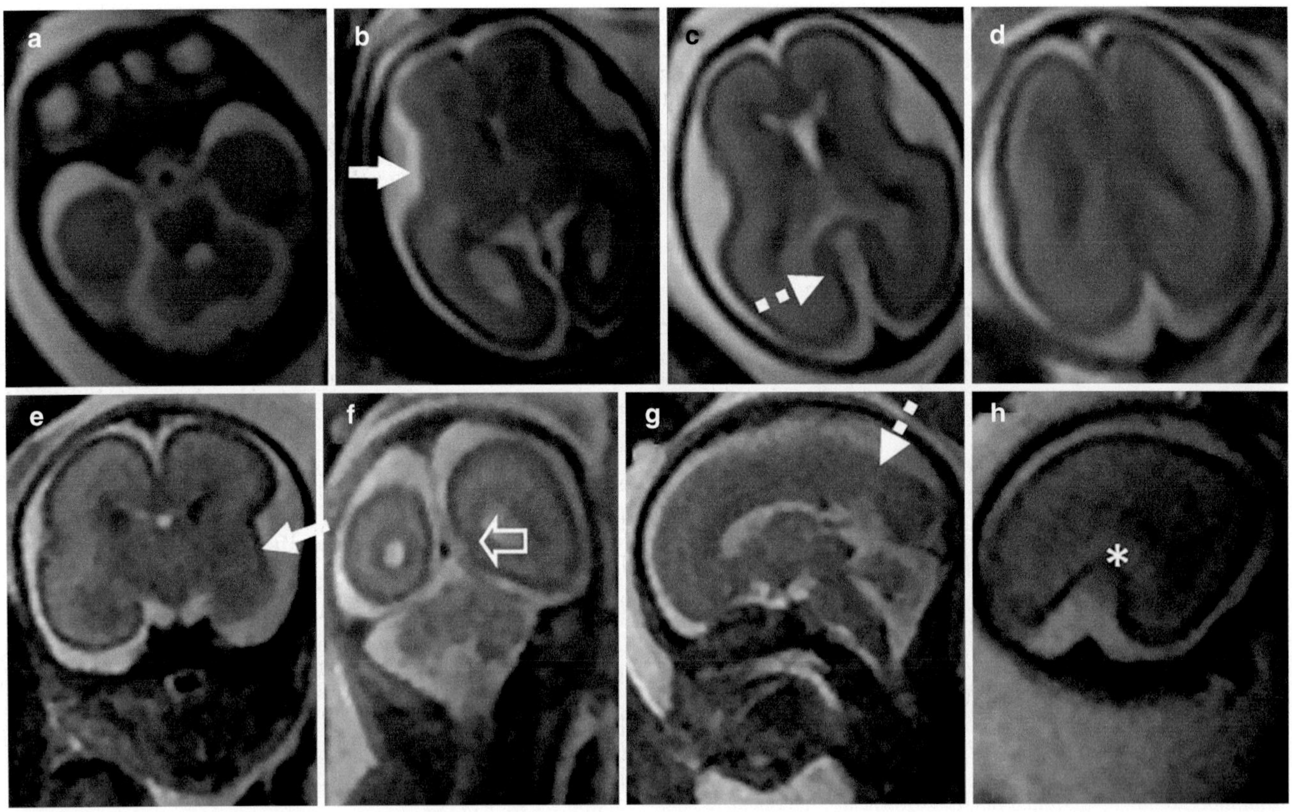

Fig. 3.5 (**a**, **b**, **c**, **d**) Axial T2W images of a 22-week fetus at the level of cerebellum, III ventricle, CSP and centrum semiovale. (**e**, **f**) coronal images at the level of sella, occipital region. (**g**, **h**) Sagittal images at the level of midline and parasagittal region. The Sylvian fissure (arrow), parieto occipital fissure (dotted arrow) lateral sulcus(asterisk), and calcarine fissure (open arrows) are identified

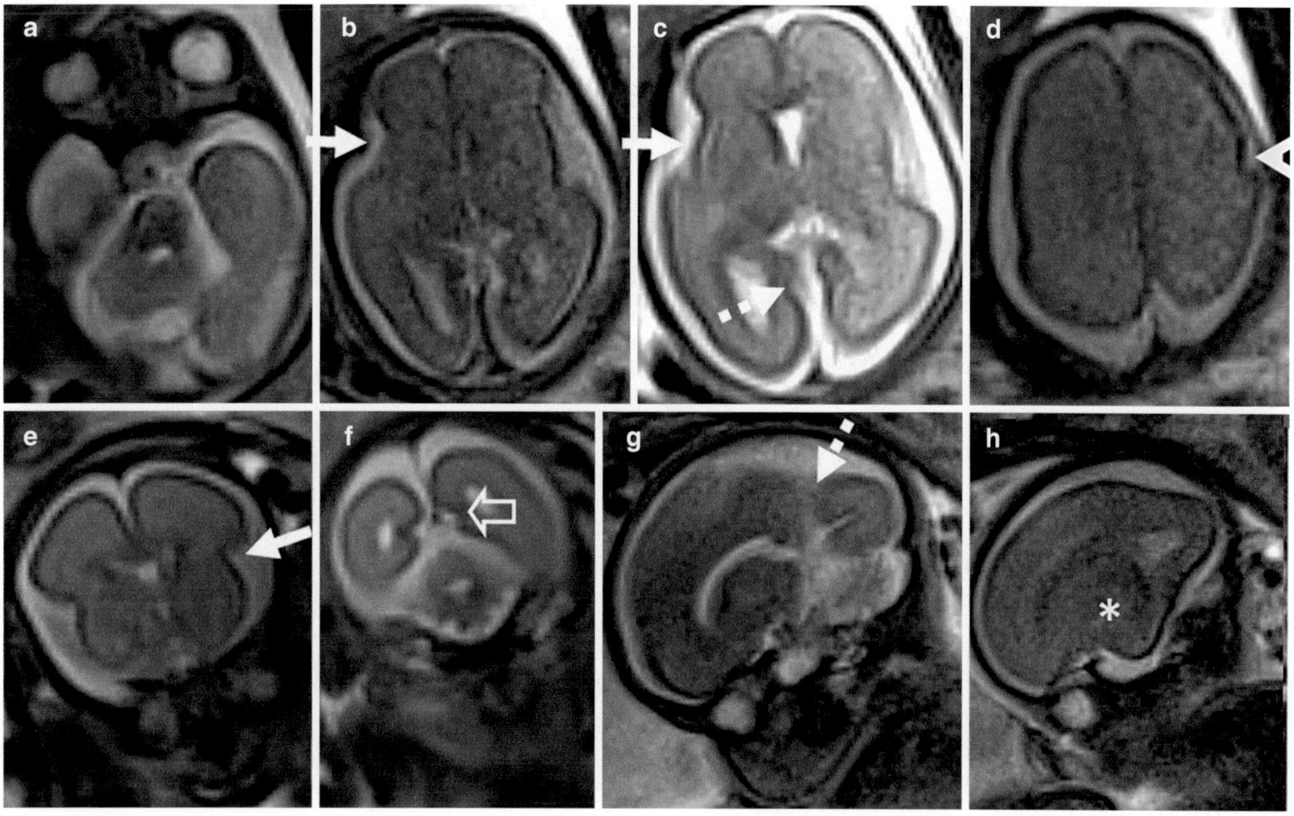

Fig. 3.6 (**a**, **b**, **c**, **d**) Axial T2W images of a 24-week fetus at the level of cerebellum, III ventricle, CSP and centrum semiovale. (**e**, **f**) coronal images at the level of sella, occipital region. (**g**, **h**) Sagittal images at the level of midline and parasagittal region. The Sylvian fissure (arrow), parieto occipital fissure (dotted arrow) lateral sulcus(asterisk), central sulcus (arrowhead) and calcarine fissure (open arrows) are identified

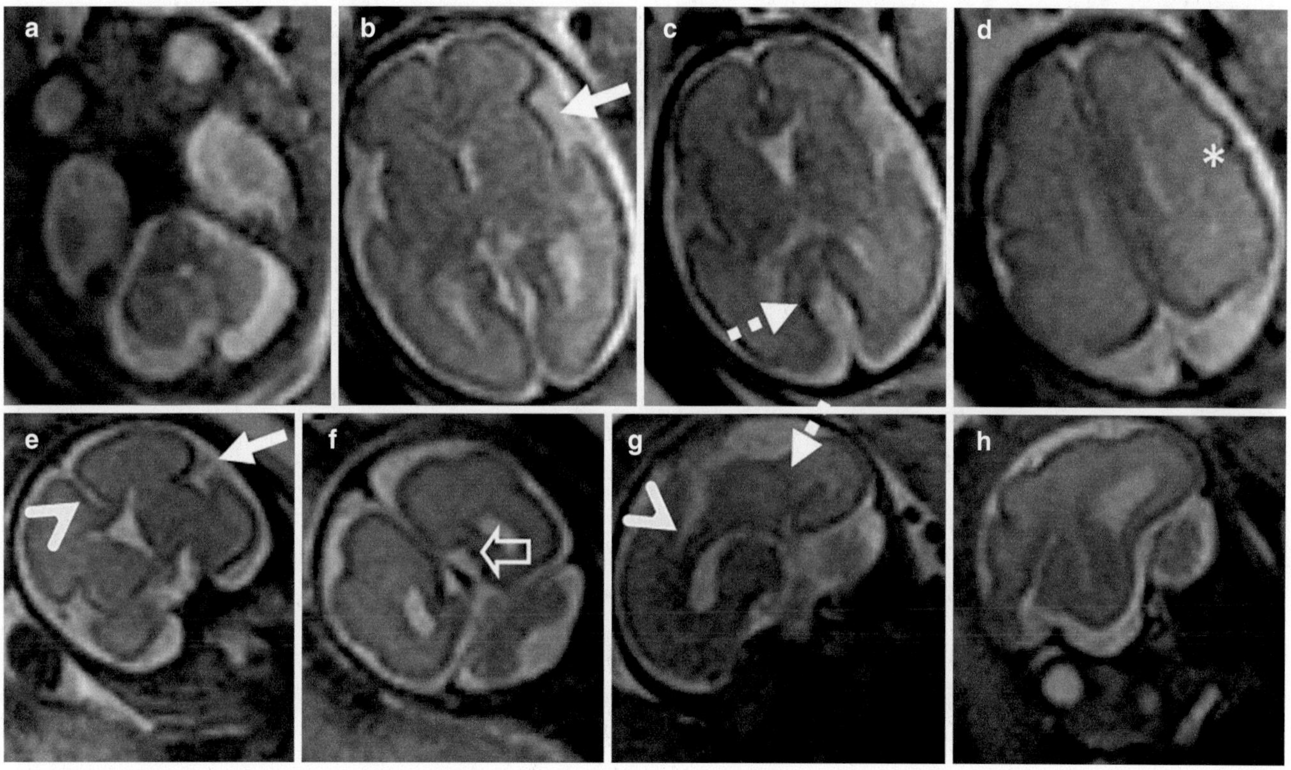

Fig. 3.7 (**a**, **b**, **c**, **d**) Axial T2W images of a 26-week fetus at the level of cerebellum, III ventricle, CSP, and centrum semiovale. (**e**, **f**) coronal images at the level of sella, occipital region. (**g**, **h**) Sagittal images at the level of midline and parasagittal region. The Sylvian fissure (arrow), parieto occipital fissure (dotted arrow), central sulcus (asterisk), calcarine fissure (open arrows), and cingulate sulcus (arrowhead) are identified

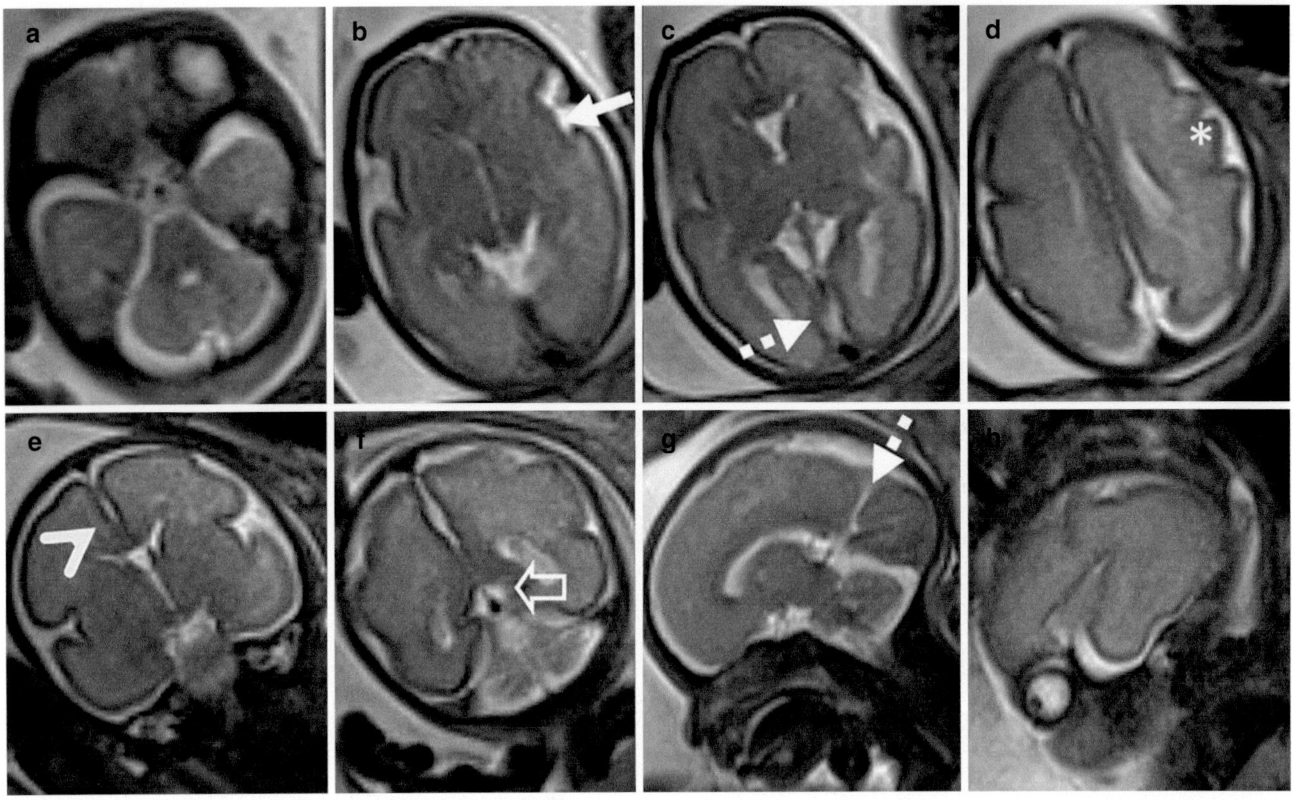

Fig. 3.8 (**a**, **b**, **c**, **d**) Axial T2W images of a 28-week fetus at the level of cerebellum, III ventricle, CSP, and centrum semiovale. (**e**, **f**) coronal images at the level of sella, occipital region. (**g**, **h**) Sagittal images at the level of midline and parasagittal region. The Sylvian fissure (arrow), parieto occipital fissure (dotted arrow) central sulcus (asterisk), calcarine fissure (open arrows), and cingulate sulcus (arrowhead) are identified

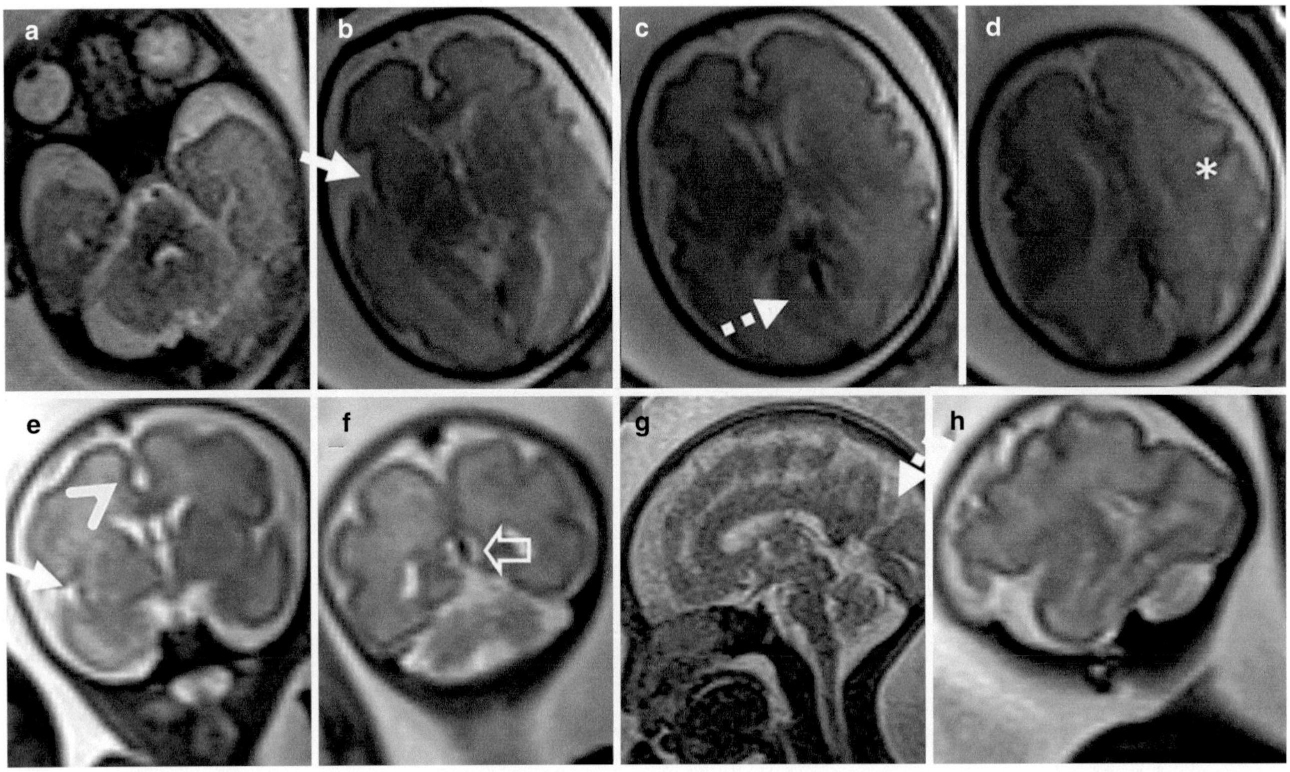

Fig. 3.9 (**a**, **b**, **c**, **d**) Axial T2W images of a 30-week fetus at the level of cerebellum, III ventricle, CSP, and centrum semiovale. (**e**, **f**) coronal images at the level of sella, occipital region. (**g**, **h**) Sagittal images at the level of midline and parasagittal region. The Sylvian fissure (arrow), parieto occipital fissure (dotted arrow) central sulcus (asterisk), calcarine fissure (open arrows) and cingulate sulcus (arrowhead) are identified

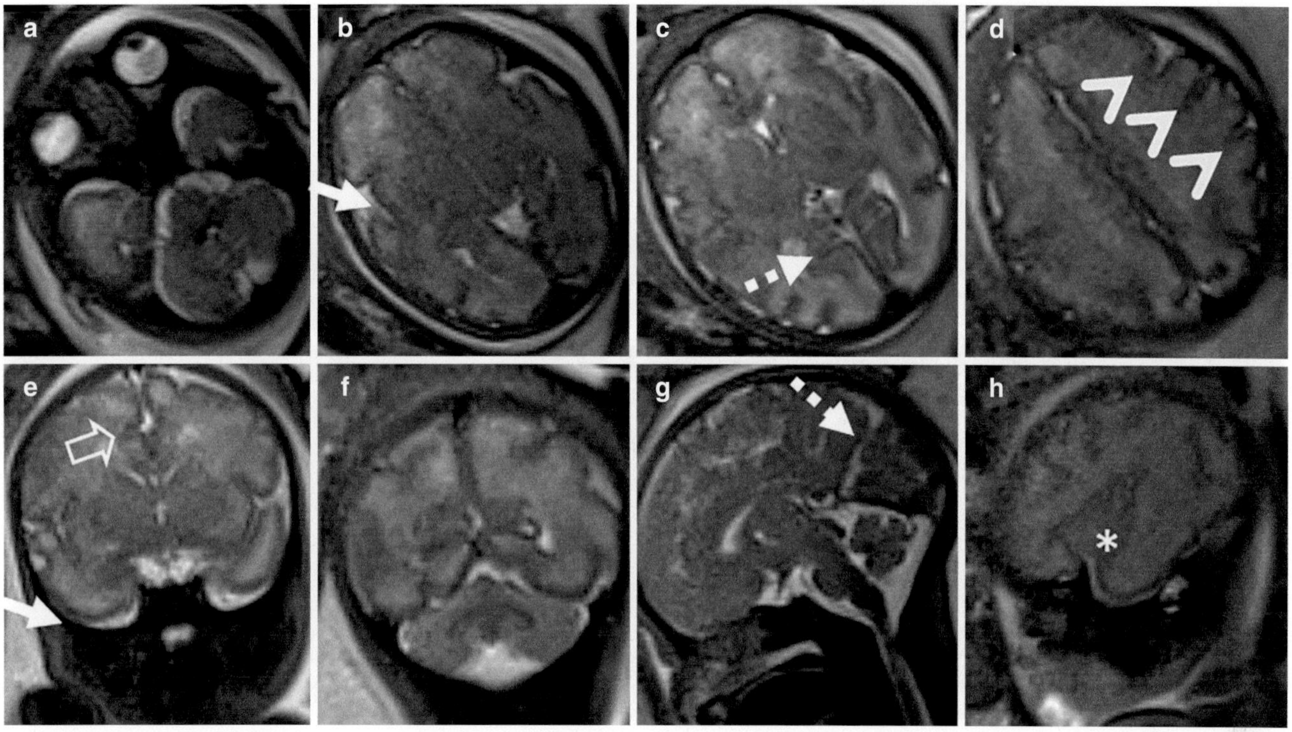

Fig. 3.10 (**a**, **b**, **c**, **d**) Axial T2W images of a 32-week fetus at the level of cerebellum, III ventricle, CSP, and centrum semiovale. (**e**, **f**) Coronal images at the level of sella, occipital region. (**g**, **h**) Sagittal images at the level of midline and parasagittal region. The Sylvian fissure (arrow), parieto occipital fissure (dotted arrow) lateral sulcus(asterisk), cingulate sulcus (open arrows), and cortical sulci (arrowhead) are identified

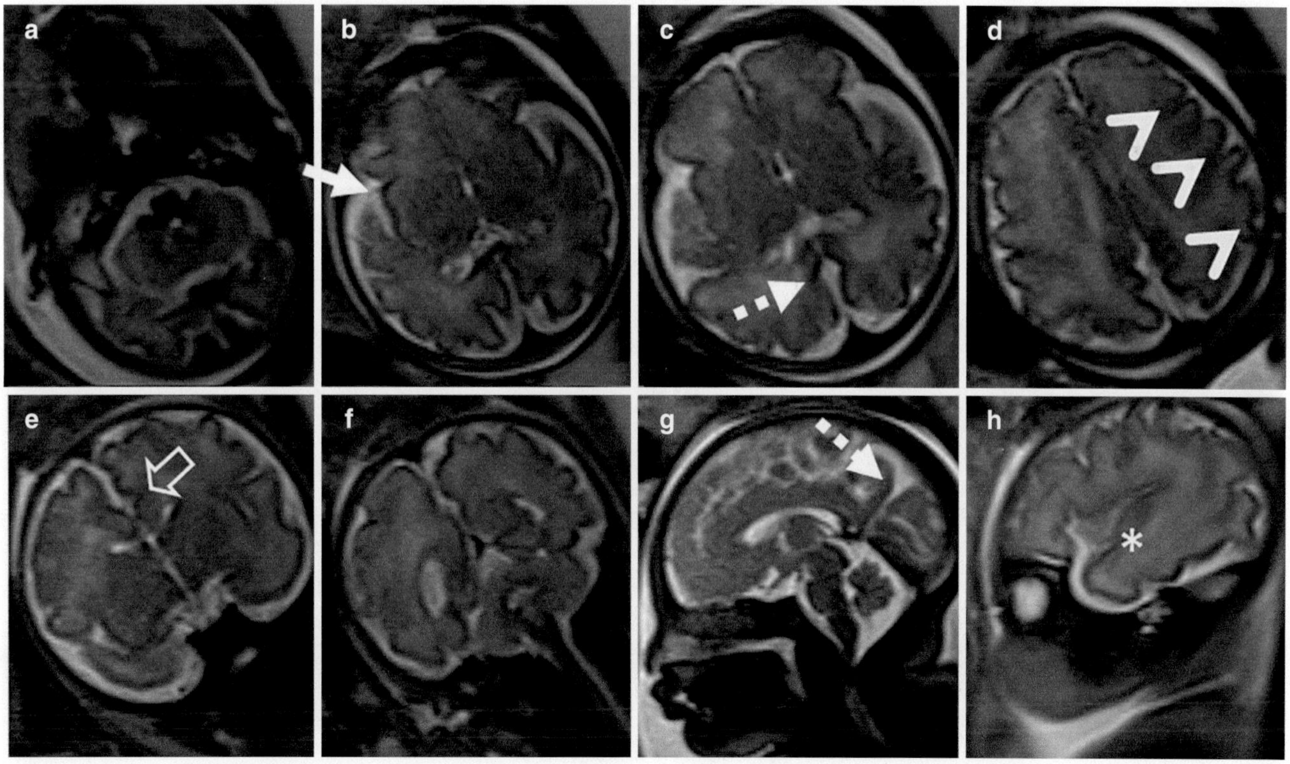

Fig. 3.11 (**a**, **b**, **c**, **d**) Axial T2W images of a 34-week fetus at the level of cerebellum, III ventricle, CSP, and centrum semiovale. (**e**, **f**) Coronal images at the level of sella, occipital region. (**g**, **h**) Sagittal images at the level of midline and parasagittal region. The Sylvian fissure (arrow), parieto occipital fissure (dotted arrow) lateral sulcus (asterisk), cingulate sulcus (open arrows), and cortical sulci (arrowhead) are identified

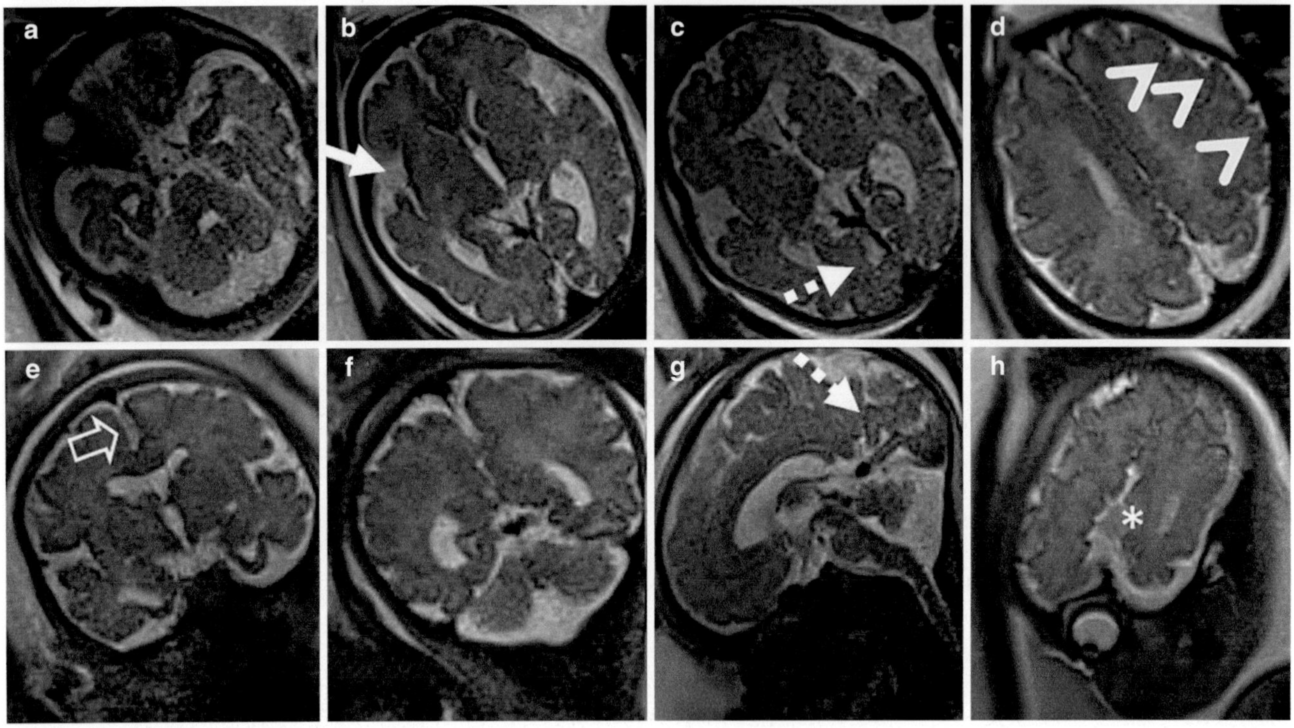

Fig. 3.12 (**a**, **b**, **c**, **d**) Axial T2W images of a 36-week fetus at the level of cerebellum, III ventricle, CSP, and centrum semiovale. (**e**, **f**) Coronal images at the level of sella, occipital region. (**g**, **h**) Sagittal images at the level of midline and parasagittal region. The Sylvian fissure (arrow), parieto occipital fissure (dotted arrow) lateral sulcus (asterisk), cingulate sulcus (open arrows), and cortical sulci (arrowhead) are identified

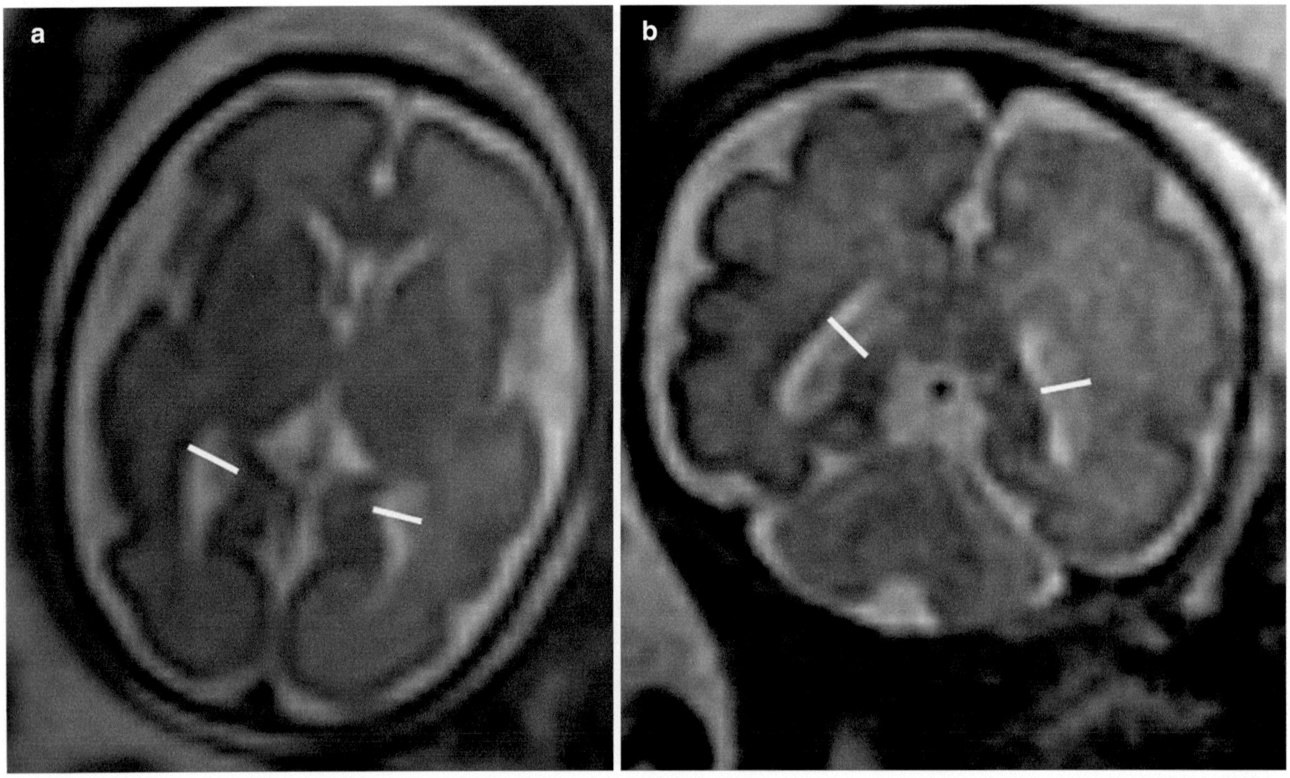

Fig. 3.13 Axial (**a**) and coronal (**b**) T2W Image of a normal 31-week fetal brain. The method of measuring the lateral ventricular width is demonstrated

3.3 The Normal Fetal Spine on MRI

Spinal development consists of three embryologic stages [19].

1. Gastrulation (2–3 weeks of embryonic development). The pluripotent cells differentiate to form three germ layers—ectoderm, mesoderm, and endoderm. The ectoderm develops to form the skin and the nervous system.
2. Primary neurulation (3–4 weeks). The notochord and the overlying ectoderm form the neural plate. The neural plate folds to form the neural tube, which closes bidirectionally in a zipperlike manner.
3. Secondary neurulation (5–6 weeks). A secondary neural tube is formed by the caudal cell mass eventually forming the tip of the conus medullaris and filum terminale by a process called retrogressive differentiation.

Between 13 and 18 weeks gestation, the conus medullaris is at the level of the L4 or caudal to it. There is ascent of the conus due to relatively faster growth of the spinal column. At term, the conus is seen above L2 (Fig. 3.14) [20–23]. The fetal spine is examined in three planes. On sagittal sections the spine shows a parallel contour with widening toward the fetal head and gradual tapering in the sacral region. The vertebral bodies appear hypointense and the discs appear hyperintense on T2WI (Fig. 3.15). The sacral spine may not be fully ossified before 22 weeks' gestational age. In suspicious cases where the sacrum is not fully visualized and when the mother is diabetic or the fetus is at high risk for developing neural tube defects, imaging needs to be repeated at or after 24 weeks. Counting of the vertebra is easily done on US using the 12th rib as a landmark. However, in MRI, the last bright disk space is supposed to be L5-S1 and based on this the vertebrae are counted [24].

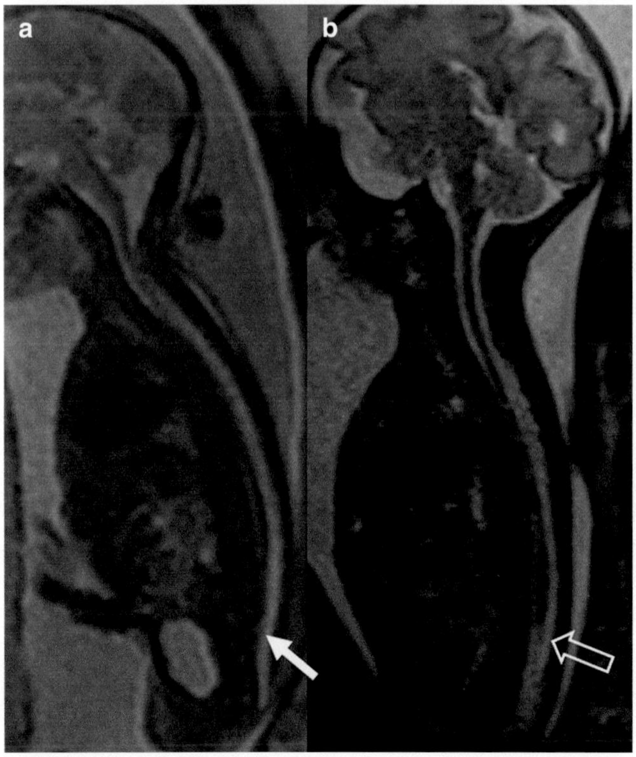

Fig. 3.14 Sagittal T2W image (**a**) of 21-week fetus showing normal spinal cord ending in lower lumbar region (arrow). Sagittal T2 image (**b**) of 29-week fetus showing normal spinal cord ending in mid-lumbar region (open arrow). The bony spine shows a parallel contour

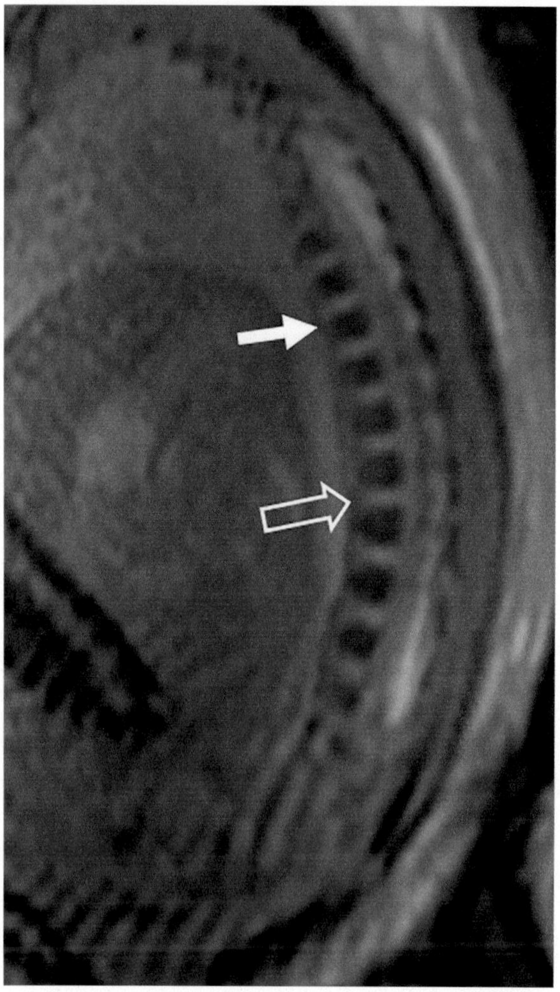

Fig. 3.15 Sagittal image obtained using true FISP sequence shows well delineation of hypointense vertebral bodies (arrow) and hyperintense intervertebral discs (open arrows)

Though US is the primary modality to identify spinal malformations, MRI is an important complementary tool. There may be limitations to US examination due to fetal position, e.g., when the fetal spine is positioned posteriorly, or the back of the fetus is close to the placenta/uterine wall. Similarly, oligohydramnios and large maternal body habitus may further limit image detail. MRI provides additional information due to its high contrast resolution [23].

References

1. Sadler TW. Embryology of neural tube development. Am J Med Genet Part C Semin Med Genet. 2005;135:2–8.
2. Acharya UV, Pendharkar H, Varma DR, Pruthi N, Varadarajan S. Spinal dysraphism illustrated; Embroyology revisited. Indian J Radiol Imaging. 2017;27(4):417–26. https://doi.org/10.4103/ijri.IJRI_451_16.
3. Kanekar S, Kaneda H, Shively A. Malformations of dorsal induction. Semin Ultrasound CT MR. 2011;32:189–99.
4. van der Knaap MS, Valk J. Classification of congenital abnormalities of the CNS. AJNR. 9:315–26.
5. Kanekar S, Shively A, Kaneda H. Malformations of ventral induction. Semin Ultrasound CT MR. 2011;32:200–10.
6. Abdel razek AA, Kandell AY, Elsorogy LG et-al. Disorders of cortical formation: MR imaging features. AJNR Am J Neuroradiol. 2009;30(1):4–11.
7. Barkovich AJ, Kuzniecky RI, Jackson GD, et-al. Classification system for malformations of cortical development: update 2001. Neurology. 2001;57(12):2168–78.
8. Barkovich AJ, Kuzniecky RI, Jackson GD, et-al. A developmental and genetic classification for malformations of cortical development. Neurology. 2005;65(12):1873–87.
9. Barkovich AJ, Guerrini R, Kuzniecky RI, et-al. A developmental and genetic classification for malformations of cortical development: update 2012. Brain. 2012;135(5):1348–69.
10. Griffiths PD, Morris J, Larroche JC, et al. Sectional anatomy of the fetal brain. In: Griffiths PD, Morris J, Larroche JC, Reeves M, editors. Atlas of fetal and postnatal brain MRI. Philadelphia, PA: Mosby, Elsevier; 2010.
11. Glenn OA, Barkovich AJ. Magnetic resonance imaging of the fetal brain and spine: an increasingly important tool in prenatal diagnosis, part 1. Am J Neuroradiol. 2006;27:1604–11.
12. Lan LM, Yamashita Y, Tang Y, Sugahara T, Takahashi M, Ohba T, Okamura H. Normal fetal brain development: MR imaging with a half-Fourier rapid acquisition with relaxation enhancement sequence. Radiology. 2000;215(1):205–10.
13. Ghai S, Fong KW, Toi A, Chitayat D, Pantazi S, Blaser S. Prenatal US and MR imaging findings of lissencephaly: review of fetal cerebral sulcal development. Radiographics. 2006;26:389–405.
14. Manor C, Rangasami R, Suresh I, Suresh S. Magnetic resonance imaging findings in fetal corpus callosal developmental abnormalities: a pictorial essay. J Pediatr Neurosci. 2020;15:352–7.
15. Nunez S, Mantilla MT, Bermúdez S. Midline congenital malformations of the brain and skull. Neuroimaging Clin N Am. 2011;21(3):429–82, vii. https://doi.org/10.1016/j.nic.2011.05.001
16. Garel C. MRI of the fetal brain. Berlin: Springer; 2004. p. 267.
17. Garel C, Chantrel E, Elmaleh M, Brisse H, Sebag G. Fetal MRI: normal gestational landmarks for cerebral biometry, gyration and myelination. Childs Nerv Syst. 2003;19:422–5.
18. Salomon LJ, Garel C. Magnetic resonance imaging examination of the fetal brain. Ultrasound Obstet Gynecol. 2007;30:1019–32.
19. Tortori-Donati P, Rossi A, Cama A. Spinal dysraphism: a review of neuroradiological features with embryological correlations and proposal for a new classification. Neuroradiology. 2000;42(7):471–91.
20. Zalel Y, Lehavi O, Aizenstein O, Achiron R. Development of the fetal spinal cord. J Ultrasound Med. 2006;25:1397–401.
21. Naidich TP, McLone DG. Congenital pathology of the spine and spinal cord. In: Taveras JM, Ferrucci JT, editors. Radiology: diagnosis-imaging intervention, vol. 3. Philadelphia: Lippincott; 1986. p. 1–23.
22. Rufener SL, Ibrahim M, Raybaud CA, Parmar HA. Congenital spine and spinal cord malformations--pictorial review. Am J Roentgenol. 2010;194(3 Suppl):S26–37.
23. Huisman TAGM, et al. MRI of fetal spinal malformations. J Pediatric Neuroradiol. 2012;1:211–23.
24. Chao TT, Dashe JS, Adams RC, Keefover-Hicks A, McIntire DD, Twickler DM. Fetal spine findings on MRI and associated outcomes in children with open neural tube defects. AJR Am J Roentgenol. 2011;197(5):W956–61.

4 Midline Brain Anomalies I: Anomalies of Septum Pellucidum and Corpus Callosum

4.1 Anomalies of Septum Pellucidum

Embryology and Normal Septum Pellucidum

Between 5 and 10 weeks of gestation, from the cranial part of the neural tube, three primary vesicles viz., prosencephalon, mesencephalon, and rhombencephalon become differentiated and form the forebrain, midbrain, and hindbrain, respectively, by ventral induction. Prosencephalon further differentiates to form telencephalon and diencephalon that develop into cerebrum and thalami respectively. Cleavage and midline development also occurs in the prosencephalon. Failure to form telencephalon leads to atelencephaly. Failure to cleavage leads to the spectrum of holoprosencephaly and failure of midline development leads to septal agenesis and anomalies of the corpus callosum [1–4].

Septum pellucidum is visualized as two layers of membranes between the lateral ventricles at 18–37 weeks, i.e., when biparietal diameter is between 44 and 88 mm. Since it contains a cavity of fluid between the membranes it is called Cavum Septum pellucidum (CSP). It starts developing by 10–12 weeks of gestation and acquires an adult form by 17 weeks. It measures between 2 and 10 mm, the diameter increasing with gestational age from 19 weeks, and reaches a plateau at 28 weeks (Fig. 4.1). Typically, the leaflets begin to close from back to front after 6 months of gestation. After 37 weeks, the cavity of fluid is absorbed and the septum is often seen as a single thin layer of membrane. Rarely the cavum persists into adult life appearing small and measuring less than 4 mm in transverse dimension [5]. The AP length of fetal CSP is directly proportional to the length of CC. However, normal CC with absent CSP can occur in septal agenesis. The USG measurements of CSP can be found in the article by Jou et al. [6]. The important septal abnormalities are summarized in Fig. 4.2.

4.1.1 Absent Septum Pellucidum

There is partial or complete absence of septum pellucidum. This may occur as a developmental anomaly or may be secondary to any destructive process [7].

Incidence 2 or 3 per 100,000.

Pathogenesis and genetics

A. *Developmental type*:
   Association: Holoprosencephaly (HPE), septo-optic dysplasia (SOD), agenesis of the corpus callosum, schizencephaly.
B. *Acquired type*: Due to hydranencephaly and congenital hydrocephalus.

Imaging features

- The septum pellucidum is not visualized with both frontal horns communicating with each other (Fig. 4.3).
- The frontal horns appear squared.
- The frontal horns show inferior pointing.
- Sometimes the fornix-internal cerebral veins may give a "pseudo septum" appearance which can be resolved by observing the coronal sections [8, 9].

Differential diagnosis

1. Septo-optic dysplasia—Besides septal agenesis, there is associated hypoplasia of optic chiasm/optic nerves or globes. However, the optic pathway involvement may be difficult to demonstrate antenatally.
2. Narrow cavum septum pellucidum—The transverse diameter is less than 2 mm and CSP are better demonstrated on coronal sections when the axial sections are deceptive.

R. Rajeswaran, *MR Imaging of the Fetus*, https://doi.org/10.1007/978-981-16-9209-3_4

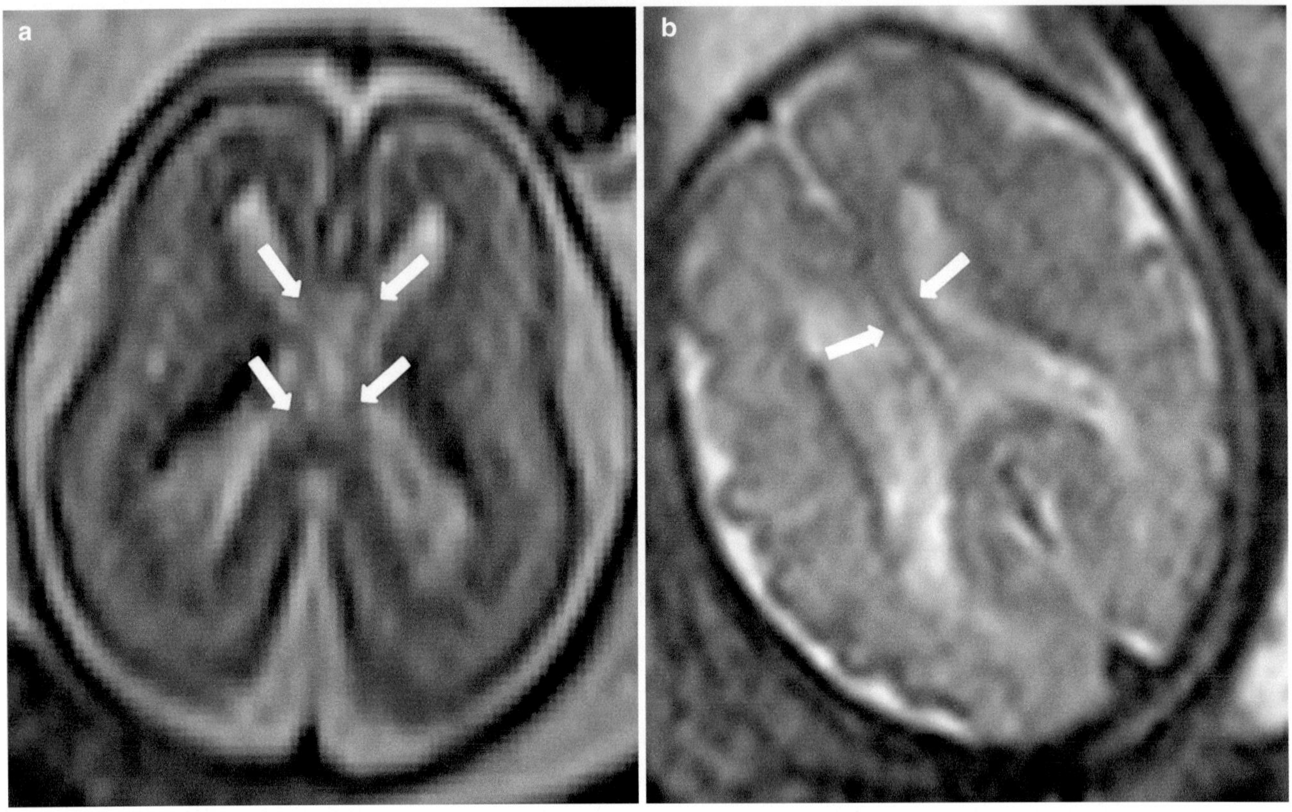

Fig. 4.1 Axial MR images showing a normal CSP at (**a**) 20 weeks, (**b**) 31 weeks

Prognosis Prognosis is often good when it is isolated (>75%) [5].

Postnatal problems like behavioral changes, learning difficulties, seizures, and reduced vision are seen in a few cases.

4.1.2 Septo-Optic Dysplasia (SOD)

Synonym: de Morsier syndrome

Septo-optic dysplasia is characterized by septal agenesis, Optic nerve hypoplasia, and with or without hypopituitarism.

Incidence prevalence of ~1:50,000.

Types

A. *Not associated with schizencephaly*
   - Visual pathway severely affected.
   - Hypothalamic-pituitary dysfunction may be present—leading to deficiency of hormones/hypoglycemia.
   - Absent olfactory bulbs (Kallmann syndrome).

B. *Associated with schizencephaly (septo-optic dysplasia plus)*
   - Optic pathway is less severely affected.
   - Cortical abnormalities like polymicrogyria and cortical dysplasia.

Imaging features

- Absent septum pellucidum—The frontal horns appear squared, communicating with each other and show inferior pointing (Fig. 4.4). There may be associated schizencephaly (Fig. 4.5).
- Pituitary hypoplasia leading to deficiency of hormones/hypoglycemia. Sometimes absent infundibulum with presence of ectopic posterior pituitary may be observed.
- Hypoplastic optic chiasm/optic nerves and globes. The optic nerve sheath diameter at 22 and 36 weeks is approximately 1.2 mm and 2.6 mm, respectively. In the third trimester, optic nerve may be seen as hypointense linear structure in the background of hyperintense orbital fat. The thickness of optic nerve approximately equals the extraocular muscle thickness [10, 11].

Association

- Rhombencephalosynapsis
- Chiari II malformation
- Aqueductal stenosis

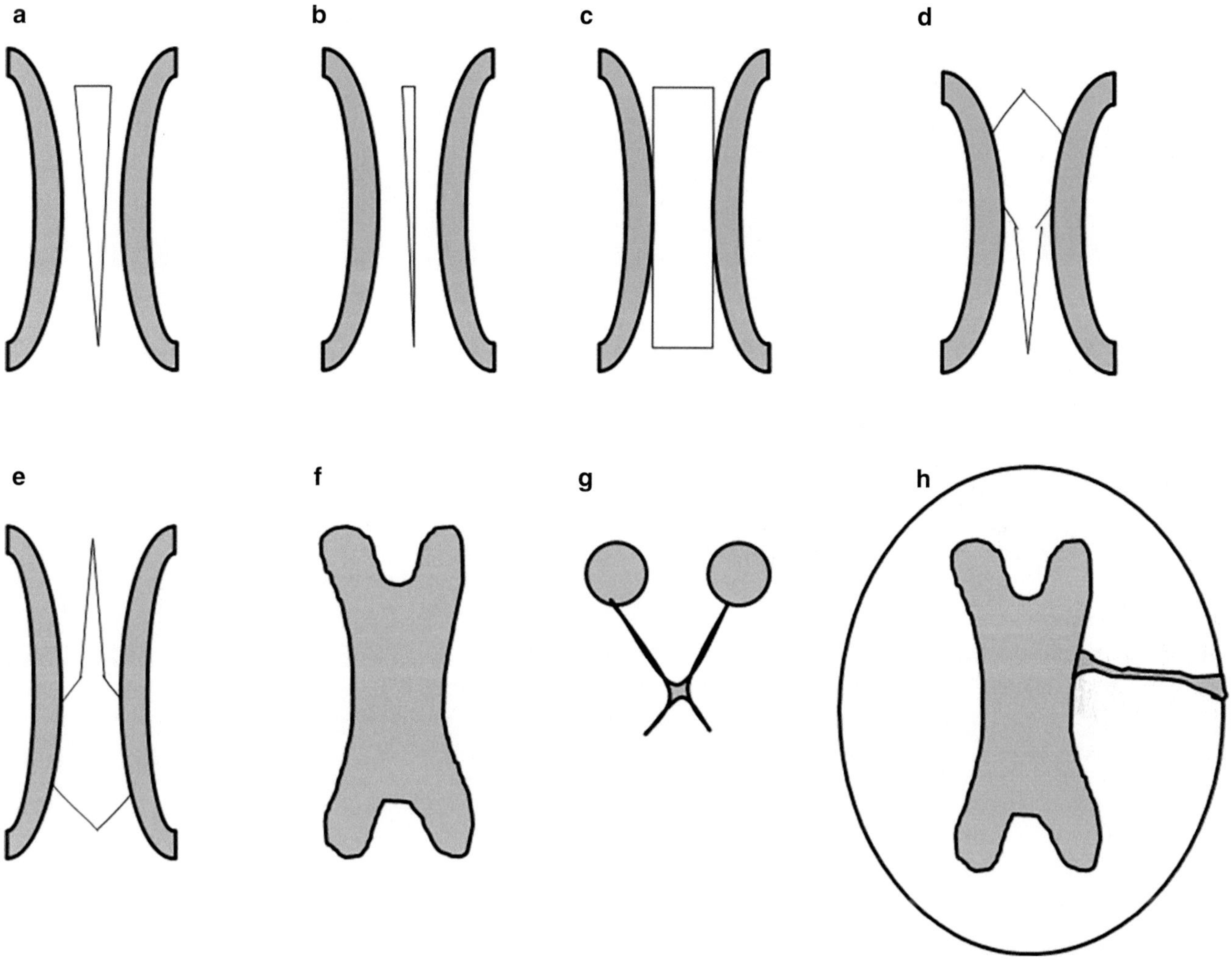

Fig. 4.2 Graphic representation of Septal anomalies. (**a**) Normal (**b**) Narrow CSP (**c**) Wide CSP (**d**) Cavum spetum pellucidum cyst (**e**) Cavum vergae cyst (**f**) Absent CSP (**g**) Hypoplasic optic nerves, chiasm and tracts (**h**) SOD with schizencephaly

Differential diagnosis

1. Lobar holoprosencephaly—the optic pathway is not affected and the anterior cerebral artery is displaced anteriorly. Fetal MRI is diagnostic.
2. Isolated septal agenesis.
3. Agenesis of corpus callosum.

Prognosis While some children with SOD have normal intelligence, others have learning disabilities and show delayed development. There may be associated visual impairment, seizures, or neurological problems.

Treatment Postnatal clinical and imaging assessment is done. Supportive and symptomatic treatment and physical therapy are given wherever it is needed.

4.1.3 Narrow CSP

CSP is labeled as narrow when its transverse diameter is less than 2 mm. Commonly they are diagnosed on fetal MRI when being referred to as non-visualized CSP on USG (Fig. 4.6). When it is an isolated finding, it carries a good prognosis [12].

Differential diagnosis Septal agenesis

4.1.4 Enlarged CSP

CSP is labeled as enlarged when its transverse diameter is greater than 10 mm (Fig. 4.7). When it is an isolated finding in the fetus, it carries a good prognosis in the majority [12].

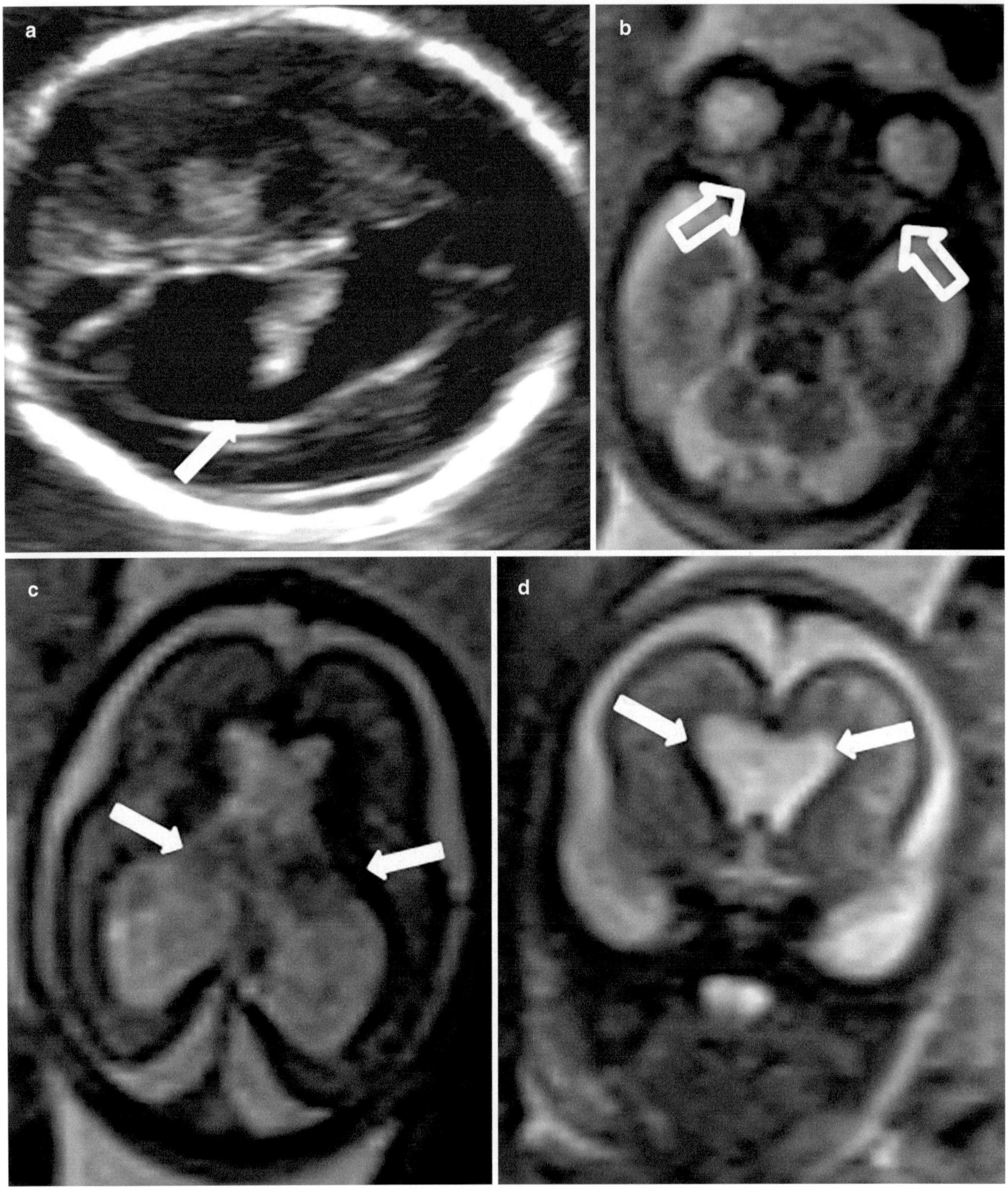

Fig. 4.3 (**a**) Sonography of a 22-week fetus shows the absence of CSP and bilateral ventriculomegaly. MRI axial images (**b**) Bilateral orbital globes and optic nerves are visualized (open arrows), axial (**c**) and coronal images (**d**) confirm absence of CSP, ventriculomegaly with bilateral ventricles communicating with each other(arrows)

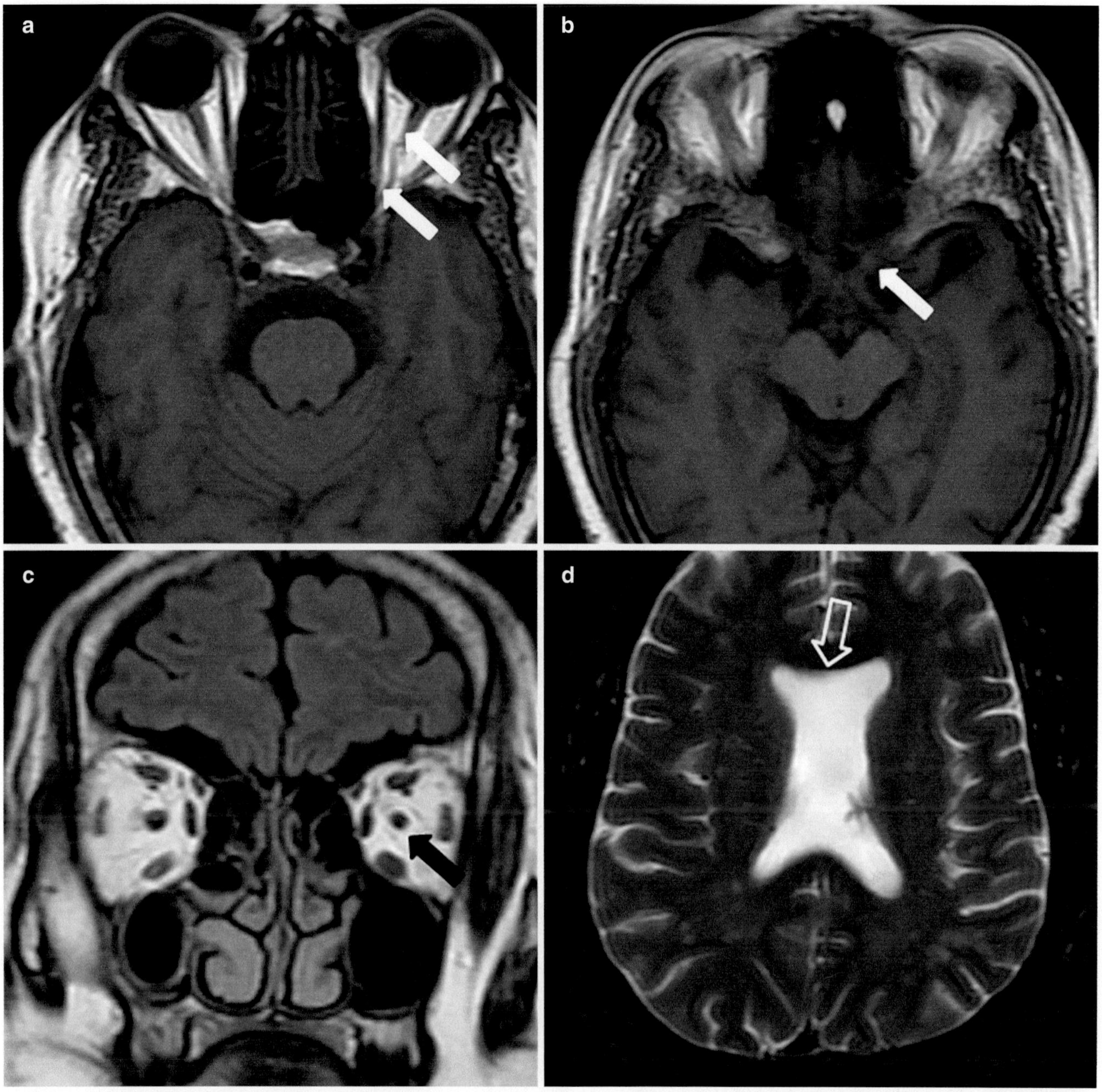

Fig. 4.4 Septo-optic dysplasia in an adult patient. T1 axial (**a**, **b**), FLAIR coronal (**c**) images show hypoplastic left optic nerve (arrows). T2 axial image (**d**) shows absent septum (open arrow)

Uncommonly it is associated with trisomy and may warrant genetic workup [5]. However, persistence of a wide cavum septi pellucidi beyond infancy has been associated with mental retardation, developmental delay, and psychiatric disturbance (schizophrenia) [13–15].

Differential diagnosis Enlarged third ventricle, vein of Galen malformation, and cyst of CSP.

4.1.5 Cyst of Cavum Septi Pellucidi

Cyst of CSP may mimic an enlarged CSP, but shows some mass effect (Fig. 4.8). Sometimes the foramen of Monro is obstructed causing dilatation of bilateral lateral ventricles. They are commonly seen incidentally on postnatal imaging. Rarely they are associated with headaches, syncope, emesis, papilledema, cognitive impairment, behavioral dis-

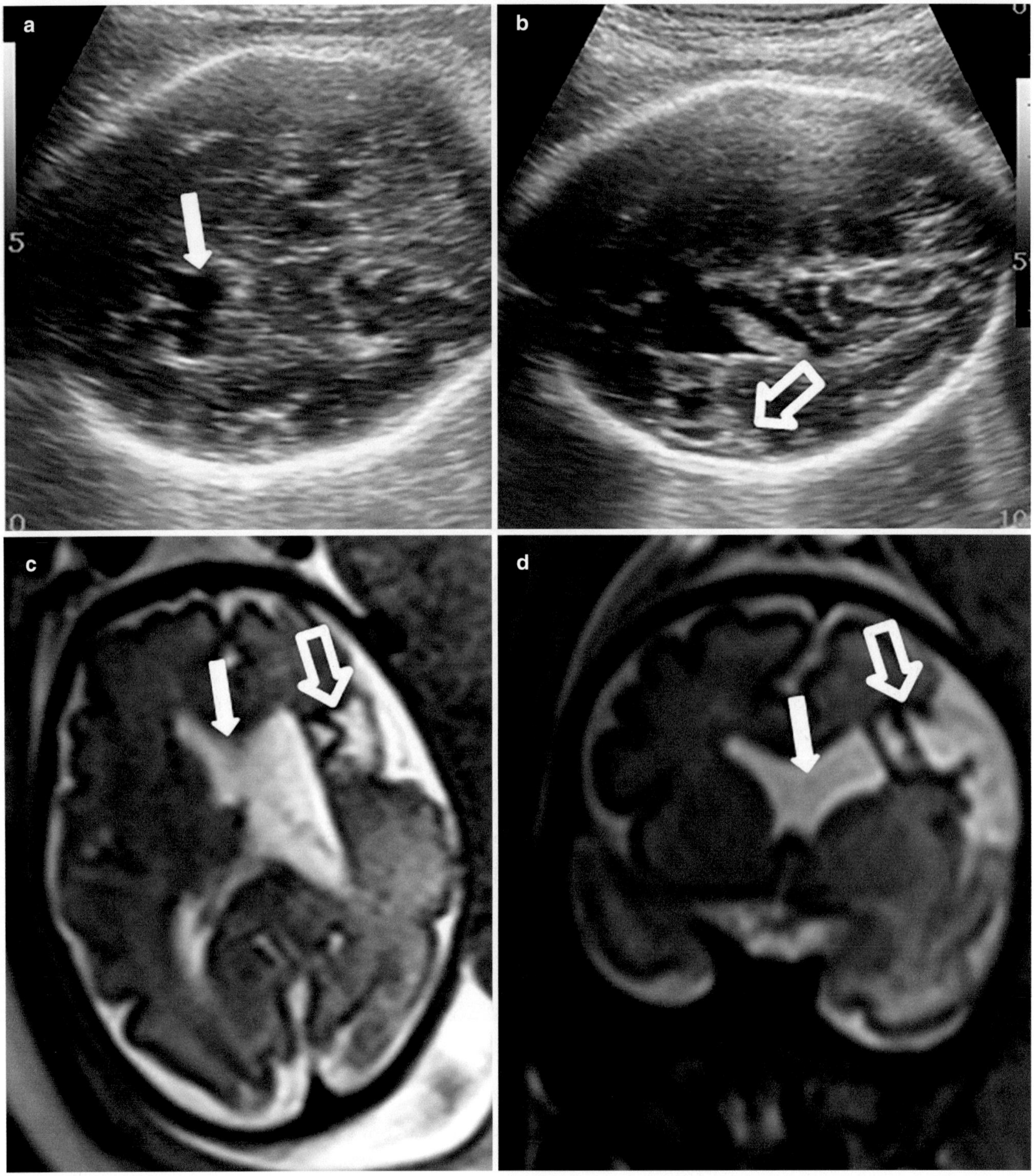

Fig. 4.5 US of fetal brain at 31 weeks showing (**a**) absent CSP (arrows) (**b**) cortical abnormality in the left frontal region (open arrows). MR axial (**c**) and coronal (**d**) images confirming septo-optic dysplasia with open lip schizencephaly

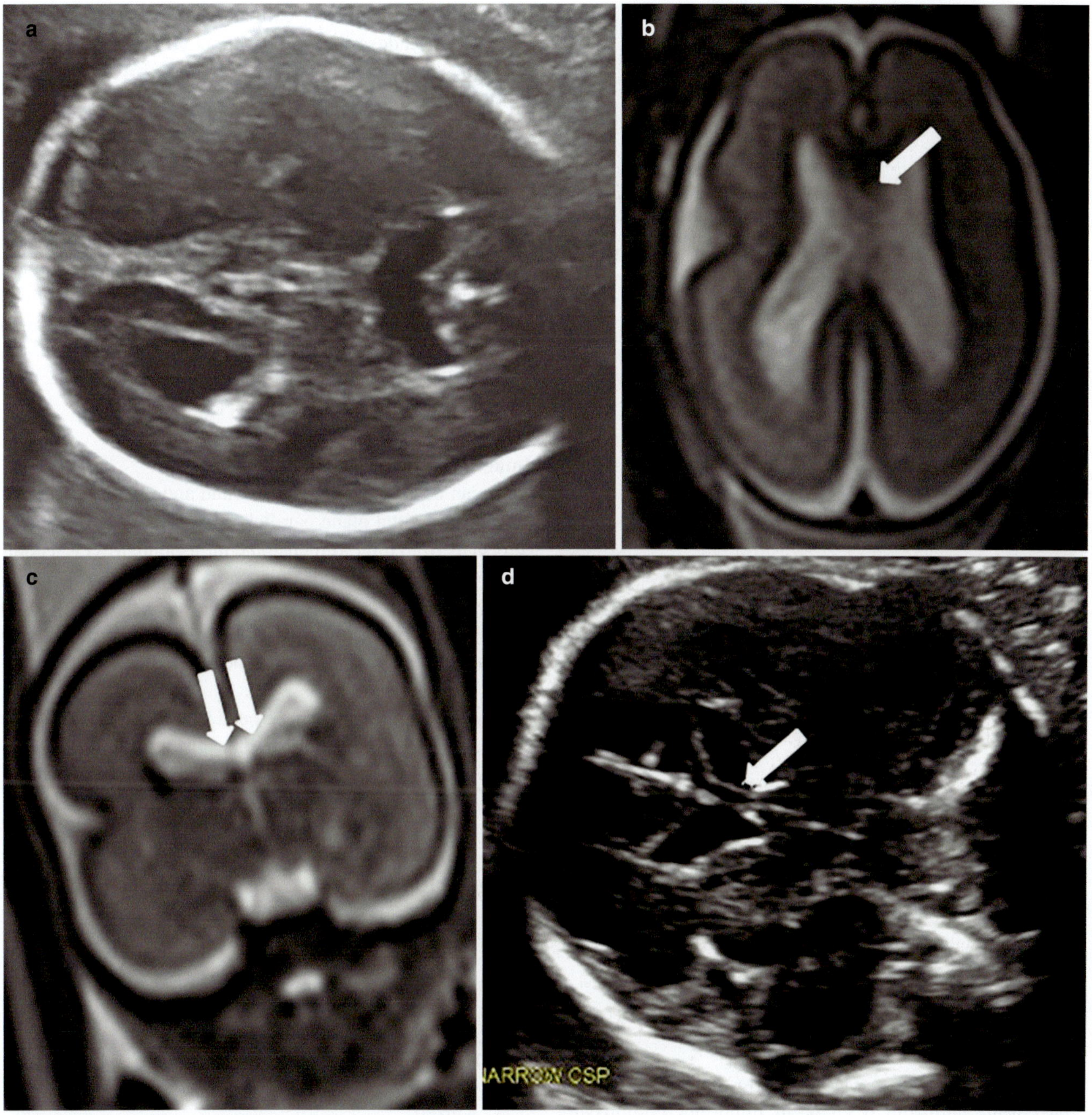

Fig. 4.6 (**a**) US of fetal brain at 23 weeks, referred to as absent CSP. MRI axial (**b**) and coronal (**c**) images showing narrow CSP measuring 2 mm (arrows) that was confirmed by follow up US (**d**) at 28 weeks

turbances, and visual findings. Surgery is indicated in case they produce a significant mass effect or neurological disturbances [16]. Few case reports are described about spontaneous resolution [16].

Differential diagnosis Enlarged CSP, Interhemispheric cyst [5].

4.1.6 Cavum Vergae and Cavum Vergae Cyst

The posterior extension of cavum septum pellucidum is called Cavum vergae. It is seen anterior to splenium of the corpus callosum and superior to the columns of the fornices. Sometimes it may show a rectangular cyst with convex outer margin and producing mass effect (Fig. 4.8).

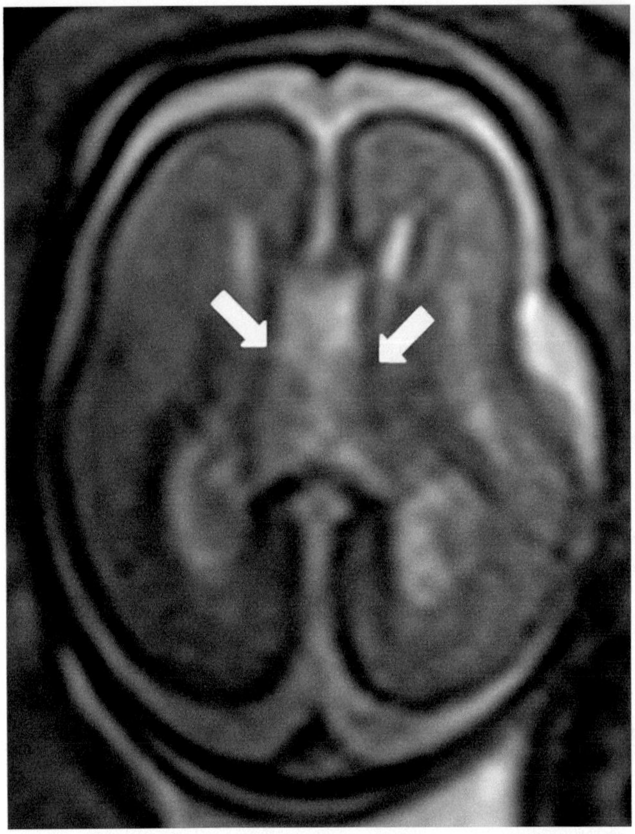

Fig. 4.7 Axial MR image of a fetus at 20 weeks showing an enlarged CSP

4.1.7 Cavum Veli Interpositi (CVI) and Cyst

CVI is a triangular space inferior to splenium and columns of the fornices. Rarely it may show as a cyst that is also triangular in shape with apex pointing anteriorly [17] (Fig. 4.9).

4.2 Corpus Callosal Abnormalities (CCA)

Embryology and normal corpus callosum

The corpus callosum (CC) is an important commissure connecting the two cerebral hemispheres. The corpus callosum consists of four parts: Rostrum, genu, body, and splenium. The CC develops from commissural plate at around 6 weeks of gestation. This is followed by crossing of fibers from one hemisphere to the other [18]. During the 8th–14th gestational weeks, callosal precursors and bilateral cerebral cortical fibers develop to form the corpus callosum. The CC develops from genu anteriorly and proceeds posteriorly to the splenium, except for the rostrum which is the last to develop [19, 20]. The final shape is attained by 19–20 weeks (Fig. 4.10). The myelination of CC occurs after birth and gets completed by adolescence. The normal measurements of corpus callosum at various gestational age have been described by Pashaj et al. [21].

Pathogenesis

Fetal corpus callosal abnormalities (CCA) may occur due to genetic causes, vitamin deficiency, maternal alcohol consumption, intrauterine infection, vascular, metabolic, and unknown causes. A number of genetic disorders in *humans* have been associated with CCA, including several X-linked diseases, metabolic disorders, and contiguous gene deletion syndromes [19, 22]. Syndromes and genetic abnormalities may be present in 40% cases of ACC and 15% cases of dysgenesis of CC (DCC) [22].

Incidence of 0.5–70 in 10,000 [18].

Imaging features

CCA can be diagnosed by ultrasound and it is mandatory to take a midsagittal plane parallel to the CC or obtain sagittal reformats from three-dimensional ultrasound. MRI is a complementary modality and depicts even the smallest CCA. It is important to view the fetal CC in all three planes to avoid errors in interpretation. MRI is also useful in diagnosing associated anomalies which can help in patient counseling.

Several terminologies have been used to describe Corpus callosal abnormalities like complete agenesis, Partial agenesis, hypogenesis, and dysgenesis. We have tried to include all subtypes based on the recent classifications [23, 24] (Fig. 4.11).

- *Hypoplastic CC*
  - Diffusely thin
  - Deficient posterior part
  - Apple core
  - Anterior remnant
- *Dysplastic CC*
- *Hypoplastic and dysplastic CC*
  - Stripe
  - Kinked
- *Complete agenesis*
- *Mega corpus callosum*

4.2.1 Hypoplastic CC

Hypoplasia consists of a diffusely thin CC or poorly developed CC in the posterior aspect. It has three subtypes—Diffusely thin CC, Apple core CC, and anterior remnant CC [23]. The AP length of CSP decreases with decreasing length of CC. The CSP length-to-width ratio decreases in hypoplasia and is an important marker on USG [25].

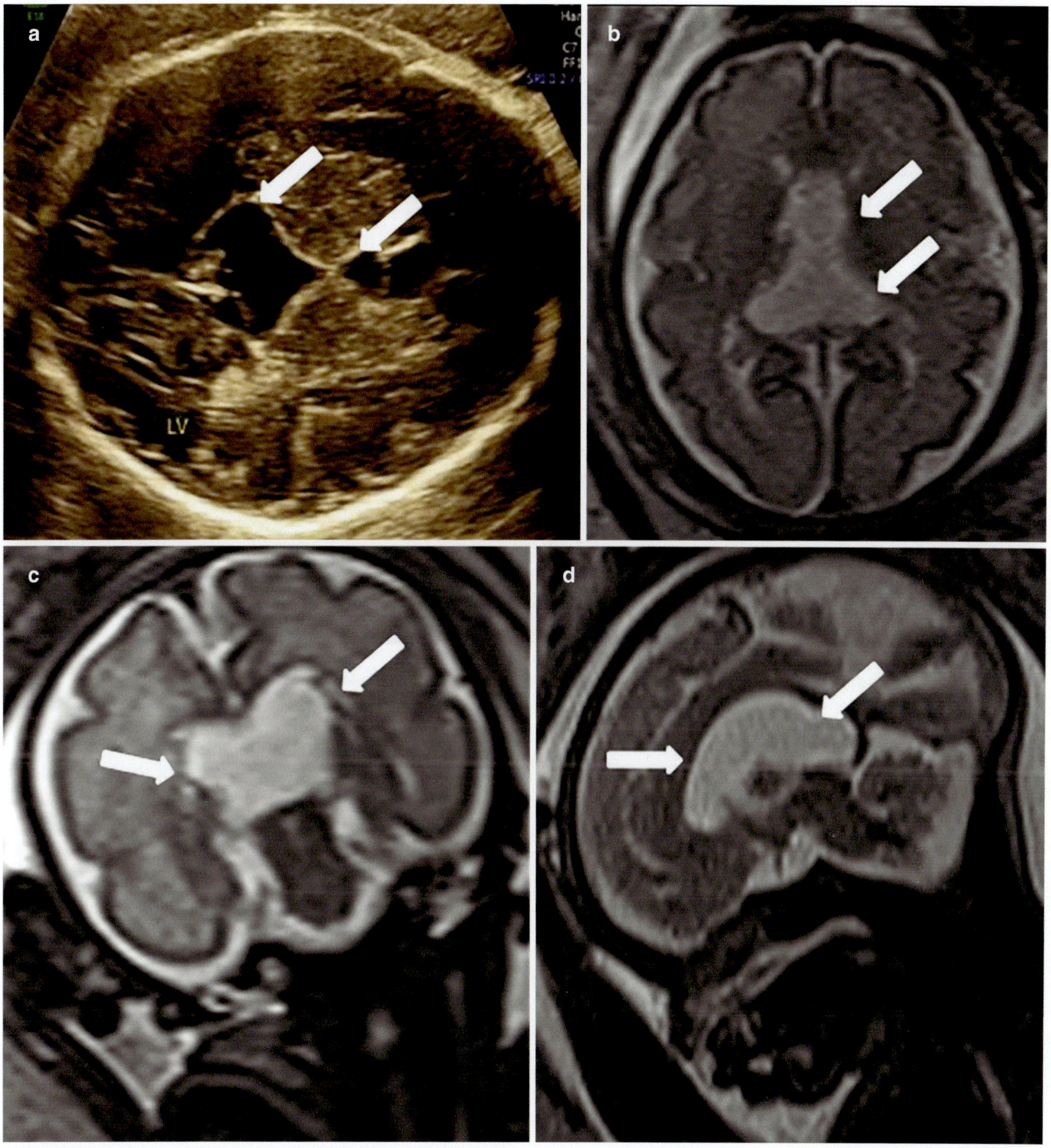

Fig. 4.8 US of fetal brain at 31 weeks (**a**), showing a Cavum Septum pellucidum–vergae cyst (arrows) that was confirmed on axial (**b**) coronal (**c**) and sagittal (**d**) MR images. The fetus was conservatively managed

a. *Diffusely thin CC*

In this, the thickness of the corpus callosum is uniformly reduced but has all anatomic landmarks—rostrum, genu, corpus, and splenium [23].

b. *Deficient posterior part*

There is progressive loss of the posterior parts (corpus or splenium) of the CC. The posterior part is deficient and foreshortened (Fig. 4.12a).

c. *Apple core CC*

The posterior part may be constricted resembling apple core (Fig. 4.12b).

d. *Anterior remnant CC*

In this type, there is agenesis of the majority of the posterior CC (i.e., corpus and splenium) (Fig. 4.12c).

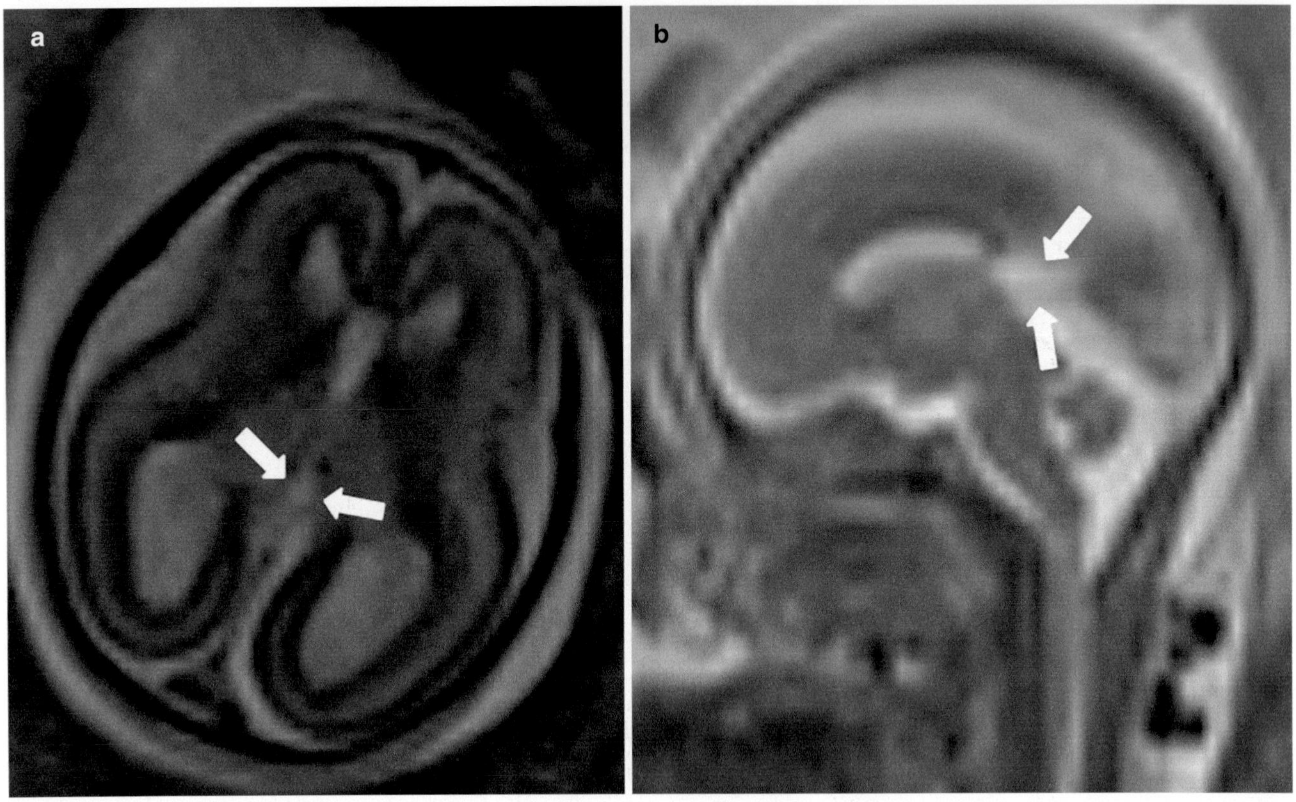

Fig. 4.9 MRI of a fetus at 20 weeks: axial (**a**), sagittal (**b**) images show a cyst inferior to the splenium (arrows)—cavum veli interpositii cyst

4.2.2 Dysplastic CC

There is abnormal shape of the CC, though the size may be roughly preserved (Fig. 4.12d).

4.2.3 Hypoplastic and Dysplastic CC

There is reduced size of the CC with associated abnormal shape. It has two subtypes—Stripe CC and Kinked CC.

Stripe CC: This type shows a uniformly thin stripe of CC and lacks anatomical landmarks (Fig. 4.12e). *Kinked CC*: This type shows a CC that is thin as well as kinked at one or more locations (Fig. 4.12f).

4.2.4 Complete Agenesis

The CC is completely absent (Fig. 4.13). The uncrossed fibers remain along the superomedial region of the lateral ventricles and parallel to the interhemispheric fissure to form the Probst bundles [26, 27]. The other features are:

- Absent CSP.
- High-riding third ventricle, which opens into the interhemispheric fissure superiorly.
- Absent CC is seen on a midline sagittal MR image as a radial or "spoke-like" configuration of the sulci and gyri around the third ventricle is seen on the medial hemispheric surface. It may be associated with the presence of a dorsal cyst.
- Disproportionate dilatation of the occipital horns of the bilateral lateral ventricles called as colpocephaly [28].
- Absent or malformed cingulate gyrus and sulcus depending on the degree of malformation of CC.

4.2.5 Mega Corpus Callosum (MCC)

Unlike hypoplasia and agenesis, MCC is very rare and presents as a CC with uniformly increased dimensions (Fig. 4.14). This enlargement of corpus callosum is due to the persistent longitudinal midline supracallosal fibers. These fibers usually disappear during axonal migration [29]. It may occur as an isolated anomaly or be associated with anomalies like polymicrogyria and megalencephaly.

4.2.6 CCA with Interhemispheric Cyst

Interhemispheric cysts are seen in 7% of the patients diagnosed with corpus callosal agenesis [27]. Suggested possible

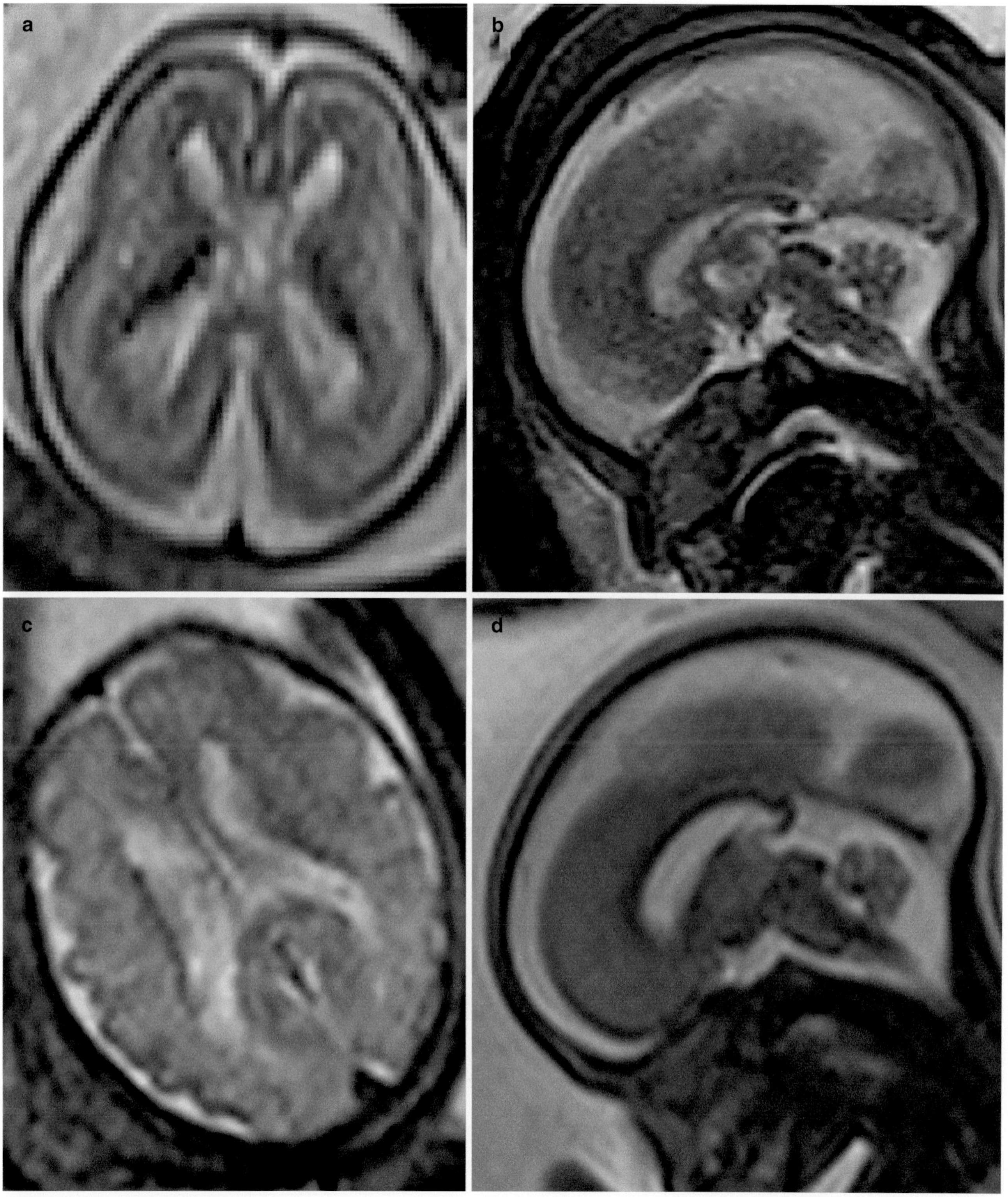

Fig. 4.10 Axial (**a**) and sagittal (**b**) MR images showing a normal corpus callosum at 20 weeks. Axial (**c**) and sagittal (**d**) MR images showing a normal corpus callosum at 31 weeks

causes are ependymal, arachnoid, and neurenteric cysts. Barkovich et al. classified interhemispheric cysts into two major types. Type 1 cysts are unilocular and are thought to be a diverticulum of the lateral or third ventricle. Type 2 cysts are multilocular and show no communication with the ventricular system (Fig. 4.15) [30].

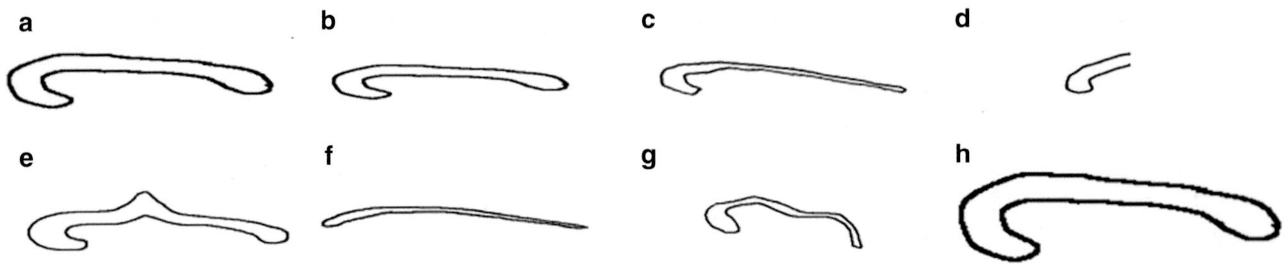

Fig. 4.11 Graphic representation of CC anomalies (**a**) Normal (**b**) Diffuse hypoplastic CC (**c**) Hypoplasia with deficiency in posterior end (**d**) Anterior Remnant hypoplasia (**e**) Dysplastic CC (**f**) Hypoplasic and dysplasic—Stripe type (**g**) Hypoplasic and dysplasic—Kinked type (**h**)—Mega Corpus callosum

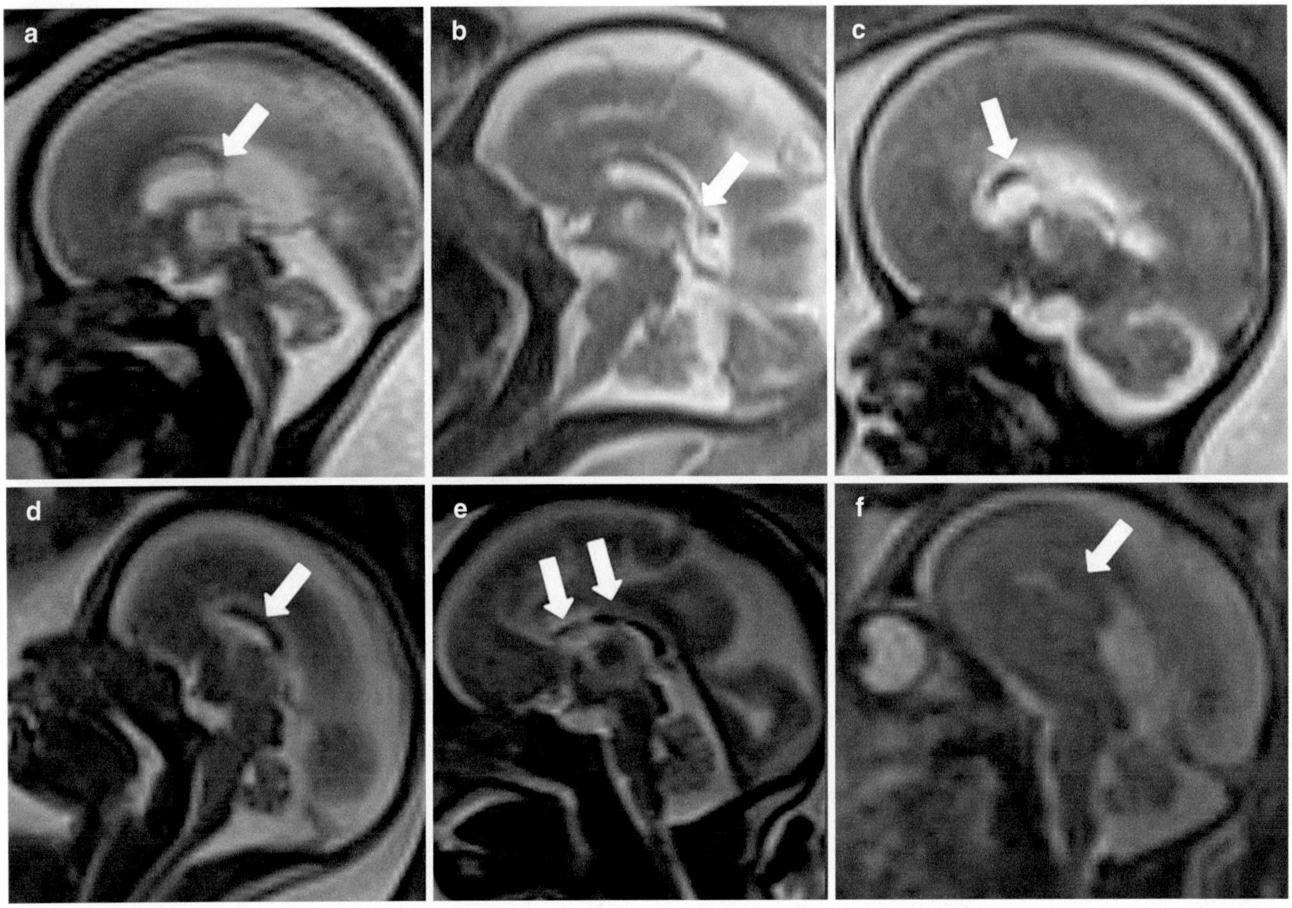

Fig. 4.12 Sagittal MR images showing corpus callosal anomalies. (**a**) Hypoplasia with deficiency in posterior end (**b**) Hypoplastic—Apple core type (**c**) Anterior Remnant hypoplasia (**d**) Dysplastic CC (**e**) Hypoplasic and dysplasic—Stripe type (**f**) Hypoplasic and dysplasic—Kinked type

4.2.7 CCA with Pericallosal Lipoma

Peri callosal lipoma is sometimes seen in partial or complete agenesis of the corpus callosum (Fig. 4.16). It is seen as a thin streak or an ovoid mass or as two longitudinal columns [31]. The lipoma is seen along the normal anatomical site of the CC and does not infiltrate it. A large lipoma may cause mass effect on the residual corpus callosum and lateral ventricles. In corpus callosum agenesis, on MRI, the lipoma of the corpus callosum is seen as well-marginated T1 hyperintense fat signal intensity masses which show attenuation on fat suppression sequences.

4.2.8 Association

Corpus callosal abnormalities may be isolated or be associated with other anomalies like sulcal abnormality, ventriculomegaly, cerebellar hypoplasia, cerebellar vermian hypoplasia, Dandy–Walker malformation, and holoprosencephaly [32, 33].

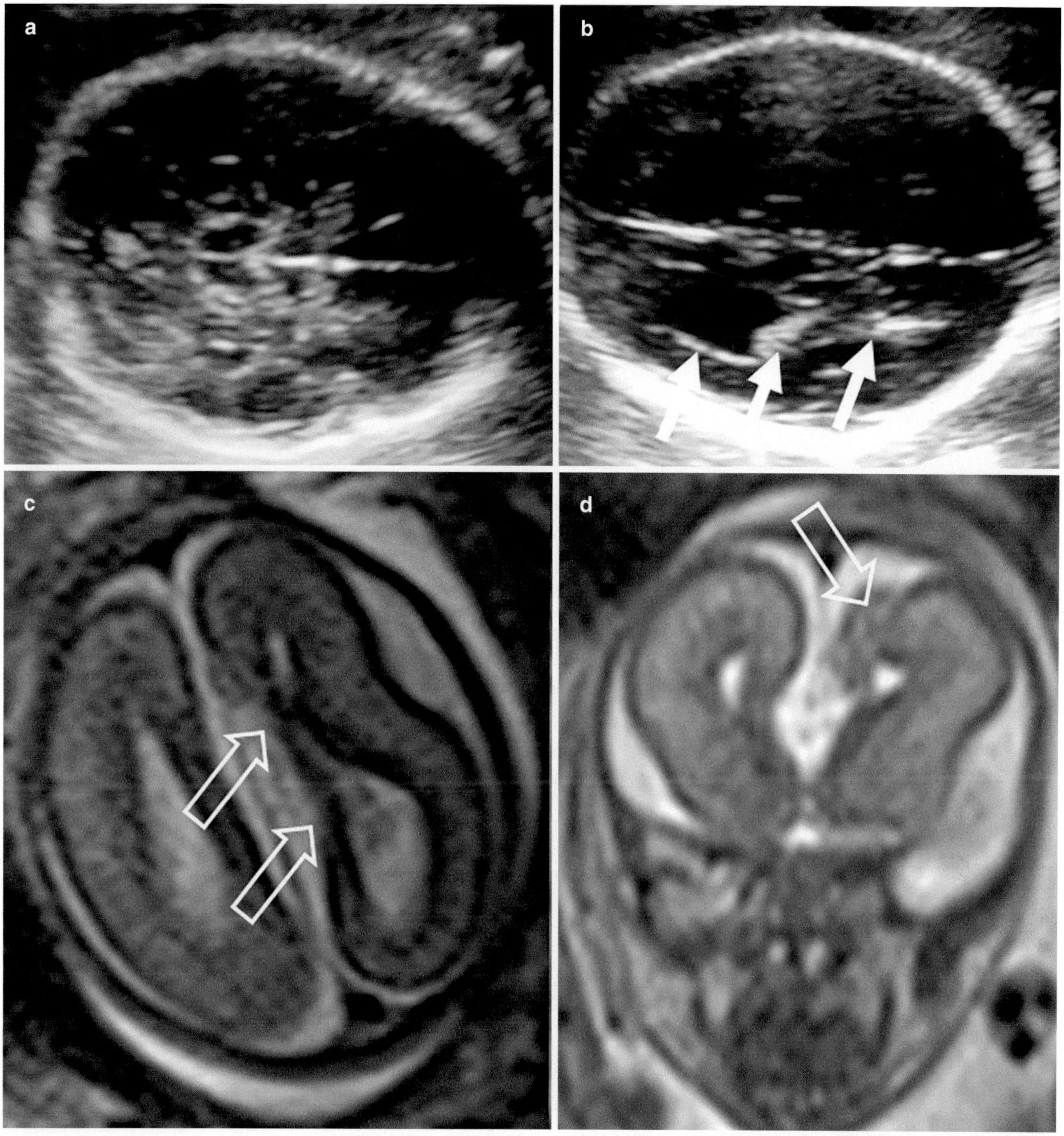

Fig. 4.13 Sonography of a 20-week fetus (**a**, **b**) shows colpocephaly (arrows) and nonvisualization of CSP favoring ACC. MRI axial (**c**) and coronal (**d**) images confirm ACC. In addition, sulcal abnormality is seen on the left cerebral hemisphere (open arrows)

Corpus callosal agenesis is the most frequently encountered anomaly coexisting in Dandy–Walker syndrome [32]. Dandy–Walker syndrome is characterized by vermian hypoplasia, enlarged fourth ventricle communicating with cisterna magna, torcular-lambdoid inversion, and commonly shows neuronal migration anomalies and corpus callosal dysgenesis. Callosal agenesis can also be seen in association with semi-lobar holoprosencephaly [33]. A dorsal interhemispheric commissure, which can mimic the splenium can be seen on sagittal images. It is also called "pseudo-splenium," since it mimics the splenium. Syntelencephaly, which was initially thought to be semi-lobar holoprosencephaly is a middle interhemispheric variant type of holoprosencephaly. Cleavage failure of the dorsal regions of the brain is the clas-

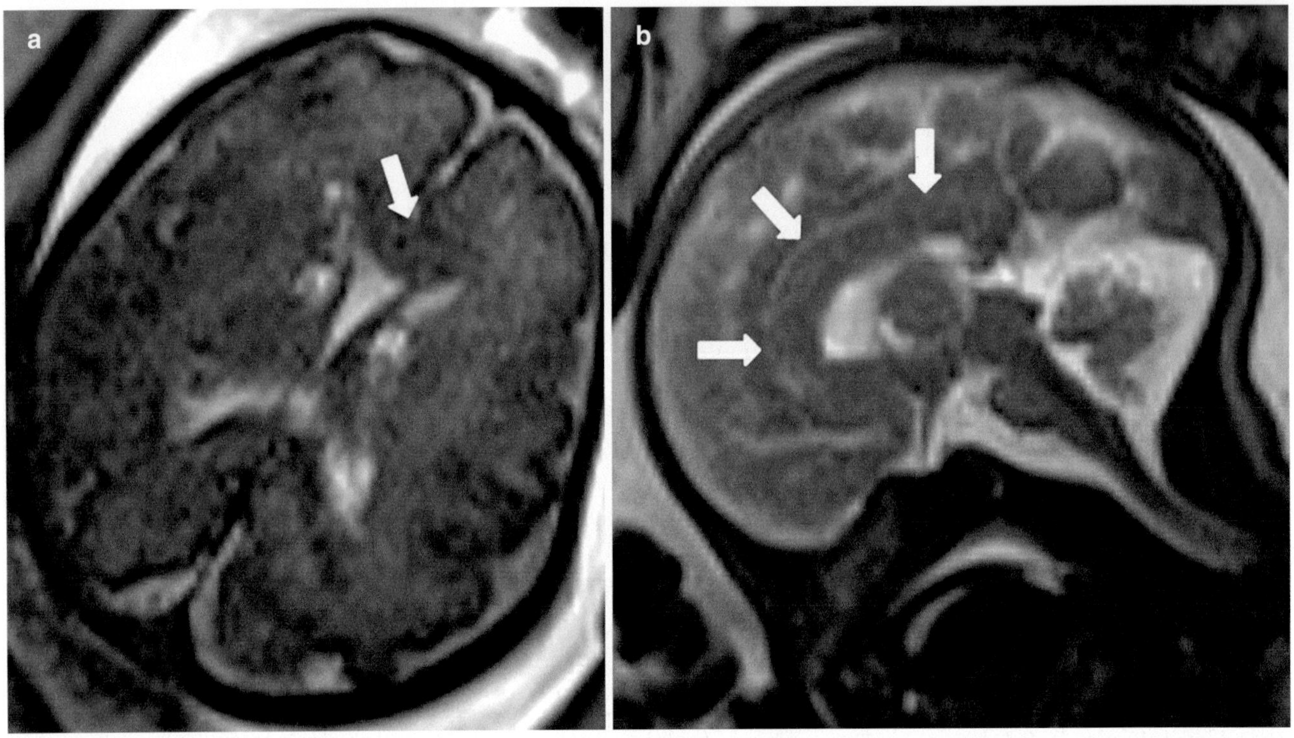

Fig. 4.14 MRI axial (**a**) and sagittal (**b**) images of a 32-week fetus show a diffusely thickened corpus callosum-Mega corpus callosum

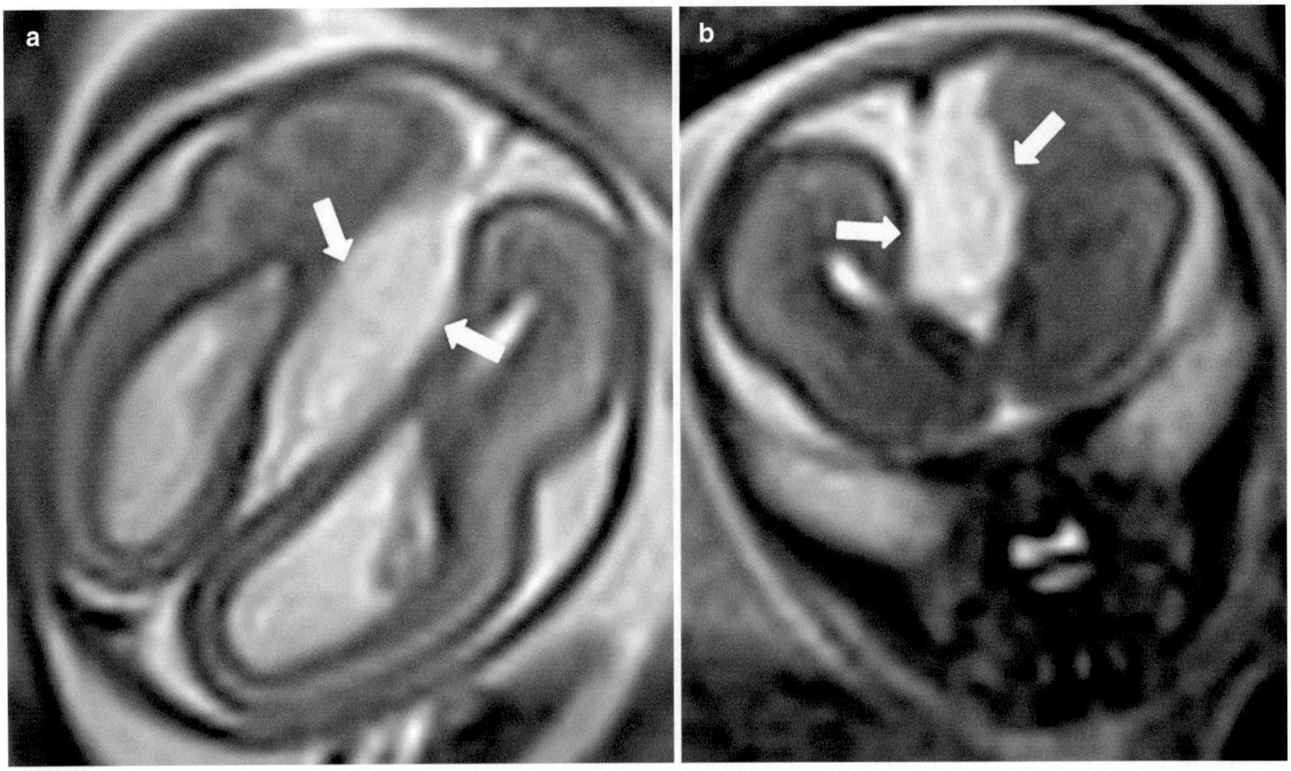

Fig. 4.15 MRI axial (**a**) and coronal (**b**) images show ACC. In addition, interhemispheric cyst is seen in the midline frontoparietal region (arrows)

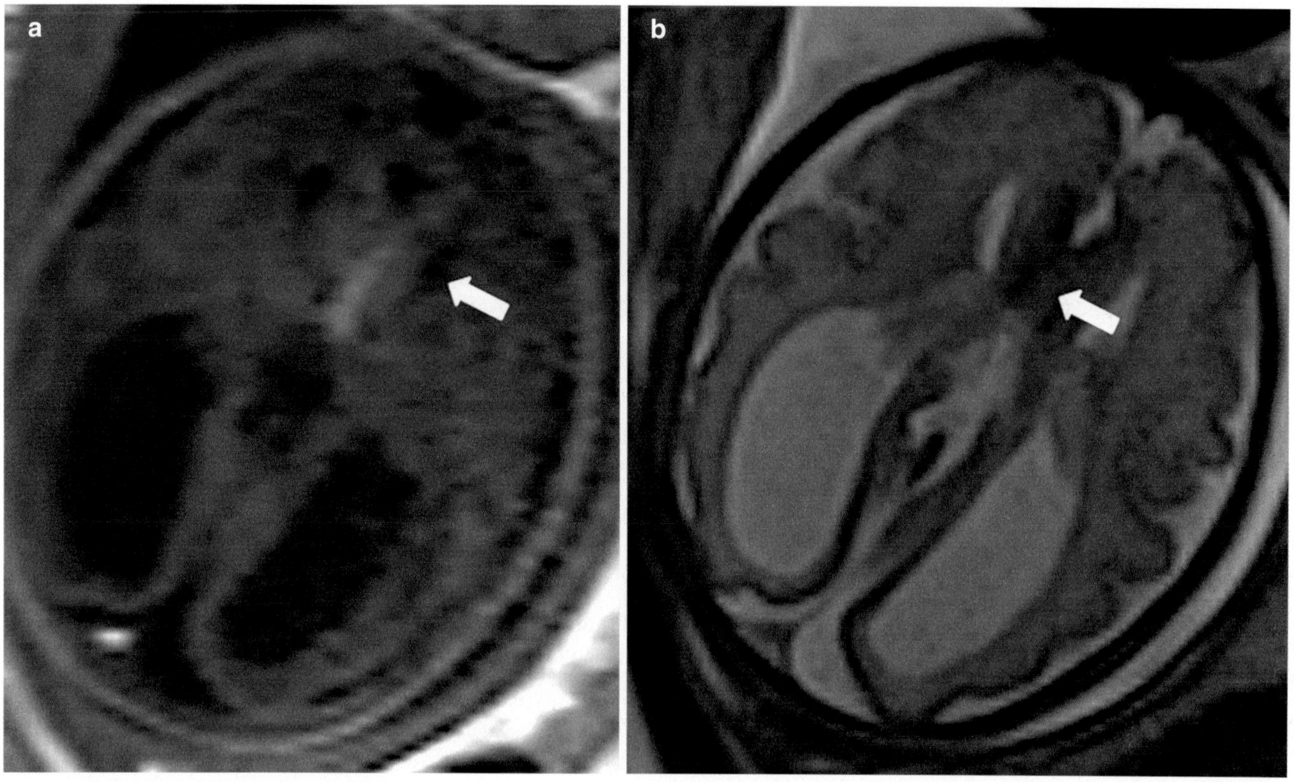

Fig. 4.16 MRI axial T1 (**a**) and T2 (**b**) weighted images show ACC. In addition, lipoma is seen in the region of the genu (arrows)

sical feature of this. Hence, on MRI the cerebral hemispheres appear fused in the dorsal region of the brain with associated varying degrees of partial agenesis of the CC [27].

Prognosis

Children may be near normal or show various neurological problems depending on the severity of abnormality and associated malformations. Mental retardation (60%), visual problems (33%), speech delay (29%), seizures (25%), abnormal muscular tone (25%), and feeding problems have been reported [32, 34]. Other associations described are mild behavioral or social problems, attention-deficit-hyperactivity disorder (ADHD), dysmorphic features, and ataxia [32–35].

Treatment

The affected children are treated symptomatically for seizures. Special education and physical therapy may be adopted depending on the severity of symptoms [34]. Hydrocephalus may be treated by shunting procedures. Genetic counseling may be done wherever necessary.

References

1. Levine LM, Bhatti MT, Mancuso AA. Septo-optic dysplasia with olfactory tract and bulb hypoplasia. J AAPOS. 2001;5(6):398–9.
2. Osborn RE. Schizencephaly and septo-optic dysplasia: separate entities. Pediatr Radiol. 1989;20(1–2):137.
3. Castillo M. Neuroradiology companion, methods, guidelines, and imaging fundamentals. Lippincott Williams & Wilkins; 2006.
4. Barkovich AJ, Norman D. Absence of the septum pellucidum: a useful sign in the diagnosis of congenital brain malformations. AJR Am J Roentgenol. 1989;152(2):353–60.
5. Nagaraj UD, Calvo-Garcia MA, Kline-Fath BM. Abnormalities associated with the cavum septi pellucidi on fetal MRI: what radiologists need to know. AJR. 2018;210(5):989–97.
6. Jou HJ, Shyu MK, Wu SC, Chen SM, Su CH, Hsieh FJ. Ultrasound measurement of the fetal cavum septi pellucidi. Ultrasound Obstet Gynecol. 1998;12(6):419–21.
7. Malinger G, Lev D, Kidron D, et-al. Differential diagnosis in fetuses with absent septum pellucidum. Ultrasound Obstet Gynecol. 2005;25(1):42–9.
8. Usman N, Rangasami R, Ramachandran R. 'Pseudo-septum' appearance in septal agenesis on fetal MRI. J Fetal Med. 2021; https://doi.org/10.1007/s40556-021-00300-y.
9. Callen PW, Callen AL, Glenn OA. Ants toi columns of the fornix, not to be mistaken for the cavum septi pellucidi on prenatal sonography. J Ultrasound Med. 2008;27:25–31.
10. Garcia-Filion P, Borchert M. Prenatal determinants of optic nerve hypoplasia: review of suggested correlates and future focus. Surv Ophthalmol. 2013;58(6):610–9. https://doi.org/10.1016/j.survophthal.2013.02.004
11. Kennedy A. Septo optic dysplasia. In: Woodward PJ, editor. Diagnostic imaging: obstetrics. 3rd ed. Philadelphia: Elsevier; 2016.
12. Cooper S, Katorza E, Berkenstadt M, Hoffmann C, Achiron R, Bar-Yosef O. Prenatal abnormal width of the cavum septum pellucidum - MRI features and neurodevelopmental outcome. J Matern Fetal Neonatal Med. 2018;31:3043–50.

13. Lewis SW, Mezey GC. Clinical correlates of septum pellucidum cavities: an unusual association with psychosis. Psychol Med. 1985;15:43–54.
14. Delisi LE, Hoff AL, Kushner M, Degreef G. Increased prevalence of cavum septum pellucidum in schizophrenia. Psychiatry Res. 1993;50:193–9.
15. Schaefer GB, Bodensteiner JB, Thompson JN. Subtle anomalies of the septum pellucidum and neurodevelopmental deficits. Dev Med Child Neurol. 1994;36:554–9.
16. Bot GM, Constantini S, Roth J. Conservative treatment of cysts of the cavum septum pellucidum presenting in childhood: report of 3 cases. J Neurosurg Pediatr. 2015;16:283–6.
17. Chen CY, Chen FH, Lee CC, et-al. Sonographic characteristics of the cavum velum interpositum. AJNR Am J Neuroradiol. 1998;19(9):1631–5.
18. Richards LJ, Plachez C, Ren T, et al. Mechanisms regulating the development of the corpus callosum and its agenesis in mouse and human. Clin Genet. 2004;66(4):276–89.
19. Lee SK, Kim DI, Kim J, et al. Diffusion-tensor MR imaging and fiber tractography: a new method of describing aberrant fiber connections in developmental CNS anomalies. Radiographics. 2005;25(1):53–65.
20. Georgy BA, Hesselink JR, Jernigan TL, et al. MR imaging of the corpus callosum. Am J Roentgenol. 1993;160(5):949–55.
21. Pashaj S, Merz E, Wellek S. Biometry of the fetal corpus callosum by three-dimensional ultrasound. Ultrasound Obstet Gynecol. 2013;42:691.
22. Schell-Apacik CC, Wagner K, Bihler M, et al. Agenesis and dysgenesis of the corpus callosum: clinical, genetic and neuroimaging findings in a series of 41 patients. Am J Med Genet A. 2008;146A(19):2501–11.
23. Hanna RM, et al. Distinguishing 3 classes of corpus callosal abnormalities in consanguineous families. Neurology. 2011;76(4):373–82.
24. Manor C, Rangasami R, Suresh I, Suresh S. Magnetic resonance imaging findings in fetal corpus callosal developmental abnormalities: a pictorial essay. J Pediatr Neurosci. 2020;15:352–7.
25. Karl K, Esser T, Heling KS, Chaoui R. Cavum septi pellucidi (CSP) ratio: a marker for partial agenesis of the fetal corpus callosum. Ultrasound Obstet Gynecol. 2017;50:336.
26. Barkovich AJ, et al. Pediatric neuroimaging. Philadelphia: Lippincott Williams & Wilkins; 2005.
27. Battal B, Kocaoglu M, Akgun, et al. Corpus callosum: normal imaging appearance, variants and pathologic conditions. J Med Imaging Radiat Oncol. 2010;54(6):541–9.
28. Singh S, Garge S, et al. Agenesis of the corpus callosum. J Pediatr Neurosci. 2010;5(1):83–5.
29. Jaisankar PK, Rangasami R. MR imaging and MR diffusion tensor imaging in mega corpus callosum. Neurol India. 2015;63: 997–8.
30. Barkovich AJ, Simon EM, Walsh CA, et al. Callosal agenesis with cyst: a better understanding and new classification. Neurology. 2001;56:220–7.
31. Nordin W, Tesluk H, Jones R, et al. Lipoma of the corpus callosum. Arch Neurol Psychiatr. 1955;74:300–6.
32. Curnes JT, Laster DW, Koubek TD, et al. MRI of corpus callosal syndromes. AJNR. 7:617–22.
33. Bourekas EC, Varakis K, Bruns D, et al. Lesions of the corpus callosum: MR imaging and differential considerations in adults and children. AJR. 2002;179:251–7.
34. Kumar P, Burton BK. Congenital malformations, evidence-based evaluation and management. McGraw-Hill Professional; 2007.
35. Schilmoeller G, Schilmoeller K. Filling a void: facilitating family support through networking for children with a rare disorder. Family Sci Rev. 2000;13:224–33.

5 Midline Brain Anomalies II: Holoprosencephaly

5.1 Embryology

During neural development, after primary neurulation, the cranial end of the neural tube forms three vesicles—the prosencephalon (forebrain), mesencephalon (midbrain), and rhombencephalon (hindbrain) [1–3]. The prosencephalon develops from the process of ventral induction, which consists of three interconnected events—formation, cleavage, and midline development. Prosencephalon further differentiates to form telencephalon that develops into cerebrum-lateral ventricles and diencephalon which forms the thalami-III ventricle. There is also cleavage and midline development occurring in prosencephalon. Abnormalities of formation result in aprosencephaly and atelencephaly. Abnormalities of cleavage lead to holoprosencephaly. Abnormalities of midline development result in agenesis of the corpus callosum, septo-optic dysplasia, and isolated septal agenesis [1].

5.2 Aprosencephaly, Atelencephaly

Aprosencephaly refers to failure to form prosencephalon.

Atelencephaly refers to failure to form telencephalon. It refers to abnormal division of prosencephalon into telencephalon/diencephalon leading to rudimentary diencephalic structures [1, 4].

Imaging features
- Is usually diagnosed by USG
- Severe microcephaly with no normal cerebral structures. Seen as amorphous mass and fluid within the cranium
- Cerebellum may be hypoplastic
- Severe craniofacial anomalies—Micrognathia, oculofacial defects including cyclopia, Cleft palate
- Urogenital anomalies—Anorectal atresia, Renal agenesis, ambiguous genitalia
- Can show associated limb and Cardiac anomalies

Prognosis
Prognosis is bad with death occurring in the prenatal or neonatal period.

5.3 Holoprosencephaly (HPE)

Rare Spectrum of disorders arising due to incomplete separation of the two cerebral hemispheres (which usually occurs during the fifth week of gestation).

Incidence 1 per 10,000–16,000 live births [5].

The main types are listed below in the order of decreasing severity: (Modified DeMyer classification) [6–8]:

1. Alobar holoprosencephaly
2. Semilobar holoprosencephaly
3. Lobar holoprosencephaly
4. Middle Interhemispheric variant
5. Septo optic dysplaia
6. Minimal HPE [9]
7. Microform HPE [1.9]

Pathogenesis and genetics
The etiology is multifactorial. Chromosomal and genetic abnormalities have been implicated including trisomy 13, trisomy 18, and Sonic hedgehog gene [10–12]. Maternal diabetes mellitus, retinoic acid, and alcohol use have also been implicated.

HPE may be associated with several syndromes such as Goldenhar syndrome, Meckel syndrome, Martin syndrome, Pallister–Hall syndrome, Fitch syndrome, Steinfeld syndrome, hypertelorism and ectrodactyly syndrome, velocardiofacial syndrome, Lambotte syndrome, acrocallosal syndrome, and Smith–Lemli–Opitz syndrome.

R. Rajeswaran, *MR Imaging of the Fetus*, https://doi.org/10.1007/978-981-16-9209-3_5

Non-cleavage of the telencephalic vesicle during the fifth and sixth week of gestation results in holoprosencephaly. It has three major subtypes based on the degree of cleavage between the hemispheres (Fig. 5.1). In the most severe type, alobar HPE, there is complete noncleavage of the cerebral hemispheres, leading to a single midline ventricle often communicating with a dorsal cyst (Fig. 5.1b). In semilobar HPE, the telencephalon remains uncleaved in the cranial part, whereas the posterior interhemispheric fissure is present (Fig. 5.1c). In lobar HPE, cleavage is near complete (Fig. 5.1d). Arhinencephaly and septal agenesis also belong to the HPE spectrum, although they can also exist as isolated anomalies unrelated to HPE.

Dorsal Cyst A dorsal cyst is commonly seen in alobar HPE (92% of cases). It is less frequently seen in semilobar HPE (28% of cases) and lobar HPE (9% of cases) [9, 11]. It is postulated that outflow of cerebrospinal fluid from the third ventricle is obstructed by the fusion of thalami. This results in the third ventricle ballooning out posteriorly in the suprapineal recess, at the point of least resistance.

Association
Rhombencephalosynapsis, Subcortical heterotopias. Polyhydramnios are commonly associated with HPE. Abnormal cleavage of the vesicles also leads to a large spectrum of midline anomalies of the face. Facial anomalies range from hypotelorism with a single upper central incisor, hypoplastic nose with a single nostril (cebocephaly), median cleft lip and palate, to cyclopia (with proboscis and synophthalmia).

5.3.1 Alobar HPE

It is characterised by complete or near complete non-cleavage of the forebrain [9].

Imaging features

- Is usually diagnosed by USG by demonstrating "Absent Butterfly sign." The butterfly sign is normally seen in a transverse first-trimester brain scan. The choroid plexus is narrow in the middle but broader on the lateral aspect, and when seen side by side resembles a butterfly [13].
- Head size is reduced and shows a rounded contour.
- *The following are absent*—Olfactory bulbs and tracts, cavum septum pellucidum, corpus callosum, and interhemispheric fissure (Fig. 5.2a–f).
- The lateral and III ventricles are replaced by a monoventricle (Fig. 5.2a, b).
- A dorsal cyst is often present (Fig. 5.2d–f).
- On the sagittal views, the brain may show the following shapes: *ball, cup, or pancake* (Fig. 5.3). In the ball-type, a good volume of cerebral cortex completely encircles the monoventricle (Fig. 5.3a). In the cup type, the monoventricle is partially encircled by the cortex that gives a "cup" configuration (Fig. 5.3b). In the "pancake" form, a small volume of cortex is seen at the base of the skull and appears flattened (Fig. 5.3c).
- The basal ganglia, hypothalamus, and thalami are fused in the midline (Fig. 5.2b). The optic nerves may be absent, fused, or normal.
- The anterior and middle cerebral arteries may be absent and replaced by a network of vessels originating from the internal carotid and basilar arteries [14].
- Facial malformations are severe.
- Subcortical heterotopia [15].

Differential diagnosis
Semilobar holoprosencephaly—Partial cleavage of the cerebral hemispheres is seen.

Severe hydrocephalus—Normal ventricular configuration is maintained in hydrocephalus although dilated. Midline falx is visualized.

Hydranencephaly—Midline falx is visualized.

Prognosis Mental retardation is profound and often fatal in the neonatal period.

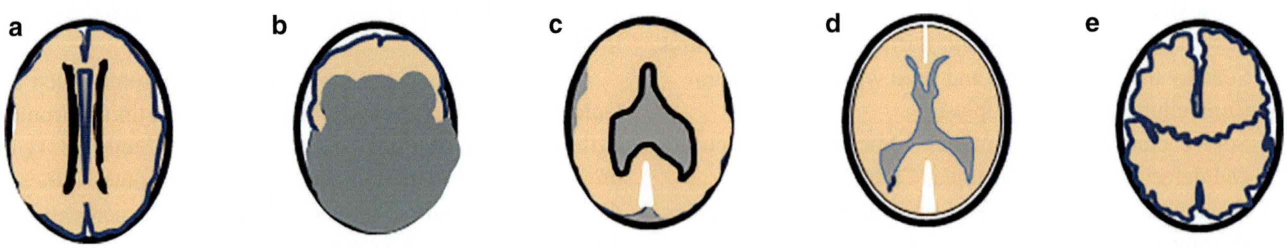

Fig. 5.1 Schematic diagram showing the types of holoprosencephaly. (**a**) Normal, (**b**) Alobar HPE (**c**) semilobar HPE, (**d**) lobar HPE, (**e**) middle hemispheric variant HPE

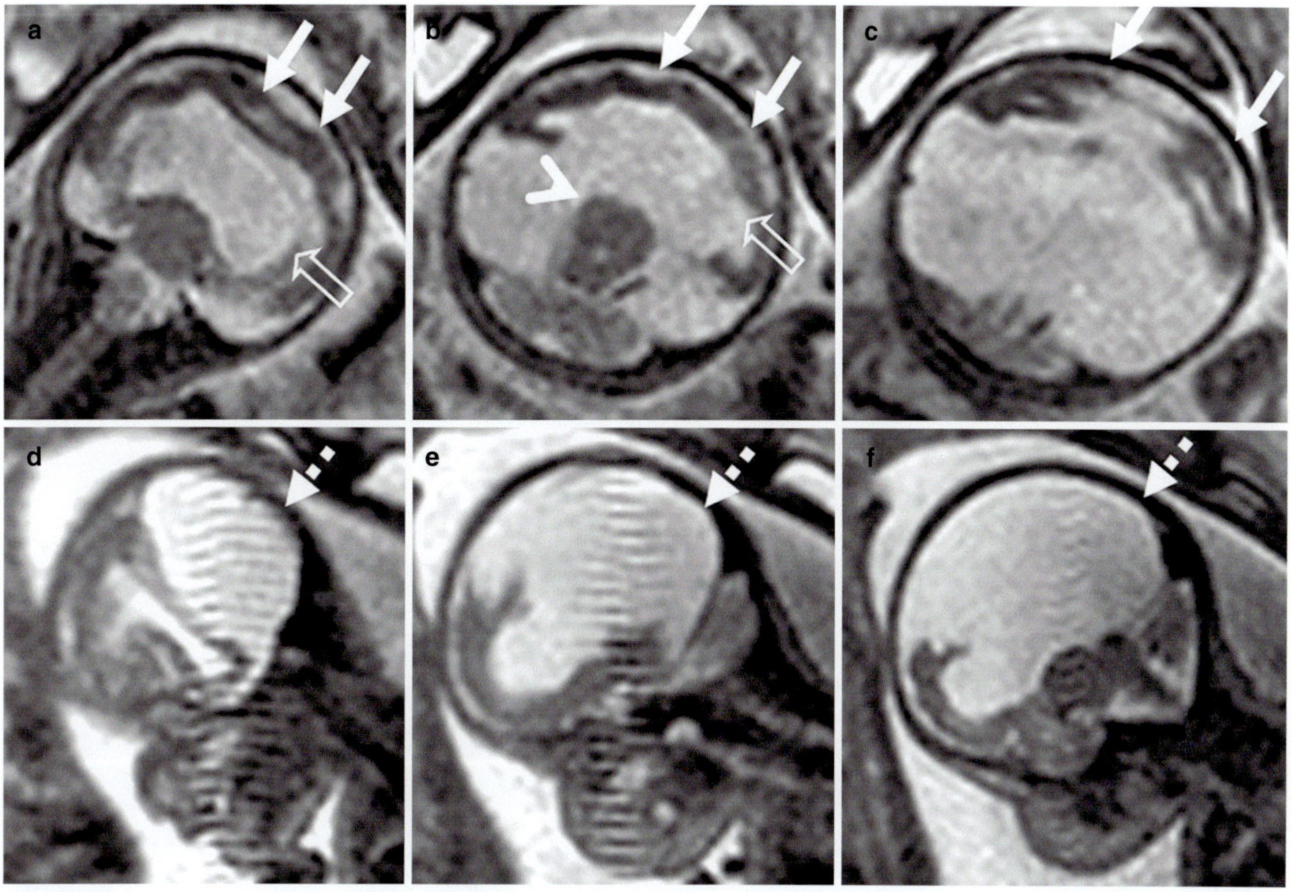

Fig. 5.2 Axial T2W images (**a**, **b**, **c**) show uncleaved cerebral hemisphere (arrows), mono ventricle (open arrows), fused thalami (arrowhead), Sagittal T2W images (**d**, **e**, **f**) show dorsal cyst (broken arrows)—features of *lobar holoprosencephaly*. The brainstem and cerebellar hemispheres are normally visualized

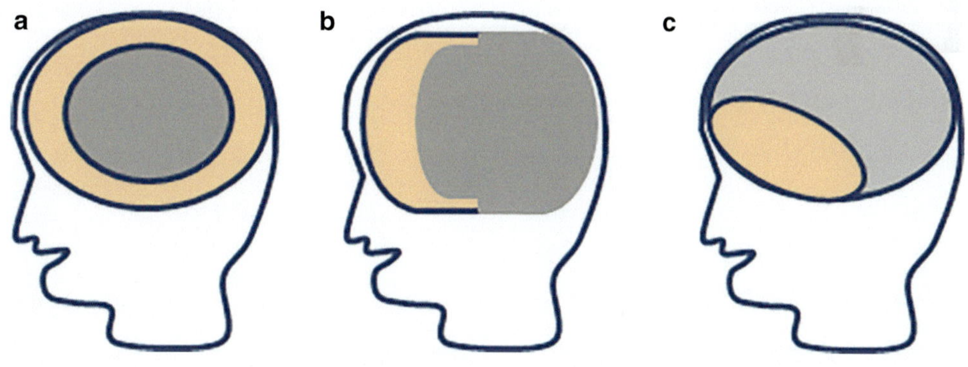

Fig. 5.3 Schematic diagram showing the shapes of the brain in alobar HPE on the sagittal view: (**a**) ball, (**b**) cup, (**c**) pancake

5.3.2 Semilobar HPE

It is characterized by incomplete cleavage of the forebrain, the frontal regions being affected [11, 16].

Imaging features

- In some cases, inability to detect the CSP may be the only obvious finding on USG at the 18–20-week anomaly scan [17] whereas it is a straightforward diagnosis on MRI
- Absent septum pellucidum, olfactory tracts, and bulbs
- Complete or partial non-cleavage of the thalami (Fig. 5.4a)
- Non-cleavage of more than 50% of frontal lobes (Fig. 5.4b, c)
- Mono-ventricle with partially formed temporal and occipital horns
- Partially formed falx cerebri and interhemispheric fissure
- Absent or hypoplastic corpus callosum
- Dorsal cyst may be present (Fig. 5.4d)
- Facial malformations are mild or absent

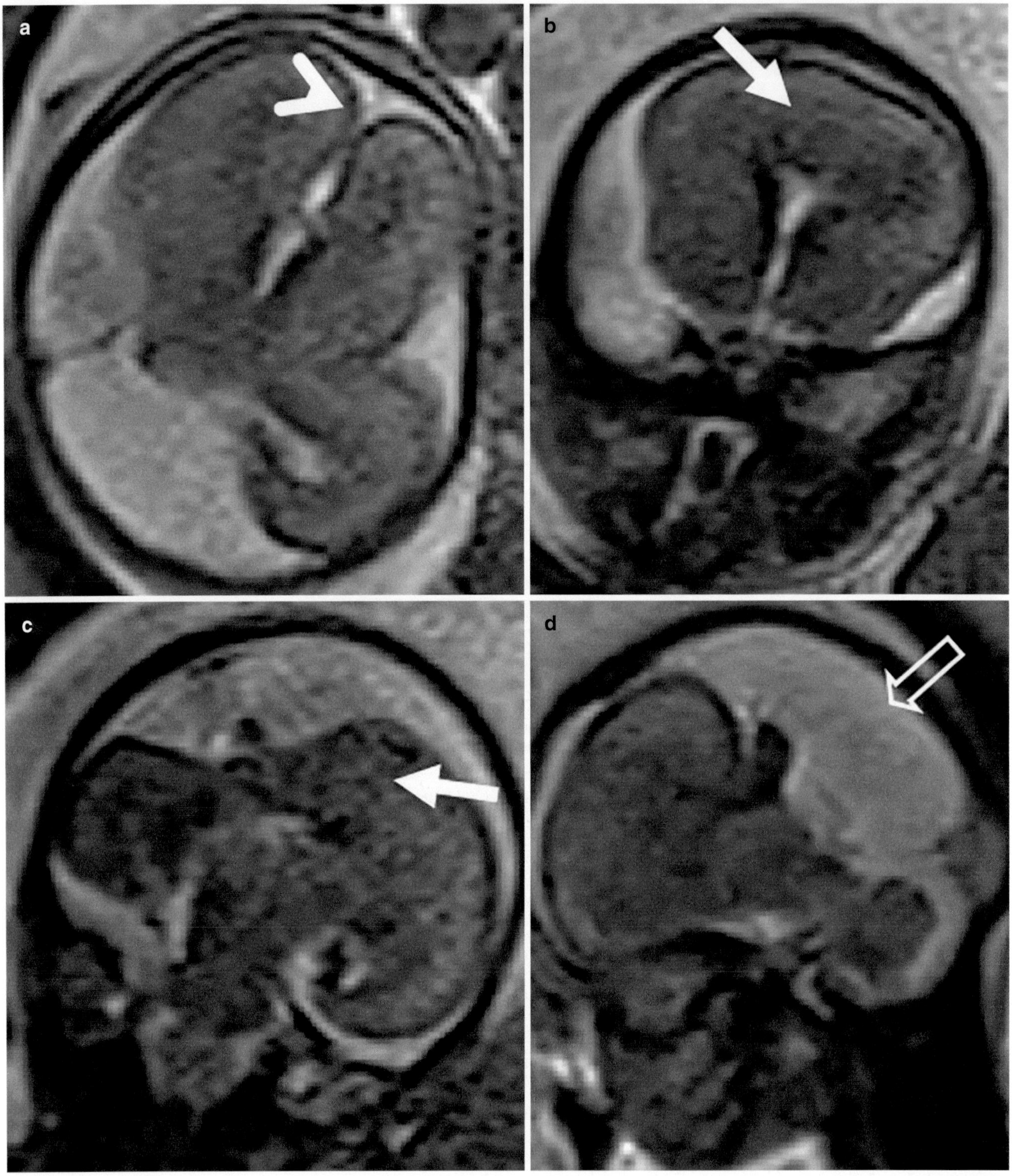

Fig. 5.4 Axial (**a**), coronal (**b**, **c**), sagittal (**d**) images of a 21-week fetus showing partial fusion of bilateral frontal and parietal lobes (arrows), the septum is not visualized, cystic area is seen in the parieto-occipital region (open arrows) with the diencephalic ventricle, the midline falx cerebri is not fully formed (arrowhead)—features of *Semilobar holoprosencephaly*

Differential diagnosis Alobar holoprosencephaly, Lobar holoprosencephaly, Arachnoid cyst.

Prognosis Mental retardation is profound and often fatal in the early childhood.

5.3.3 Lobar HPE

It is characterised by incomplete cleavage of the forebrain (but better than that of Semilobar HPE), the basi frontal regions being more affected. The interhemispheric fissure, falx are formed and the thalami are separated (Fig. 5.5a, b).

Imaging features

- Absent septum pellucidum.
- The frontal horns of bilateral lateral ventricles are fused. The fused segment is seen to communicate with the third ventricle.
- Noncleavage of the fornices [18].
- Normal or hypoplastic corpus callosum.
- The interhemispheric fissure is completely or near completely formed.
- The thalami are completely or almost completely separated.
- The inferior most portions of the frontal lobes are fused (Fig. 5.5a, b).
- Anterior cerebral artery is seen inferior to the frontal bones (snake under the skull sign) [19].

Differential diagnosis Semilobar holoprosencephaly, SOD.

Prognosis and management
Children with lobar HPE may survive into adulthood. Common causes of death include respiratory infections, intractable seizures, dehydration secondary to uncontrolled and diabetes insipidus. Death due to improper control of respiration and heart rate due to brainstem malfunction have also been described [20].

Medical management includes correction of hypothalamic and endocrinologic dysfunction, appropriate therapy for motor/developmental/visual impairment, seizures, and hydrocephalus. Genetic testing, determination of any associated syndromes, and appropriate genetic counseling may also be offered.

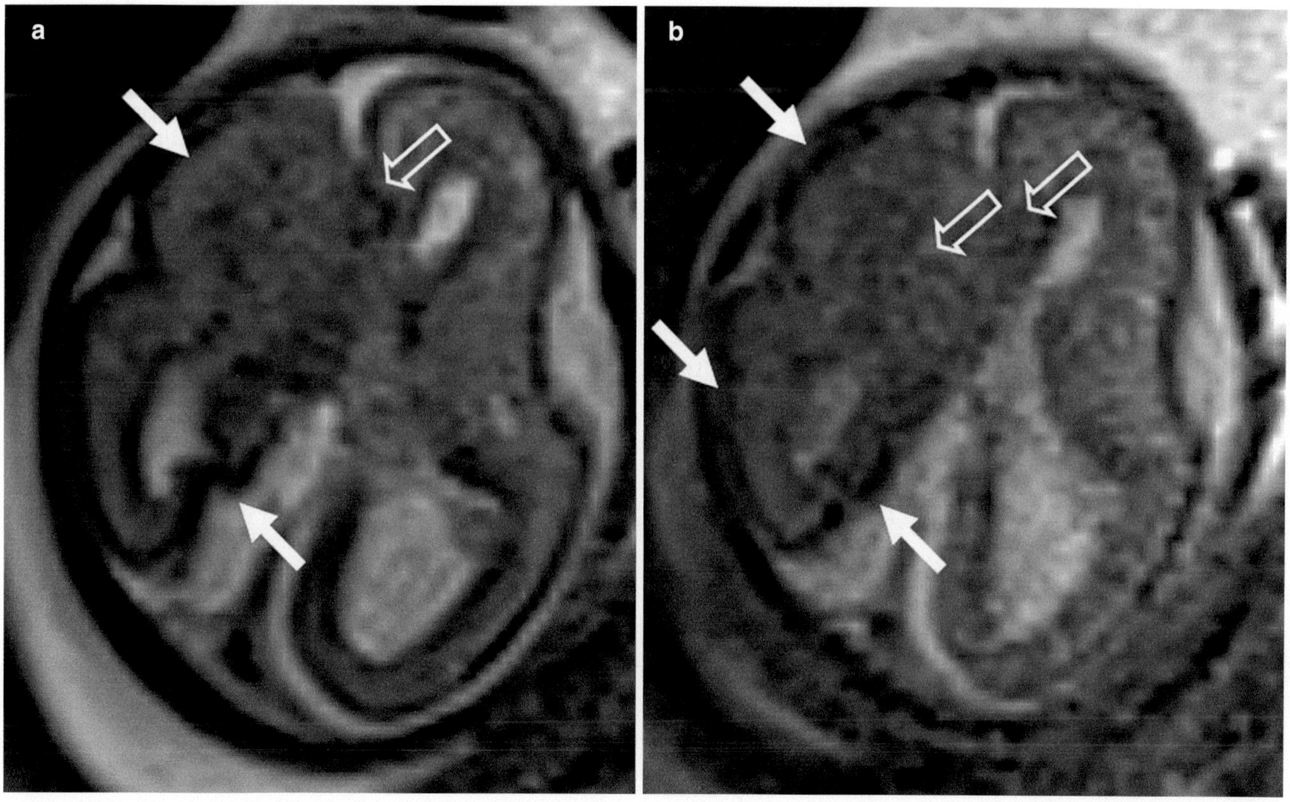

Fig. 5.5 Axial T2W images (**a**, **b**) of a 22-week fetus show a small right cerebral hemisphere with cortical abnormality (arrows). There is partial fusion of the cerebral hemispheres at the level of basal ganglia and in the frontal region (open arrows)—*lobar type of holoprosencephaly*. Mild ventriculomegaly of left lateral ventricle is also seen

5.3.4 Middle Interhemispheric Variant (MIH)

It is mild form of HPE where the cleavage has not occurred in the posterior frontal and parietal lobes (Fig. 5.1e).

Synonym—Syntelencephaly.

Imaging features [21–24]

- Absent septum pellucidum
- Agenesis or hypoplasia of the body of corpus callosum
- Dorsal cyst may be present
- Vertically oriented Sylvian fissures which are abnormally connected across midline over the vertex of the brain
- Cortical dysplasia or subcortical heterotopias may be present
- Mild craniofacial abnormalities
- There are fairly well-developed frontal and occipital lobes and the intervening interhemispheric fissure. However, the interhemispheric fissure and falx are absent in the middle interhemispheric region

Differential diagnosis

1. Lobar HPE—In lobar HPE, the most severely noncleaved part is the basal forebrain, whereas, in MIH, the non-cleaved part is in the posterior frontal and parietal lobes.
2. Schizencephaly—There is no non-cleavage abnormality.

Prognosis Developmental delay, mental retardation, seizures, and Spasticity or hypotonia may be present in postnatal life.

Children with MIH may walk with support and show mild impairment in speech and motor functions. Developmental outcome of Children with MIH is similar to that in lobar HPE [25–27].

5.3.5 Septo Optic Dysplaia

Is discussed in Chap. 4.

5.3.6 Minimal HPE

Is characterized by trivial craniofacial malformations, non-cleavage in the preoptic (suprachiasmic) area, thickened or dysplastic fornix, and absent or hypoplastic anterior part of the corpus callosum. These patients also had single unpaired anterior cerebral artery [28].

Prognosis Patients often manifested mild developmental delay in the form of language delay, learning disabilities, or behavioral disturbances, while motor function was relatively spared [11].

5.3.7 Microform HPE

Microform HPE occur in relatives of patients affected by HPE, exhibit craniofacial anomalies and do not show brain involvement [28, 29].

References

1. Volpe P, Campobasso G, De Robertis V, Rembouskos G. Disorders of prosencephalic development. Prenat Diagn. 2009;29(4):340–54.
2. Fotos J, Olson R, Kanekar S. Embryology of the brain and molecular genetics of central nervous system malformation. Semin Ultrasound CT MR. 2011;32(3):159–66.
3. Blaas HG, Eik-Nes SH. Sonoembryology and early prenatal diagnosis of neural anomalies. Prenat Diagn. 2009;29(4):312–25.
4. Pasquier L, et al. First occurrence of aprosencephaly/atelencephaly and holoprosencephaly in a family with a SIX3 gene mutation and phenotype/genotype correlation in our series of SIX3 mutations. J Med Genet. 2005;42(1):e4.
5. Dubourg C, Bendavid C, Pasquier L, et al. Holoprosencephaly Orphanet. J Rare Dis. 2007;2(1):8. https://doi.org/10.1186/1750-1172-2-8.
6. DeMyer W, Zeman W. Alobar holoprosencephaly (arhinencephaly) with median cleft lip and palate: clinical, electroencephalographic and nosologic considerations. Confin Neurol. 1963;23:1–36.
7. DeMyer W, Zeman W, Palmer CG. Familial alobar holoprosencephaly (arhinencephaly) with median cleft lip and palate: report of patient with 46 chromosomes. Neurology. 1963;13:913–8.
8. DeMyer W, Zeman W, Palmer CG. The face predicts the brain: diagnostic significance of median facial anomalies for holoprosencephaly (arhinencephaly). Pediatrics. 1964;34:256–63.
9. Hahn JS, Barnes PD. Neuroimaging advances in holoprosencephaly: refining the spectrum of the midline malformation. Am J Med Genet C Semin Med Genet. 2010;154C(1):120–32.
10. Tekendo-Ngongang C, Muenke M, Kruszka P. Holoprosencephaly overview. 2000 Dec 27 [Updated 2020 Mar 5]. In: Adam MP, Ardinger HH, Pagon RA, et al., editors. GeneReviews® [Internet]. Seattle (WA): University of Washington, Seattle; 1993–2020. Available from: https://www.ncbi.nlm.nih.gov/sites/books/NBK1530/
11. Winter TC, Kennedy AM, Woodward PJ. Holoprosencephaly: a survey of the entity, with embryology and fetal imaging. Radiographics. 2015;35:275–90.
12. Orioli IM, Castilla EE. Epidemiology of holoprosencephaly: prevalence and risk factors. Am J Med Genet C Semin Med Genet. 2010;154C(1):13–21.
13. Timor-Tritsch IE, Monteagudo A, Santos R. Three-dimensional inversion rendering in the first- and early second-trimester fetal brain: its use in holoprosencephaly. Ultrasound Obstet Gynecol. 2008;32(6):744–50.
14. Kathuria S, Gregg L, Chen J, Gandhi D. Normal cerebral arterial development and variations. Semin Ultrasound CT MR. 2011;32(3):242–51.
15. Barkovich AJ, Simon EM, Clegg NJ, Kinsman SL, Hahn JS. Analysis of the cerebral cortex in holoprosencephaly with attention to the sylvian fissures. AJNR Am J Neuroradiol. 2002;23(1):143–50.
16. Cayea PD, Balcar I, Alberti O, et-al. Prenatal diagnosis of semilobar holoprosencephaly. AJR Am J Roentgenol. 1984;142(2):401–2.
17. Winter TC, Kennedy AM, Byrne J, Woodward PJ. The cavum septi pellucidi: why is it important? J Ultrasound Med. 2010;29(3):427–44.

18. Pilu G, Ambrosetto P, Sandri F, et al. Intraventricular fused fornices: a specific sign of fetal lobar holoprosencephaly. Ultrasound Obstet Gynecol. 1994;4(1):65–7.
19. Bernard JP, Drummond CL, Zaarour P, Molho M, Ville Y. A new clue to the prenatal diagnosis of lobar holoprosencephaly: the abnormal pathway of the anterior cerebral artery crawling under the skull. Ultrasound Obstet Gynecol. 2002;19(6):605–7. https://doi.org/10.1046/j.1469-0705.2002.00729.x.
20. Raam MS, Solomon BD, Muenke M. Holoprosencephaly: a guide to diagnosis and clinical management. Indian Pediatr. 2011;48(6):457–66. https://doi.org/10.1007/s13312-011-0078-x.
21. Simon EM, Hevner RF, Pinter JD, et-al. The middle interhemispheric variant of holoprosencephaly. AJNR Am J Neuroradiol. 2002;23(1):151–6.
22. Pulitzer SB, Simon EM, Crombleholme TM, et-al. Prenatal MR findings of the middle interhemispheric variant of holoprosencephaly. AJNR Am J Neuroradiol. 2004;25(6):1034–6.
23. Barkovich AJ, Quint DJ. Middle interhemispheric fusion: an unusual variant of holoprosencephaly. AJNR Am J Neuroradiol. 1993;14(2):431–40.
24. Picone O, Hirt R, Suarez B, et al. Prenatal diagnosis of a possible new middle interhemispheric variant of holoprosencephaly using sonographic and magnetic resonance imaging. Ultrasound Obstet Gynecol. 2006;28(2):229–31.
25. Lewis AJ, Simon EM, Barkovich AJ, et al. Middle interhemispheric variant of holoprosencephaly: a distinct cliniconeuroradiologic subtype. Neurology. 2002;59(12):1860–186.
26. Stashinko EE, Clegg NJ, Kammann HA, et al. A retrospective survey of perinatal risk factors of 104 living children with holoprosencephaly. Am J Med Genet A. 2004;128A(2):114–9.
27. Barr M Jr, Cohen MM Jr. Holoprosencephaly survival and performance. Am J Med Genet. 1999;89(2):116–20.
28. Solomon BD, Mercier S, Vélez JI, et al. Analysis of genotypephenotype correlations in human holoprosencephaly. Am J Med Genet C Semin Med Genet. 2010;154C(1):133–41.
29. Della Giustina E, Iodice A, Spagnoli C, et al. "Minimal" holoprosencephaly in a 14q deletion syndrome patient. Am J Med Genet Part A. 2017;173A:3216–20. https://doi.org/10.1002/ajmg.a.38378.

6 Neural Tube Defects

During 3–5 weeks of gestation, there is formation and closure of neural tube, also termed as dorsal induction. The primary neurulation process is responsible for the development of brain and spinal cord up to S2 from the neural tube. Secondary neurulation occurs later and results in the formation of caudal part of the neural tube that develops into sacral and coccygeal segments. The cranial segment of the neural tube develops into the forebrain, midbrain, and hindbrain. The caudal segment of the neural tube develops into the spinal cord and spine. Partial or complete failure of closure of the neural groove leads to neural tube defects (or defects of dorsal induction) and multiple causes have been identified. These include folic acid deficiency, maternal diabetes, exposure to teratogens, and karyotype/genetic defects [1, 2].

During neural tube closure, the overlying epidermal cells form the ectodermal layer of the skin. The neural tube then separates from the superficial ectoderm, by a process called dysjunction. Maternal alphafeto protein is elevated in many of the neural tube defects. The incidence of Neural tube defects (NTDs) ranges from 1 to 11 per 1000 live births and shows a geographic variation [3]. The NTDs are broadly classified as in Box 6.1.

Box 6.1 The Broad Classification of Neural Tube Defects

Anomalies arising due to failure of closure of cranial neuropore-anterior wall of the neural tube

- Acrania
- Exencephaly
- Anencephaly
- Encephalocele

Anomalies arising due to failure of closure of cranial and caudal neuropore

- Craniorachischisis

Anomalies arising due to failure of closure of caudal neuropore

- Myeloschisis
- Spinal dysraphism
- Chiari malformation

6.1 Cranial Neuropore Defects

6.1.1 Anencephaly

There is failure of closure of the cranial part of the NTD. This leads to acrania—exencephaly—anencephaly sequence. Acrania is characterized by partial or complete absence of the ossified cranial vault above the orbits. This results in exposure of brain tissue to aminiotic fluid (exencephaly) with subsequent degeneration leading to anencephaly.

Imaging features The frontal, parietal, and occipital bones are deficient with exposure of neural tissue to the amniotic fluid leading to loss of brain tissue. There is absence of bilateral cerebral hemispheres, cranial vault, and part of the midbrain. This gives a frog-like appearance to the fetal head (Figs. 6.1 and 6.2a). It is usually associated with polyhydramnios and elevated alpha-fetoproteins [4].

Associations Diaphragmatic hernia, spinal dysraphism, and amniotic band syndrome.

Differential diagnosis

Extreme microcrania—The calvarium is intact and is not interrupted.

Large encephaloceles—Defect is present in the cranium through which the brain herniates.

R. Rajeswaran, *MR Imaging of the Fetus*, https://doi.org/10.1007/978-981-16-9209-3_6

Amniotic band syndrome—Can lead to destruction of the cranial vault, often accompanied by other abnormalities like limb amputation.

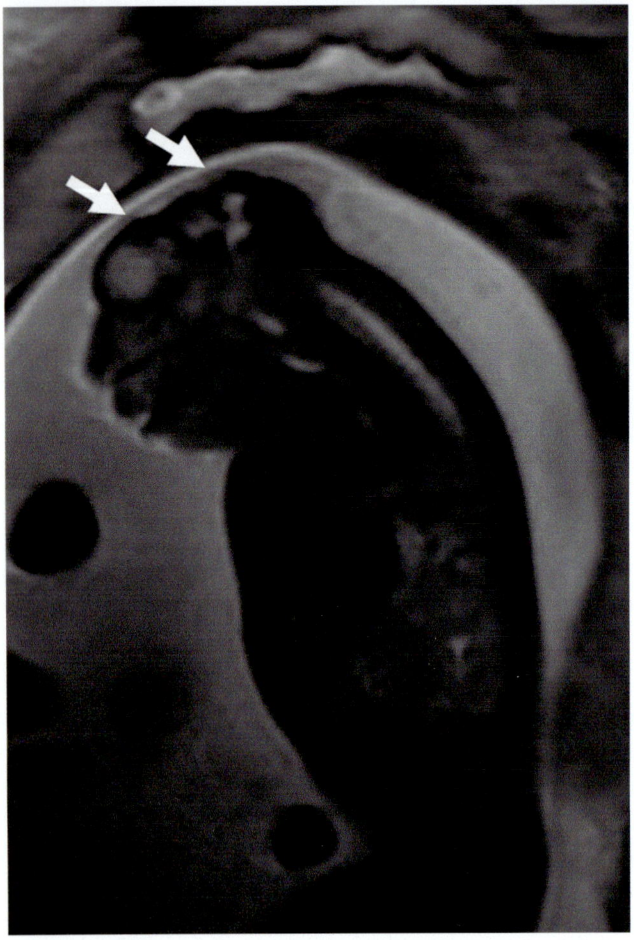

Fig. 6.1 Sagittal image showing anencephaly (arrows)

Prognosis A majority are stillborn while others die in the neonatal period. It can be diagnosed in the first trimester by USG. NTDs can recur in subsequent pregnancies.

Treatment NTDs can be prevented with dietary folate supplements to the pregnant mother.

6.1.2 Encephalocele

Synonym-Meningo encephalocele.

There is failure of closure of the anterior aspect of the neural tube leading to herniation of brain tissue through deficiency in the developing neurocranium [5]. The common sites are occipital, cervico-occipital and frontal/fronto-ethmoidal region. Less common sites are temporal, sphenoidal, parietal, and nasopharyngeal regions.

Prevalence 1 in 4000 live births. Increased incidence of fronto-ethmoidal encephaloceles are seen in south and south-east Asia.

Imaging features
There is herniation of brain tissue through the defect in the cranium (Figs. 6.2b and 6.3). It may present as a cystic lesion (meningocele) with or without brain tissue. MRI is useful to identify the presence of brain tissue, especially when the encephalocele is small or when the base of skull is involved. Larger encephalocele may be associated with microcephaly.

Associations
- Dandy–Walker malformations
- Chiari malformations
- Complete or partial agenesis of corpus callosum

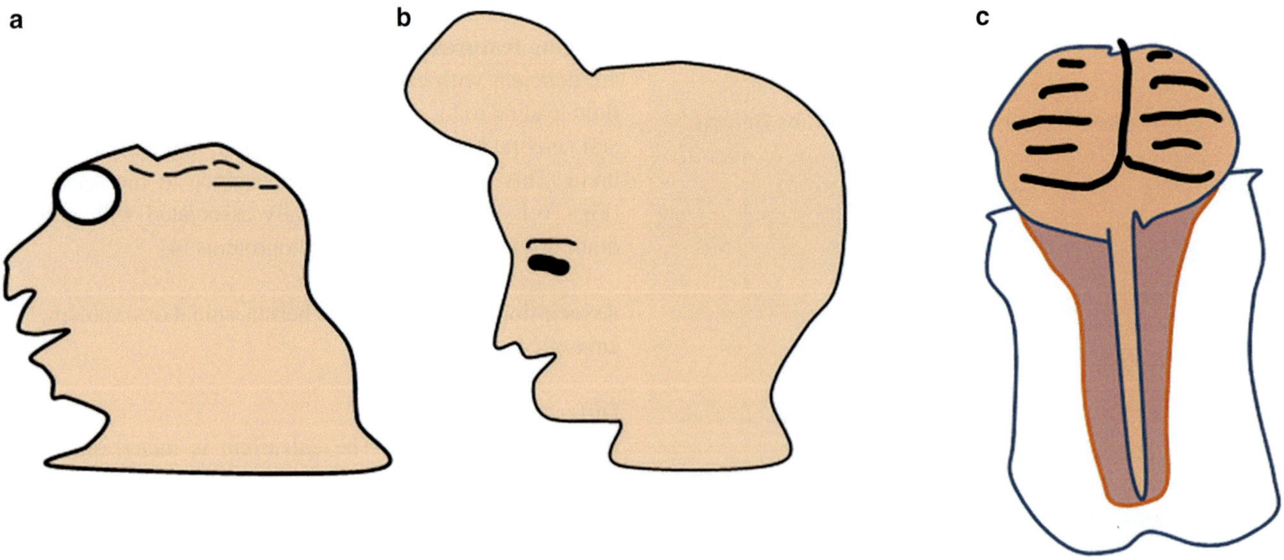

Fig. 6.2 Schematic diagram showing (**a**) Anencephaly (**b**) Encephalocele (**c**) Craniospinal rachischisis

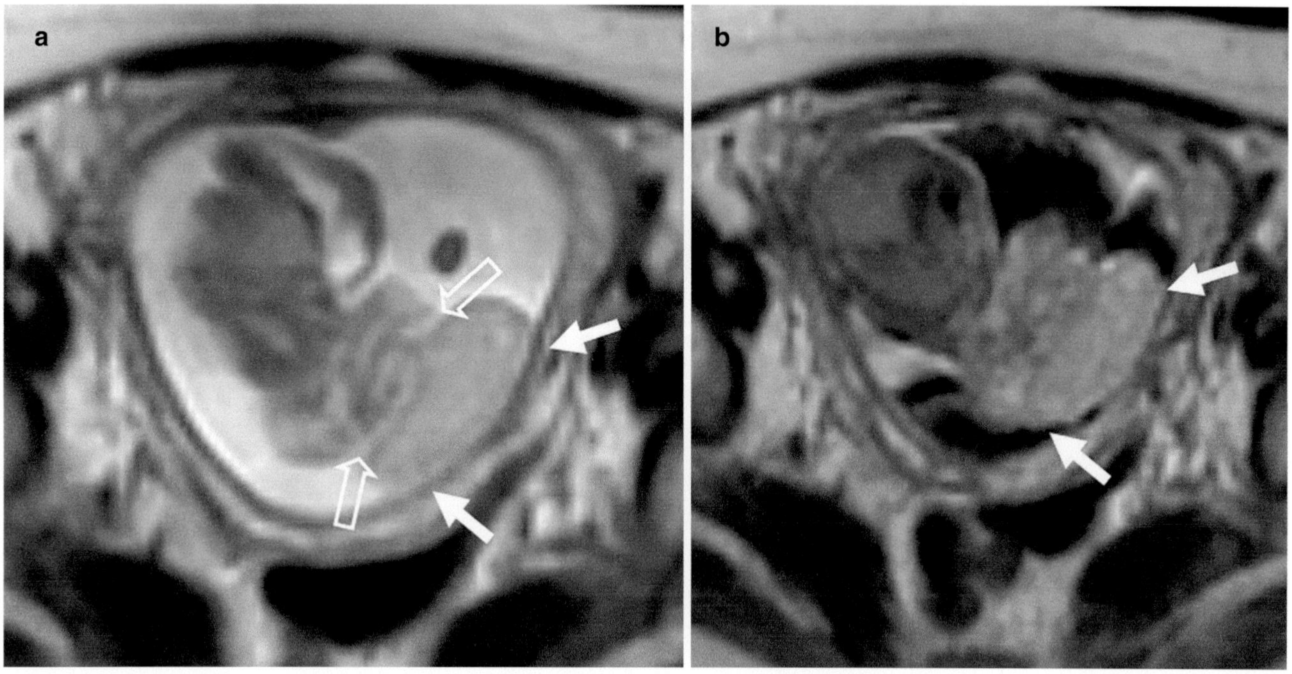

Fig. 6.3 T2W Images (**a**, **b**) show herniated brain tissue (arrows) due to defect in the calvarium (open arrows)—Encephalocele

- Venous malformations
- Meckel–Gruber syndrome

Differential diagnosis

1. *Meningocele*: Fetal MRI can identify the neural contents better and its continuation with the intracranial brain. MRI can identify its continuation with the intracranial brain–spine.
2. *Lymphangioma when it is cervico occipital*: Lymphangioma is seen in the skin—subcutaneous plane does not show any communication with the CNS.

Prognosis This depends on the accompanying anomalies. Encephaloceles with microcephaly show poor outcome. Cesarean delivery may be needed to reduce injury to the encephalocele. Temporal encephalocele may be associated with seizure disorder. Postnatally surgery may be needed in many of them. Anterior meningoceles perform better than the posterior ones. Surgery may not be the option for very large encephaloceles and those with severe microcephaly [5]. Mental retardation and motor deficits are seen in nearly 50% of the cases [5].

6.2 Cranial and Caudal Neuropore Defects

6.2.1 Craniorachischisis Totalis

Craniospinal rachischisis is characterized by anencephaly and open spinal dysraphism. It is a very rare and severe form of neural tube defect with the brain and spinal cord being open to varying degrees [6].

Imaging features

There is anencephaly with associated absence of posterior elements at multiple levels (Figs. 6.2c and 6.4) resulting in exposure of neural tissue to the amniotic fluid It is usually associated with polyhydramnios.

Prognosis It is always fatal and can be diagnosed in the first trimester by USG. NTDs can recur in the subsequent pregnancies.

Treatment NTDs can be prevented with dietary folate supplements to the pregnant mother.

6.3 Caudal Neuropore Defects

6.3.1 Myeloschisis

There is failure of closure of the posterior aspect of the neural tube. It occurs at 3–4 weeks of gestation. The affected infants may be stillborn. Its features may merge with that of myelomeningocele [5]. There is deficiency of meninges and skin resulting in the exposure of spinal cord to the aminotic fluid/environment.

Spinal Malformations

The spinal malformations include (1) Spinal dysraphism; (2) Vertebral anomalies; and (3) Sacrococcygeal teratoma.

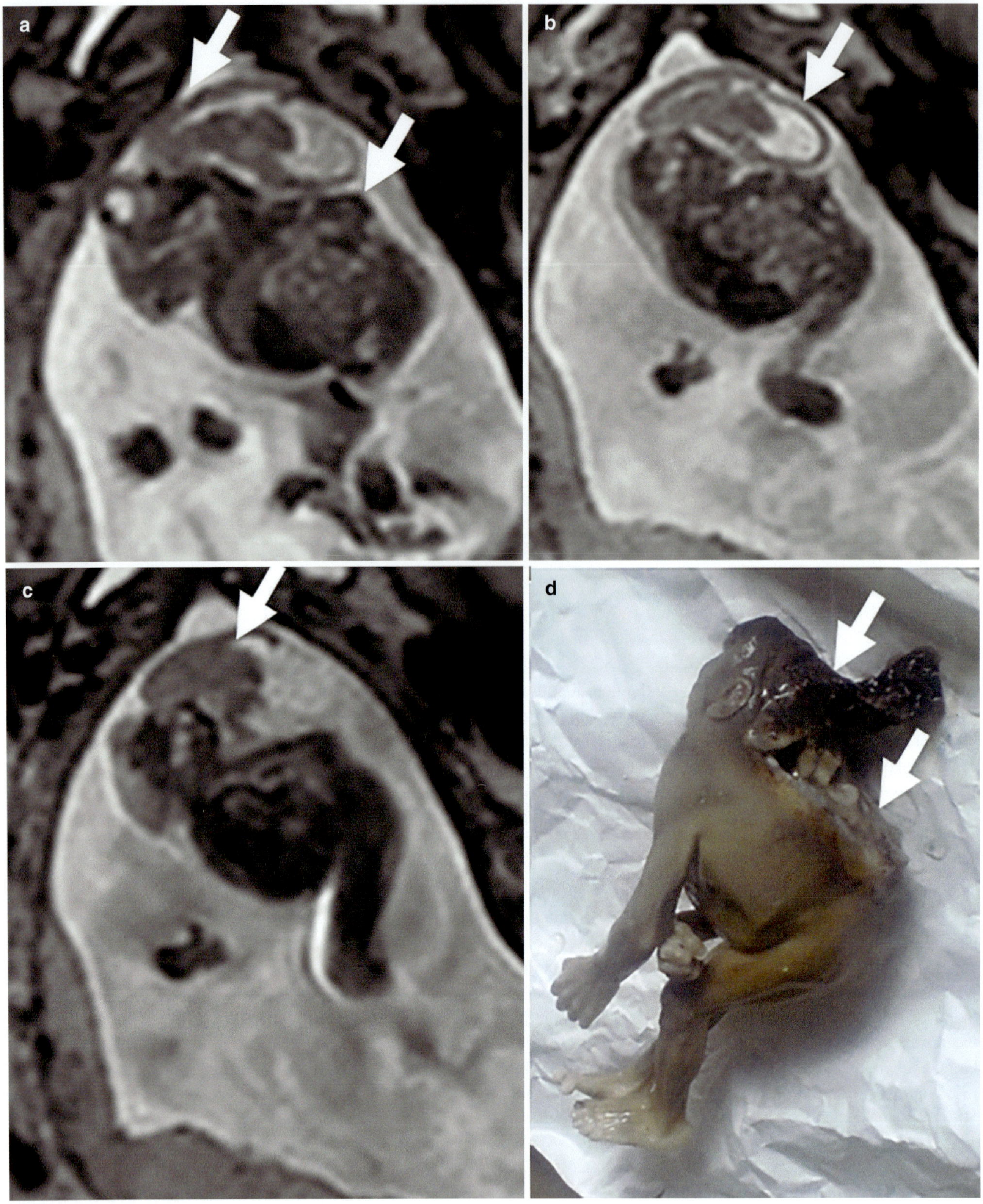

Fig. 6.4 Sagittal images (**a**, **b**, **c**) of a 20-week fetus showing defective cranium, Spine (arrows)—Cranio spino rachis. Clinical photograph (**d**) confirms the diagnosis

Common vertebral anomalies include congenital scoliosis, hemivertebra and butterfly vertebra.

Spinal Dysraphism

Spinal dysraphism refers to congenital anomalies affecting the spinal cord and spine [7]. Spinal dysraphisms can be classified into open and closed spinal dysraphism. In open spinal dysraphism, there is exposure of the neural tissue to the amniotic fluid/environment due to a deficiency in the overlying skin. In the closed type, the neural tissue is covered by skin.

Open Spinal Dysraphisms

Synonym—Spina bifida aperta or cystica

The spinal cord and its covering membrane communicate with the outside. There are no tissues or skin covering the sac. The important subtypes of open spinal dysraphism are enumerated in Box 6.2.

Box 6.2 The Important Subtypes of Open Spinal Dysraphism

- Myelomeningocele (98% of open spinal dysraphism)
- Myelocele
- Hemimyelocele
- Hemimyelomeningocele

6.3.2 Myelomeningocele (Syn—Spina Bifida Cystica)

Prevalence 1:500 of live births with female preponderance [8]. Sites of occurrence in the decreasing frequency are lumbo sacral, dorso-lumbar, lumbar and cervical region. Myelomeningoceles account for 98% of open spinal dysraphism [9].

Embryology/Pathogenesis During 4th week of gestation, there is inadequate closure of the dorsal part of the neural tube resulting in herniation of neural contents [5].

Imaging features

There are deficient and splayed posterior elements leading to herniation of part of the spinal cord with the meninges and subarachnoid space (Figs. 6.5c and 6.6). There may be deficient skin, covering the swelling exposing the contents into the amniotic fluid/environment There may be associated tethering of the spinal cord, hydrocephalus, and syringomyelia [7]. MRI is useful to differentiate myelomeningocele from meningocele and in the identification of associated spinal cord abnormalities like tethering.

Other Associations

Trisomy 18, 13, Chiari II malformation, arachnoid cysts, diastematomyelia.

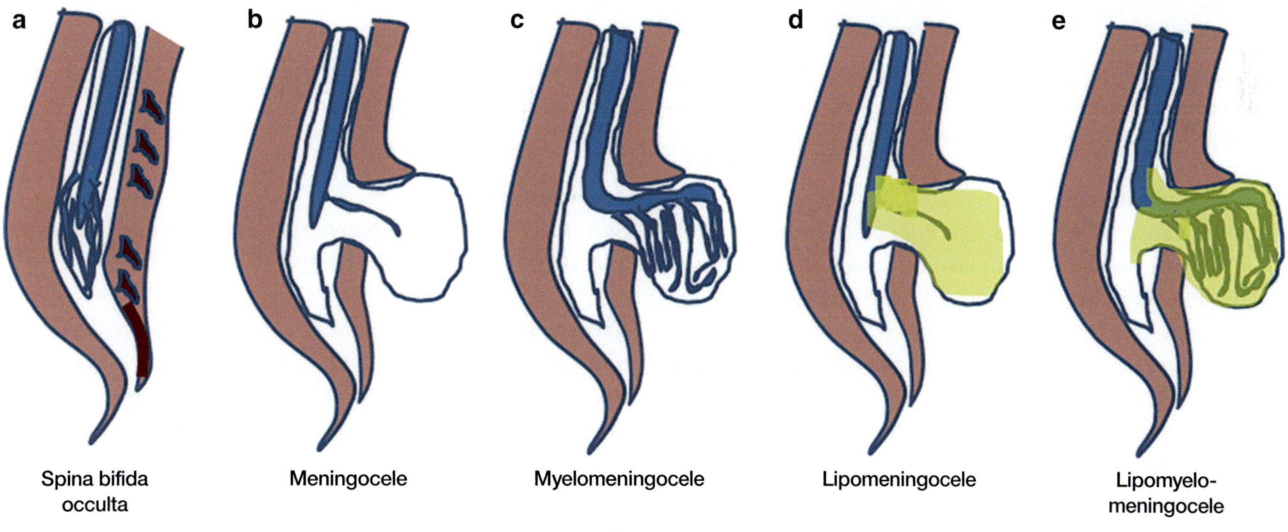

Fig. 6.5 Schematic diagram showing different types of spinal dysraphism. (**a**) Spina bifida occulta (**b**) Meningocele (**c**) Myelomeningocele (**d**) Lipomeningocele (**e**) Lipomyelomeningocele

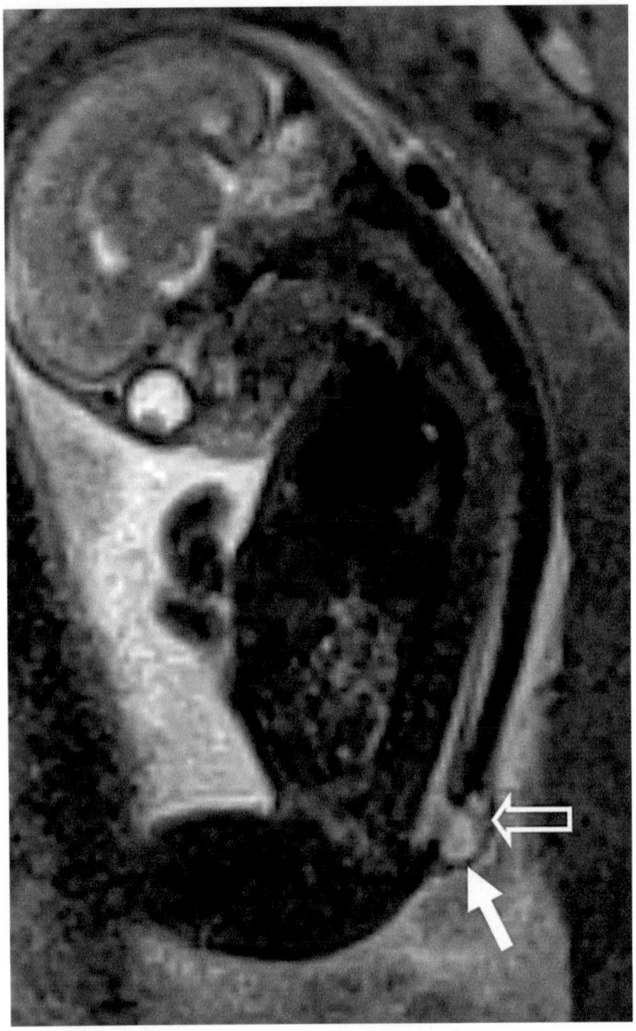

Fig. 6.6 Sagittal T2W image showing spina bifida in the lumbar region with the spinal cord (open arrow) extending into the subcutaneous-cutaneous cyst (arrow) suggesting myelomeningocele

Differential diagnosis

1. *Myeloceles*—They are a rare type of open spinal dysraphism where the neural placode is seen flush with skin surface. (cf in Myelomeningocele the neural placode protrudes beyond the skin surface).
2. *Meningocele*—Part of the spinal cord is not the content of the cystic swelling.
3. Lipomeningocele—the contents are meninges, CSF, and fat and there is absence of spinal cord within the cystic swelling.

6.3.3 Hemimyelomeningocele and Hemimyelocele

They are very rare occurring in one of the hemicords of diastematomyelia [7]. One of the hemicord is normally covered and the other hemicord shows features of myelo meningocele/myelocele.

6.3.4 Chiari Malformation

It is a group of disorders arising due to descent of the brainstem and cerebellum [5, 10, 11].

Embryology/Pathogenesis

In Chiari I and 1.5 malformation, there is a small posterior fossa leading to inferior herniation of brainstem, IV ventricle and cerebellum. Chiari 1.5 malformation is considered as a progression of Chiari I malformation.

In Chiari II malformation, there is a myelomeningocele with tethering and CSF leak leading to inferior herniation of brainstem, IV ventricle and cerebellum. The posterior fossa may be small in size.

Chiari III malformation: There is Inferior herniation of posterior fossa contents with associated occipital or high cervical encephalocele.

Chiari IV malformation: There is severe cerebellar hypoplasia without inferior herniation into foramen magnum, occipital encephalocele [12]. This terminology is no longer being used.

Chiari I malformation

Antenatal diagnosis of Chiari I malformation is extremely rare [13]. They are commonly diagnosed incidentally in children and adults, though they may occasionally present with neck pain, giddiness, muscle weakness, or numbness.

Imaging features

There is presence of peg-like tonsils (triangular and not rounded), 6–12 mm below the foramen magnum. There is crowding of structures in the posterior fossa with obliterated cisterns. It may be associated with syrinx involving the spinal cord.

Associations

Syrinx, hydrocephalus, bony craniovertebral junction anomalies, Crouzon syndrome, Klippel–Feil syndrome.

Treatment Surgical treatment is usually done for the symptomatic group and those with brainstem compression or syrinx. The posterior fossa is decompressed by removing inferior part of the occipital bone and the posterior arch of atlas. An additional duroplasty is also performed.

Differential diagnosis

Low lying tonsil or benign tonsillar ectopia (<5 mm).

Tonsillar herniation due to raised intracranial pressure.

Chiari 1.5 malformation [14].

Chiari 1.5 Malformation

Imaging features

There is inferior herniation of peg-like tonsils, >12 mm below the foramen magnum. There is crowding of structures in the posterior fossa with obliterated cisterns. It may be associated with syrinx involving the spinal cord. The medulla is herniated inferiorly till the obex [12, 15]:

Associations
Syrinx, hydrocephalus, bony craniovertebral junction anomalies, scoliosis.

Differential diagnosis
Low lying tonsil or benign tonsillar ectopia (<5 mm)
Tonsillar herniation due to raised intracranial pressure
Chiari I malformation (tonsillar herniation of 6–12 mm)

Treatment The posterior fossa is decompressed by removing the inferior part of the occipital bone and the posterior arch of atlas. An additional duroplasty is also performed. Sometimes there may be persistence/recurrence of the syrinx after surgery.

Chiari II malformation
The features include small posterior fossa with inferior herniation of brainstem, IV ventricle, cerebellar tonsils, and myelomeningocele.

Incidence 1 in 1000 live births [16]. In 95% of the fetuses with myelomeningocele, there is associated Chiari II malformation.

Imaging features
There is inferior herniation of the medulla, cerebellar tonsils and vermis below the foramen magnum besides myelomeningocele (Fig. 6.7). This results in crowding of structures in the posterior fossa with obliterated cisterns. It may be associated with syrinx involving the spinal cord. Tectal beaking, aqueduct stenosis, and hydrocephalus may also be present. Antenatal USG of the cranium shows "lemon sign" due to indentation of the frontal bones. "Banana sign" refers to the cerebellum that is tightly wrapped around the brain stem due to inferior migration of the posterior fossa contents. This banana sign is also seen in isolated spina bifida but disappears after 24 weeks. MRI is useful when the myelomeningocele is small or when posterior fossa abnormalities are ambiguous on US and to identify associated anomalies. MRI is also recommended if inutero surgery is contemplated.

Associations
Bony craniovertebral junction anomalies, scoliosis, Klippel–Feil syndrome, diastematomyelia, Corpus callosal abnormalities, septal agenesis, polymicrogyria, and club foot.

Differential diagnosis
Isolated meningomyelocele—Posterior fossa contents are normal.
Chiari I malformation—Meningomyelocele is absent.

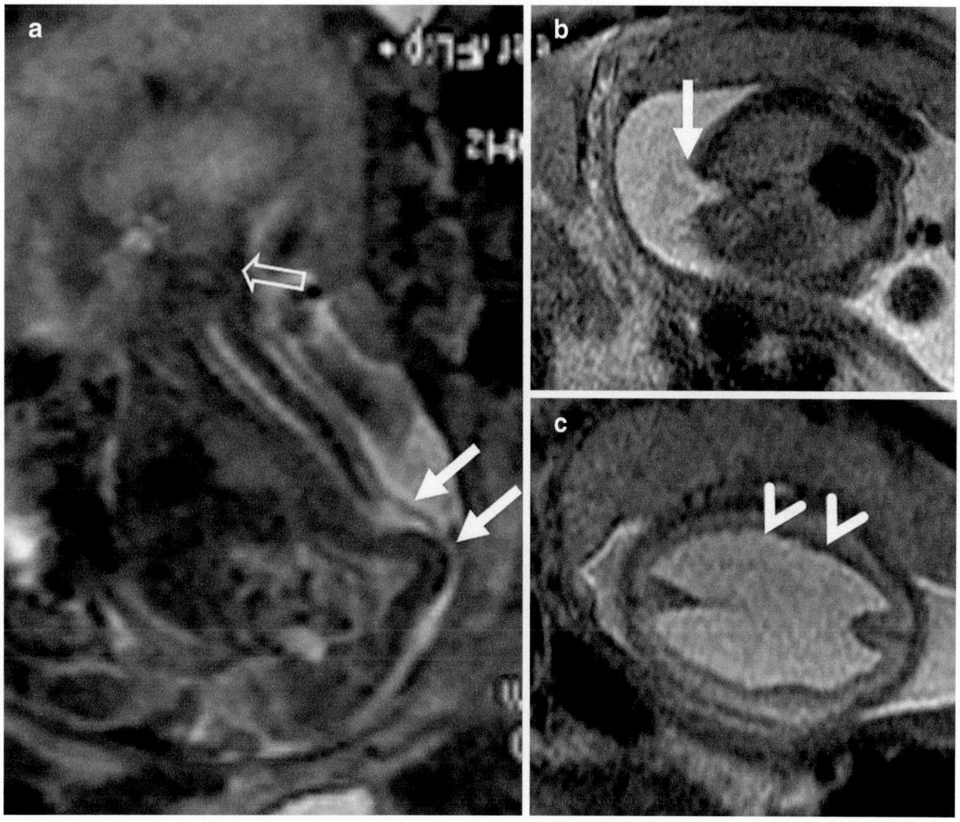

Fig. 6.7 Sagittal (**a**), axial (**b**) T2W images show spina bifida in the dorsolumbar region with the spinal canal—spinal cord communicating with a subcutaneous-cutaneous cyst (arrow) suggesting myelomeningocele. There is associated tonsillar herniation (open arrows). Axial (**c**) T2W image of brain shows hydrocephalus (arrowhead)—Chiari 2 malformation

Treatment
Meningomyelocele repair can be done in utero or postnatally. Detethering is also performed whenever needed.

Ventriculoperitoneal shunt needs to be performed when there is associated hydrocephalus.

Decompression of the posterior fossa and posterior arch of atlas may also be needed postnatally.

Chiari III Malformation
It is a very severe malformation characterized by inferior herniation of posterior fossa contents with associated occipital or high cervical encephalocele [17]. Aberrant draining veins may be seen within the encephaloceles.

Associations
- Dysgenesis of the corpus callosum.
- Hydrocephalus.
- Syringohydromyelia.

Closed Spinal Dysraphisms
In the mildest form *spina bifida occulta*, there is a defect in the neural arch with skin covering the defect (Fig. 6.5a). As there are no associated abnormalities of the spinal cord or nerve roots, the children are asymptomatic.

Closed spinal dysraphisms can be further subclassified based on the presence of an associated subcutaneous mass and presence or absence of normal mesenchymal tissue covering the cord.

Closed Spinal Dysraphisms with a Subcutaneous Mass.

The important subtypes of closed spinal dysraphisms with a subcutaneous mass are enumerated in Box 6.3.

Box 6.3 Important Subtypes of Closed Spinal Dysraphisms with a Subcutaneous Mass/Normal Mesenchymal Tissue Covering the Cord
- Lipoma with dural defect
  - Lipomyelomeningocele
  - Lipomyelocele
- Meningocele
- Myelocystocele

6.3.5 Lipomyelomeningoceles, Lipomeningocele and Lipomyelocele

They are seen as a skin-covered fatty mass in the subcutaneous plane above the intergluteal groove.

Embryology/Pathogenesis During primary neurulation, mesenchymal tissue enters the neural tube and forms a lipoma along the spinal cord. Lipomyeloceles are commoner than Lipomyelomeningoceles [7].

Imaging features
Antenatal sonography shows deficiency of posterior elements, with an elongated spinal cord with placode attached to an intrathecal echogenic fatty mass that may protrude into the dorsal subcutaneous tissue.

MRI shows spina bifida with focal enlargement of the spinal canal at the level of the placode. In the lipomyelocele, the neural placode–lipoma interface lies inside the spinal canal. In the lipomyelomeningocele, the neural placode–lipoma interface lies exterior to the spinal canal (Fig. 6.5e). Lipomeningocele is a meningocele that has some amount of fat associated with it (Figs. 6.5d and 6.8). A low ending spinal cord is commonly present.

Differential diagnosis
Spinal intradural lipoma—Posterior elements of the spine are intact and fatty tissue is present within the spinal canal (Fig. 6.9).

6.3.6 Meningocele

These are protrusions of the meninges with CSF through a defect in the skull or spine, usually covered by the skin.

Embryology/Pathogenesis Due to the presence of neural tube defect there is protrusion of meninges through a bone defect in the cranium/vertebral column.

Types
1. Cranial
2. Spinal—Dorsal, anterior, lateral thoracic and lateral sacral

Imaging features
Cranial meningocele is seen as a cystic lesion communicating with the subarachnoid space of brain through a defect in the skull. Spinal meningocele is seen as a cystic lesion communicating with the spinal canal through a defect in the posterior elements of spine, though a few thin neural elements may be present (Figs. 6.5b and 6.10). However, there is no herniation of the brain tissue or spinal cord into the sac. MRI is useful to differentiate meningocele from myelomeningocele and in the identification of associated abnormalities like spinal cord tethering.

Associations Fibrous band tethering, tight filum terminale, adhesion of spinal cord/cauda equina to the dura

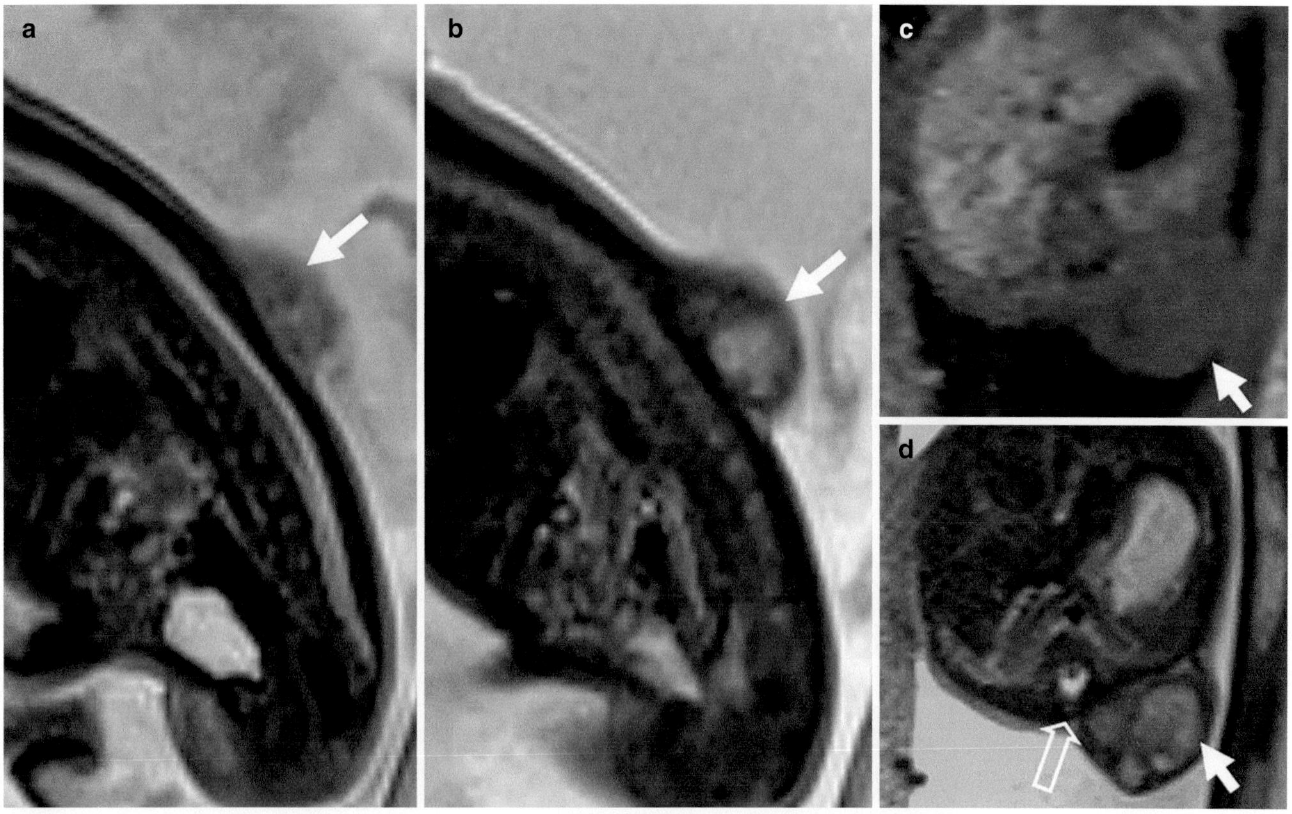

Fig. 6.8 Sagittal T2W (**a**, **b**), axial T1W (**c**), axial T2W (**d**) images of a 24 week shows a mass lesion in the left posterior paravertebral region (arrows). The lesion is seen in the muscular and subcutaneous plane and reaches up to the superficial surface of the bony spine. There is a tiny communication of the subarachnoid CSF into the mass, at the level of dorso lumbar junction—lipomeningocele

mater, low-lying conus, spinal cord lipoma, diastematomyelia, syringomyelia, arachnoid cyst, fatty filum terminale.

Differential diagnosis

- *Meningomyelocele*: The herniated cystic lesion contains spinal cord in addition to meninges and CSF.
- *Meningocele manqué*: The herniated cystic lesion contains atretic tethering neural tissue attached to the spinal cord besides meninges and CSF [18].
- *Prognosis and treatment*: Postnatal MRI is advisable to confirm the diagnosis and to identify additional findings like tethered cord. The outcome is good after repair of meningocele/meningocele manqué and the associated tethering [18, 19].

6.3.7 Myelocystocele

There is focal severe dilatation of the central canal of the spinal cord, that can herniate posteriorly through a dorsal spinal defect. This results in a skin-covered ependymal lined sac that herniates posteriorly. It is named as "terminal" myelocystocele when located in the sacral region and "non-terminal" when located elsewhere in the spinal column [20].

Closed Spinal Dysraphism Without Subcutaneous Mass The various subtypes are enumerated in Box 6.4.

Box 6.4 The Various Subtypes of Closed Spinal Dysraphism Without Subcutaneous Mass

- Disorders of notochordal formation
  - Caudal regression syndrome
  - Segmental spinal dysgenesis
- Disorders of notochordral integration
  - Dorsal dermal sinus
  - Dorsal enteric fistula
  - Neurenteric cyst
  - Split cord malformations (Diastematomyelia and Diplomyelia)
- Posterior spina bifida (isolated defect of posterior neural arch of vertebra)
- Intradural lipoma
- Filum terminale lipoma
- Tight filum terminale

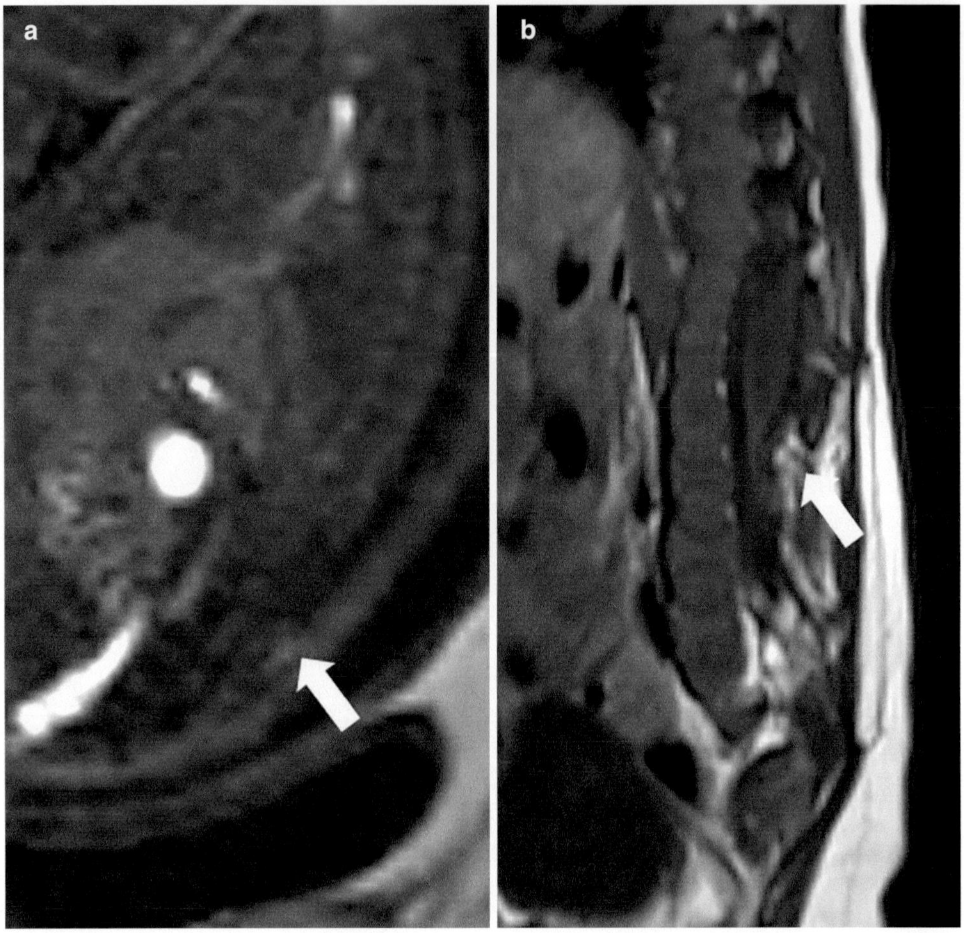

Fig. 6.9 Sagittal T1W (**a**) image of a 27-week fetus with diastematomyelia, shows intraspinal lipoma (arrow). Sagittal (**b**) T1W postnatal images confirm the diagnosis (arrow)

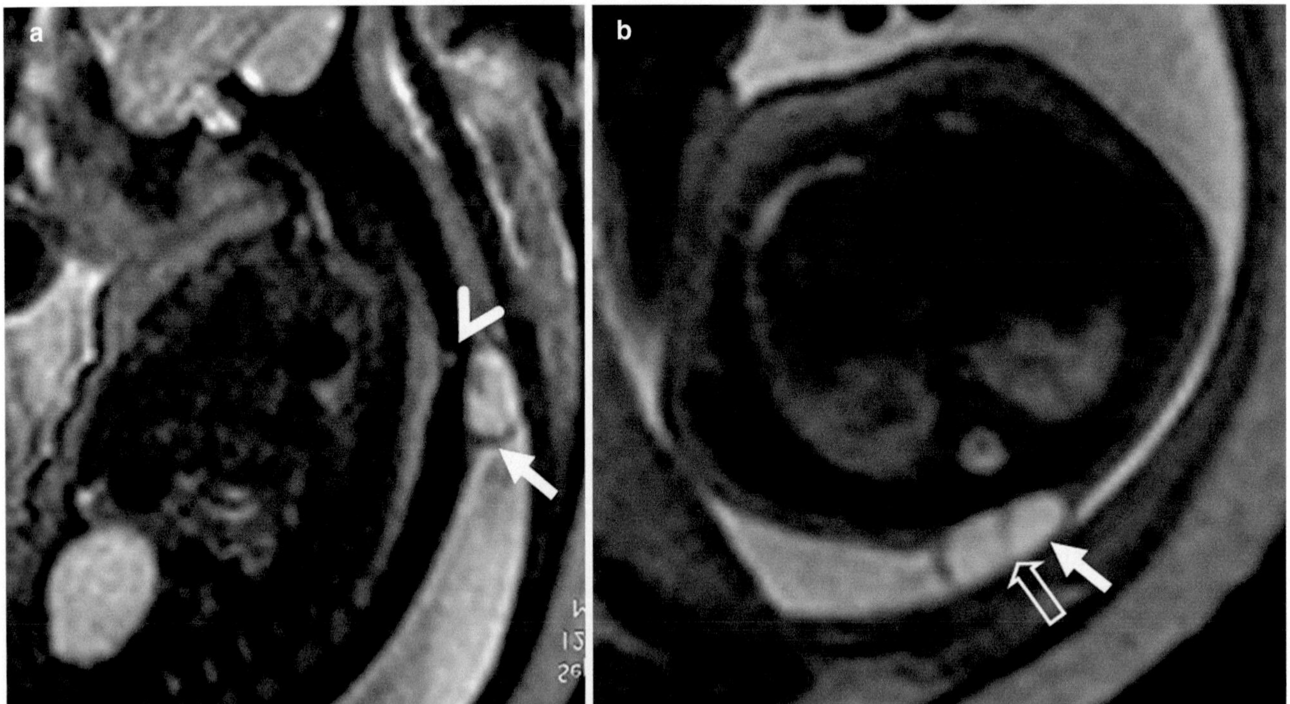

Fig. 6.10 Sagittal (**a**), axial (**b**) T2W images show spina bifida in the upper dorsal region with a subcutaneous-cutaneous cyst communicating with the spinal canal (arrowhead) suggesting meningocele. A rudimentary connecting band (open arrow) is visualized and the spinal cord appears normal

6.3.8 Caudal Regression Syndrome (CRS)

This syndrome represents developmental failure of the caudal spine ranging from lumbosacral agenesis to coccygeal agenesis. Associated abnormalities involving the corresponding segments of the spinal cord may be present

Incidence Rare, 1–10 in 100,000.

Embryology/Pathology Insult during Primary Neurulation (around 4 weeks). Possible etiologies include hyperglycemia (common in diabetic mothers). infections, toxins, and ischemia

Imaging features

- *I trimester*—Reduced crown-rump length and increased nuchal translucency.
- *II and III trimester*.
- Lumbosacral vertebral agenesis/hypogenesis/dysgenesis.
- Abrupt ending of the spine. The level of agenesis/dysgenesis is commonly below L1 or involving the sacrum.
- Abrupt ending of the spinal cord well above the vertebral defect (the conus tip is cigar-shaped or wedge shaped).
- Spinal canal narrowing inferior to the last intact vertebra.
- Hypoplastic lower extremities, club feet.
- "Crossed leg" or "Buddha position" appearance
- Polyhydramnios.
- Absence of sacral ossification centers from 17 weeks on axial scans causing opposed iliac bones—"Shield Sign":
- MRI is useful in depicting the spinal and spinal cord abnormalities better and when the position of fetus is difficult to be assessed by US.
- *Type 1*—the conus medullaris terminates above the normal level. There may be associated dilated central canal or CSF cyst at the conus and major sacral deformities. *Type 2*—the conus medullaris is low ending and tethered by a thickened filum terminale or lipoma. Sacral deformities are less commonly seen.

Associations

- VACTERL anomalies
- Cardiovascular anomalies
- GI anomalies like Anorectal agenesis, duodenal atresia
- Genitourinary anomalies like cystic renal dysplasia, hydronephrosis
- Chiari 2 malformation

Differential diagnosis

- *Sirenomelia*: Presence of lower limb fusion
- *Myelo meningocele*—There is presence of an external sac. The vertebral ossification centers are seen, but posterior elements are splayed
- *VACTERL* anomalies—Spine is present but deformed

6.3.9 Dorsal Dermal Sinus Tract (DDS)

It is a form of spinal dysraphism where an epithelialized tract exists between the skin and the arachnoid or cauda equina or spinal cord [21].

Embryology/Pathology
When there is incomplete separation of the neural ectoderm from the superficial ectoderm, the focal adhesion leads to the formation of a long, tubular dermal sinus tract.

Imaging features
DDS are commonly seen in the lumbosacral region, followed by the occipital region.

Sonography shows an echogenic tract sometimes filled with CSF between the skin and spinal cord/cauda equina. Associated findings like diastematomyelia, intraspinal mass (dermoid) may be seen MRI is complementary when sonography findings are equivocal.

Associations
Intraspinal epidermoid/dermoid, diastematomyelia.

Prognosis and treatment
Postnatally, patients can be asymptomatic or present with recurrent meningitis or intraspinal abscess.

Treatment consists of resection of the DDS/intraspinal mass and correction of the associated malformations like diastematomyelia.

Differential diagnosis
Sacral dimples are small pits (<5 mm) occurring near the anal orifice. They may exist as an incidental finding or may be associated with occult spinal dysraphism like tethered cord. Sonography/MRI may reveal the depth of the tract and any communication with the spinal canal.

Pilonidal sinuses result from a hair follicle infection in the skin—subcutaneous plane in the intergluteal cleft in the buttocks region. The sinus tract may extend up to the coccyx. Sonography/MRI can reveal the depth of the tract/abscess formation and any communication with the coccyx.

6.3.10 Diastematomyelia

Syn—Split cord malformation (SCM) includes both diastematomyelia and diplomyelia [22].

It is characterized by a longitudinal split within the spinal cord [23].

Incidence
SCM account for ~5% of congenital spinal anomalies [22]. About 50% of the cases occur at L1–L3 level followed by T7–T12 in 25% of cases.

Classification (proposed by Pang) and Imaging features

Type I: A midline osseous or fibrous spur is seen with a duplicated dural sac. MRI shows focal widening of the spinal canal with a hypointense lesion in the midline (Fig. 6.11). Associated anomalies include tethering of the cord, hydromyelia (Fig. 6.12), vertebral anomalies like scoliosis, block vertebrae, hemivertebrae, spina bifida, and butterfly vertebrae. MRI is useful in depicting spinal cord abnormalities better. There may be overlying skin changes and hypertrichosis.

Type II: Imaging shows focal widening of the spinal canal with a single dural sac that contains two hemicords. Associated anomalies include spina bifida and hydromyelia.

Prognosis and Treatment

Postnatally many children are symptomatic in Type 1 diastematomyelia. They are minimally symptomatic or asymptomatic in Type 2 diastematomyelia.

Treatment consists of, resection of the spur, dural repair, and release of the tethered cord.

Differential diagnosis

Diplomyelia—There are two spinal cords and each has two anterior and two posterior horns with their nerve roots.

6.3.11 Lipoma

Intradural lipoma

It occurs due to an error in neurulation. Before the neural folds close a small mesenchymal tissue passes into the

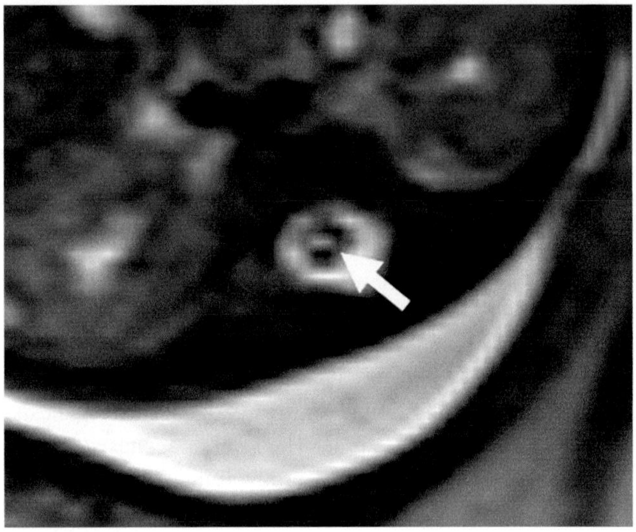

Fig. 6.12 Axial images of the spine of a 27-week fetus with diastematomyelia show syringomyelia (arrow) in the cranial aspect of the spinal cord

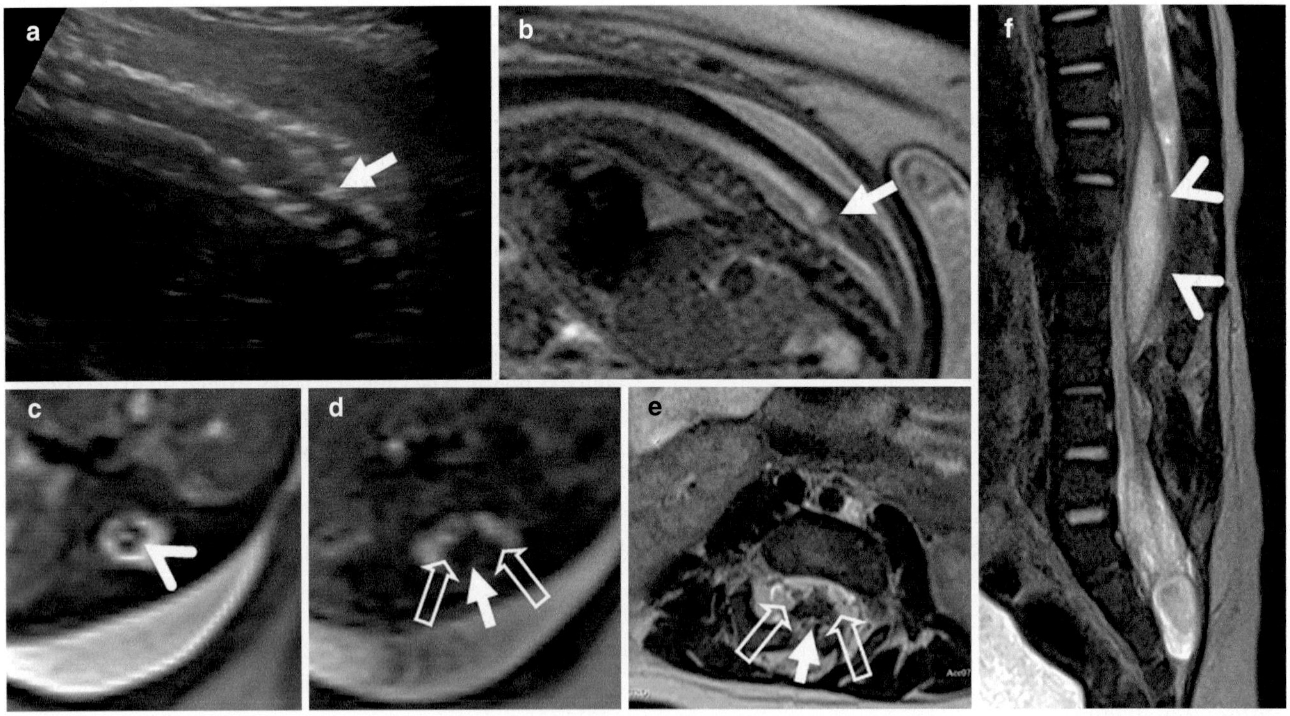

Fig. 6.11 Sagittal T2W (**a**, **b**), axial T2W (**c**, **d**) images of a 27-week fetus, shows a bony-fibrous septum (arrow) with 2 cords (open arrows) and low ending spinal cord—diastematomyelia. Axial (**e**) and sagittal (**f**) T2W postnatal images of the infant confirm the diagnosis (arrow). There is associated Syringomyelia at the dorsolumbar junction (arrowhead)

central canal (premature dysjunction) that later on forms the lipoma (Fig. 6.9).

Filar Lipoma

These are lipomas occurring along the filum terminale and are embryonal in origin. They are seen as small areas of fat along the filum terminale on MR images. They usually asymptomatic though rarely they can cause cord tethering and tight filum terminale syndrome.

6.3.12 Tethered Cord/Tight Filum Terminale Syndrome

Tethered cord is a disorder where the superior migration of the spinal cord is limited by tissue attachments [24].

Embryology/Pathogenesis The tethered cord occurs along with several types of spinal dysraphism except for neurenteric cyst and spina bifida occulta.

As the vertebral column grows faster than the spinal cord, tethered lesions can stretch the spinal cord. This can lead to ischemic changes in the spinal cord.

Imaging features

It is commonly recognized when there is an abnormally low positioned conus medullaris. Sometimes the conus may be in a normal position but may be attached by a thickened filum terminale >2 mm in thickness [25, 26].

6.4 Scoliosis

Abnormal lateral spinal curvature is scoliosis (Fig. 6.13) and abnormal anterior spinal curvature is Kyphosis. They can be diagnosed by sonography, made easy by 3D imaging. Counting of the vertebra is accomplished by using the 12th rib as the landmark. Features include short spinal length, abnormal spinal curvature, and flared vertebral arches. It is important to look for vertebral abnormalities like hemivertebra, wedge vertebra, block vertebrae (Fig. 6.14), butterfly vertebra and spinal cord abnormalities. Sometimes they are associated with anomalies in other systems (VACTERL). Fetal MRI is complementary and is very useful to visualize the spinal cord and to rule out associated spinal dysraphism [27, 28].

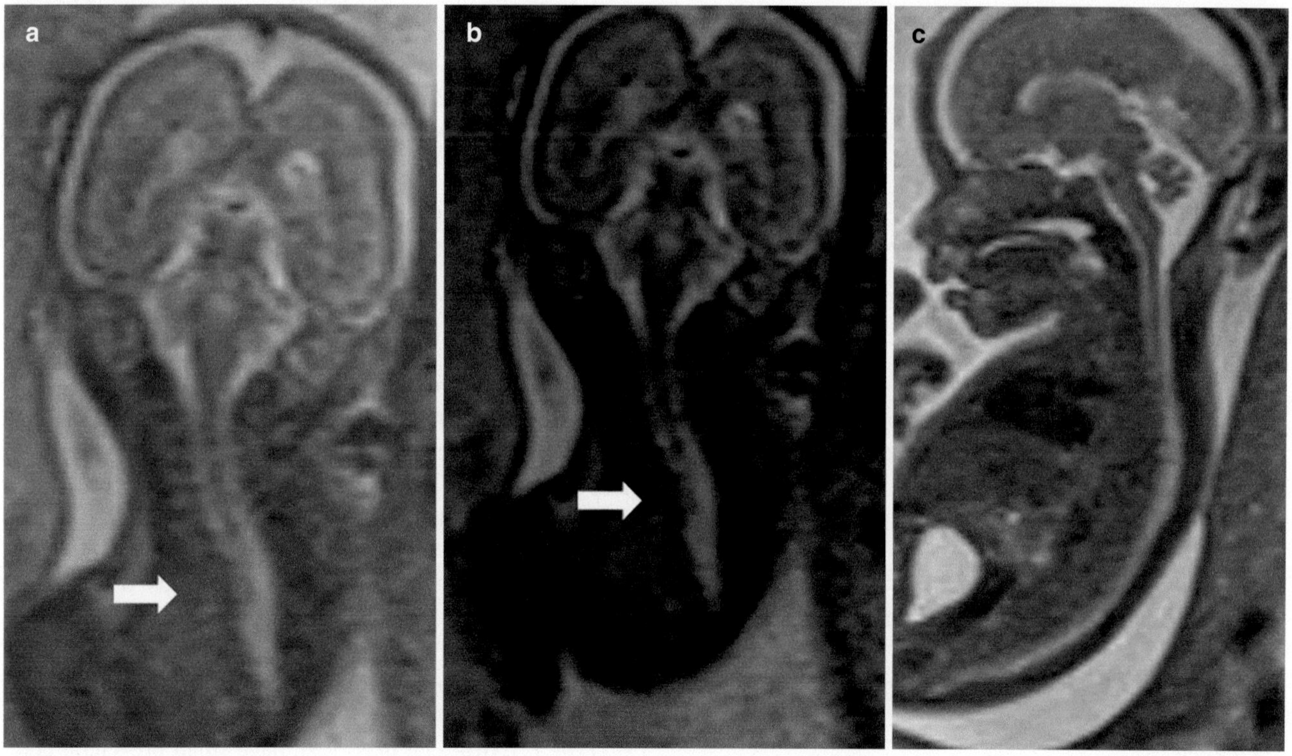

Fig. 6.13 Coronal T2W (**a**, **b**) image shows mild scoliosis cervicodorsal junction. Sagittal image (**c**) shows normal spinal cord and the fetus was managed conservatively

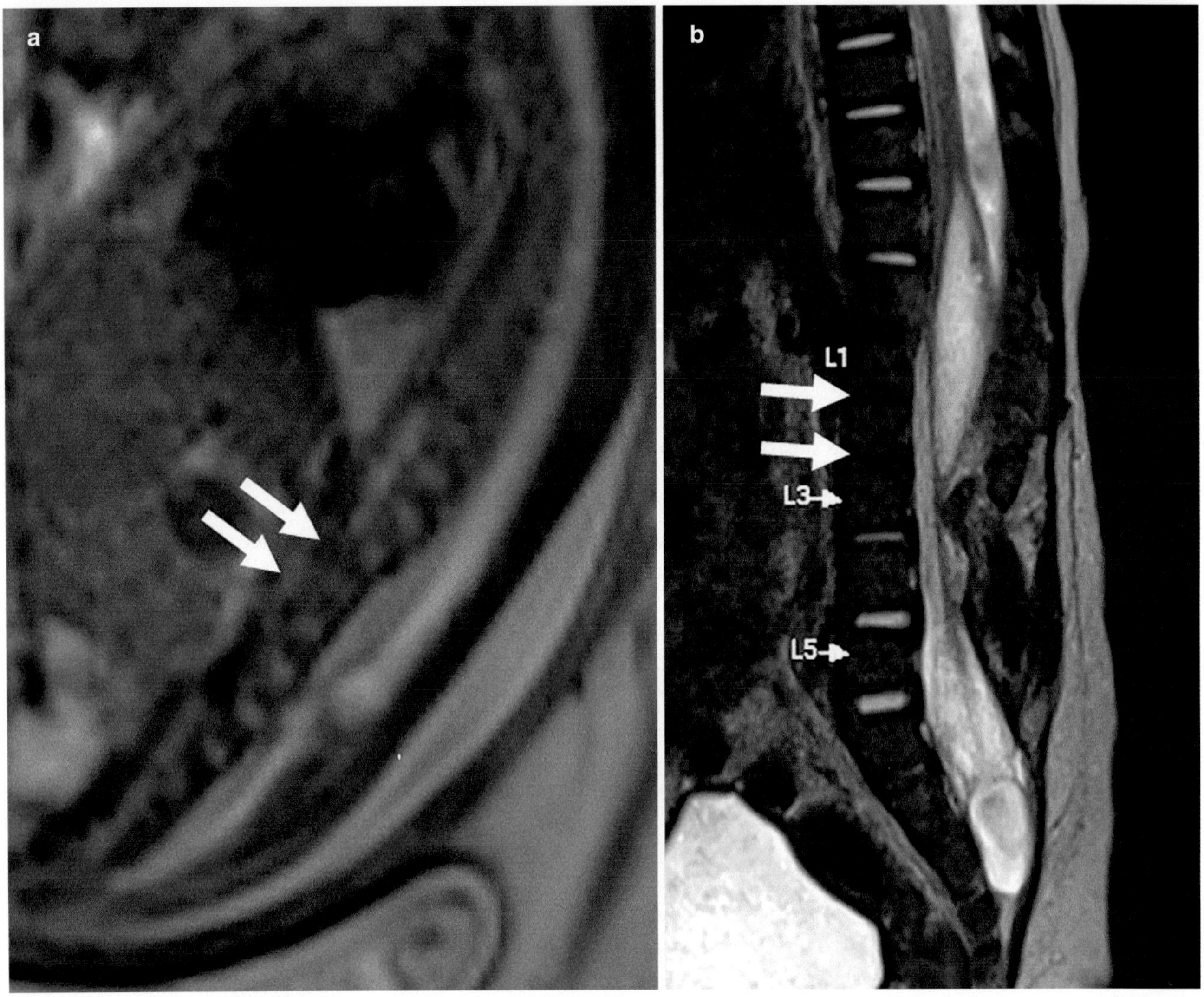

Fig. 6.14 Sagittal T2W (**a**) image of a 27-week fetus with diastematomyelia, shows reduced disc height in upper lumbar region (arrow). Postnatal sagittal image (**b**) shows partial fusion of the upper lumbar vertebrae

Prognosis and treatment

Mild isolated scoliosis has a good prognosis. Severe scoliosis may need corrective surgeries postnatally. Sometimes they are associated with open neural tube defects that may carry a poor prognosis.

6.5 Sacrococcygeal Teratoma (SCT)

Teratoma occurring in the sacrococcygeal region.

Incidence

SCT is the commonest tumor occurring in the fetus [29] with an incidence of 1 in 35,000–40,000. SCT are four times more common in female fetuses than males.

Embryology/Pathology

They arise from totipotent cells from the node of Hensen [30] that are present in the anterior aspect of the coccyx by 2nd–3rd weeks of gestation. They may have solid, cystic, or mixed components and may cause elevated serum Alpha-fetoprotein (AFP) levels in the infants. They may present as a *benign tumor—mature type* (80%) or as a *malignant tumor—immature type.*

Classification based on location (From American Academy of Pediatric Surgery)

- *Type I*: Extra-fetal mass (can have small pre-sacral component); accounts for the majority of cases, 47% [12]
- *Type II*: Extra-fetal mass with intrapelvic or presacral extension

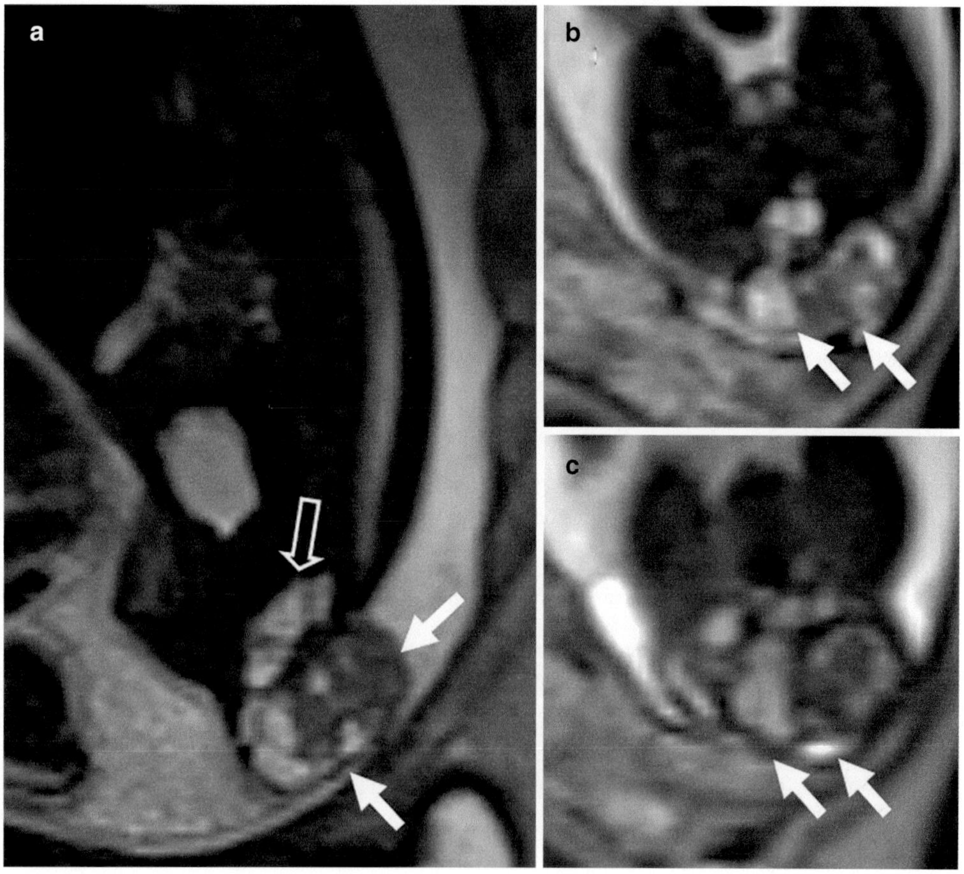

Fig. 6.15 Sagittal (**a**) and axial (**b**, **c**) T2W images show a well-defined mass inferior to sacrum-coccygeal region (arrows) with an intrapelvic component (open arrows). The rectum is displaced anteriorly by the mass—Type II Sacrococcygeal teratoma

- *Type III*: Extra-fetal mass with extension into the pelvis and abdomen
- *Type IV*: Mass entirely within the fetal pelvis

Imaging features

- Polyhydramnios
- Exophytic mass showing solid, cystic, or mixed components (Fig. 6.15). Solid tumors may show increased vascularity with AV shunting. Intrapelvic/abdominal extension may be seen
- Coccyx/sacrum are involved
- Hydrops due to cardiac failure
- MRI is superior in showing bony involvement and Intrapelvic/abdominal extension. MRI is also useful when the size of the mass is small and is difficult to be assessed on US.

Associations

- Due to mass effect on adjacent structures—urinary tract obstruction, renal dysplasia, hydrocolpos, anorectal malformation
- Myelomeningocele
- Vertebral anomalies

Differential diagnosis

Myelomeningocele—Splayed posterior elements with cystic mass and neural elements.

Terminal myelocystocoele—Hydromyelia with low lying spinal cord that traverses into a dorsal meningocele.

Prognosis and treatment

Tumor volume/fetal weight ratio (TFR) is calculated. Large mass with TFR >0.12 have a bad prognosis. Solid components with increased vascularity, intra-abdominal extension, malignant transformation, and fetal hydrops show increased morbidity and mortality.

References

1. Kanekar S, Kaneda H, Shively A. Malformations of dorsal induction. Semin Ultrasound CT MR. 2011;32:189–99.
2. Rama Murthy BS. Anomalies of dorsal induction: neural tube defects. In: Imaging of fetal brain and spine. Singapore: Springer; 2019.
3. Salih MA, Murshid WR, Seidahmed MZ. Epidemiology, prenatal management, and prevention of neural tube defects. Saudi Med J. 2015;35(Suppl 1):S15–28.
4. Mehta TS, Levine D. Ultrasound and MR imaging of fetal neural tube defects. Ultrasound Clin. 2007;2:187–201.

5. Volpe JJ. Neurology of the newborn, vol 899.
6. Jaganmohan D, Subramaniam P, Krishnan N, Mahajan P. Two cases of craniospinal rachischisis totalis: role of magnetic resonance imaging in diagnosis and review of neural tube defects in the Indian context with implications for folate fortification. J Pediatr Neurosci. 2017;12:32–5.
7. Rufener SL, Ibrahim M, Raybaud CA, et-al. Congenital spine and spinal cord malformations—pictorial review. AJR Am J Roentgenol. 2010;194(3):S26–40.
8. Dick EA, Patel K, Owens CM, et-al. Spinal ultrasound in infants. Br J Radiol. 2002;75(892):384–92.
9. Tortori-Donati P, Rossi A, Cama A. Spinal dysraphism: a review of neuroradiologicalfeatures with embryological correlations and proposal for a new classification. Neuroradiology. 2000;42:471–91.
10. El Gammal T, Mark EK, Brooks BS. MR imaging of Chiari II malformation. AJR Am J Roentgenol. 1988;150(1):163–70.
11. Osborn A, Blaser S, Salzman K. Encyclopedia of diagnostic imaging. AMIRSYS. 2008.
12. Tubbs RS, Demerdash A, Vahedi P, et al. Chiari IV malformation: correcting an over one century long historical error. Childs Nerv Syst. 2016;32:1175–9.
13. Iruretagoyena JI, Trampe B, Shah D. Prenatal diagnosis of Chiari malformation with syringomyelia in the second trimester. J Matern Fetal Neonatal Med. 2010;23(2):184–6.
14. Chiapparini L, Saletti V, Solero CL, et-al. Neuroradiological diagnosis of Chiari malformations. Neurol Sci. 2011;32(Suppl 3):S283–6.
15. Tubbs RS, Iskandar BJ, Bartolucci AA, et-al. A critical analysis of the Chiari 1.5 malformation. J Neurosurg. 2004;101(2):179–83.
16. Maixner WJ. Spina bifida, management and outcome. Springer; 2008. ISBN: 8847006511.
17. Castillo M, Quencer RM, Dominguez R. Chiari III malformation: imaging features. AJNR Am J Neuroradiol. 1992;13:107–13.
18. Shabina Banu MH, Rangasami R, Suresh I. Fetal Meningocele manqué. Neurol India. 2018;66:879–81.
19. Yun-Hai S, Nan B, Ping-Ping G, Bo Y, Cheng C. Is repair of the protruded meninges sufficient for treatment of meningocele? Childs Nerv Syst. 2015;31(11):2135–40. https://doi.org/10.1007/s00381-015-2874-4.
20. Yu JA, Sohaey R, Kennedy AM, et-al. Terminal myelocystocele and sacrococcygeal teratoma: a comparison of fetal ultrasound presentation and perinatal risk. AJNR Am J Neuroradiol. 2007;28(6):1058–60.
21. Singh I, Rohilla S, Kumar P, Sharma S. Spinal dorsal dermal sinus tract: an experience of 21 cases. Surg Neurol Int. 2015;6(Suppl 17):S429–34.
22. Özek MM, Cinalli G, Maixner WJ. The spina bifida, management and outcome. Springer; 2008. ISBN: 8847006503.
23. Cheng B, Li FT, Lin L. Diastematomyelia: a retrospective review of 138 patients. J Bone Joint Surg Br. 2012;94:365–72.
24. Yamada S, et al. Pathophysiology of tethered cord syndrome and similar complex disorders. Neurosurg Focus. 2007;23(E6):1–10.
25. Warder DE, Oakes WJ. Tethered cord syndrome and the conus in a normal position. Neurosurgery. 1993;33:374–8.
26. Unsinn KM, Geley T, Freund MC et al. US of the spinal cord in newborns: spectrum of normal findings, variants, congenital anomalies, and acquired diseases. Radiographics. 20(4):923–38.
27. Paoletti D, Robertson M, Sia SB. A sonographic approach to prenatal classification of congenital spine anomalies. Australas J Ultrasound Med. 2014;17:20–37.
28. Kaplan K, Spivak J, Bendo J. Embryology of the spine and associated congenital abnormalities [electronic version]. Spine J. 2005;5:564–76.
29. Roman AS, Monteagudo A, Timor-tritsch I, et-al. First-trimester diagnosis of sacrococcygeal teratoma: the role of three-dimensional ultrasound. Ultrasound Obstet Gynecol. 2004;23(6):612–4.
30. Avni FE, Guibaud L, Robert Y, et-al. MR imaging of fetal sacrococcygeal teratoma: diagnosis and assessment. AJR Am J Roentgenol. 2002;178(1):179–83.

7 Ventriculomegaly

7.1 Ventriculomegaly

Definition The term ventriculomegaly is used when the ventricular diameter is 10 mm or more and it can be unilateral or bilateral. The dimensions (inner wall to inner wall) of the lateral ventricle need to be measured at the level of the atrium, on the axial or coronal images, the latter being preferable (Fig. 7.1a, b).

Incidence 0.9% of all pregnancies [1].

Grades Mild—The ventricular diameter is 10–12 mm,
Moderate—The ventricular diameter is 12.1–15 mm.
Severe—The ventricular diameter is more than 15 mm.

Mild to moderate ventriculomegaly (10–15 mm diameter) is associated with a mild or no neurological disability when it is isolated. However, fetuses with ventriculomegaly may often show additional findings on MRI, such as posterior fossa abnormalities, agenesis corpus callosum, hemorrhage, encephalomalacia, and heterotopias [2, 3].

Causes of ventriculomegaly [4]

- *Ventriculomegaly due to Obstruction.*
  - Dandy–Walker Malformation.
  - Chiari II malformation.
  - Aqueductal stenosis.
  - Secondary to mass lesions such as arachnoid cyst.
- *Resulting from Dysgenesis.*
  - Agenesis of the corpus callosum.
  - Septo-optic dysplasia.
  - Schizencephaly.
- *Resulting from Destructive process.*
  - Hemorrhage.
  - Post-infection.
  - Leukomalacia.
- *Associations.*
  - Syndromes.
  - Chromosomal/Genetic disorders—Trisomy 13,18, X-linked hydrocephaly.
  - Porencephaly.
  - Cortical malformations like heterotopia.

Imaging features
MRI is useful to grade the ventriculomegaly, to identify the cause and other associated anomalies [5].

Ventriculomegaly due to Obstruction

- Dilatation of a structurally normal cerebral ventricle (Fig. 7.2a–c).
- Ventricular walls appear smooth.
- Cortex is compressed.
- The posterior fossa structures may be abnormal.
  - If normal, aqueductal stenosis is a possibility.
- CSP may be absent in severe obstructive ventriculomegaly.
- Obstructing lesion causing ventriculomegaly has to be looked for.

Ventriculomegaly Resulting from Dysgenesis

- Ventricular shape and position may be abnormal (Fig. 7.3).
- Ventricular walls appear smooth.
- CSP may be abnormal.
- The cerebral cortex is preserved (with the exception of open lip schizencephaly).
- Other CNS abnormalities may be visible (e.g., fused frontal horns).

Ventriculomegaly Resulting from Destructive Process

- Ventricular position is normal.
- Ventricular walls may appear irregular or nodular from old hemorrhage. However, the ventricular walls may

R. Rajeswaran, *MR Imaging of the Fetus*, https://doi.org/10.1007/978-981-16-9209-3_7

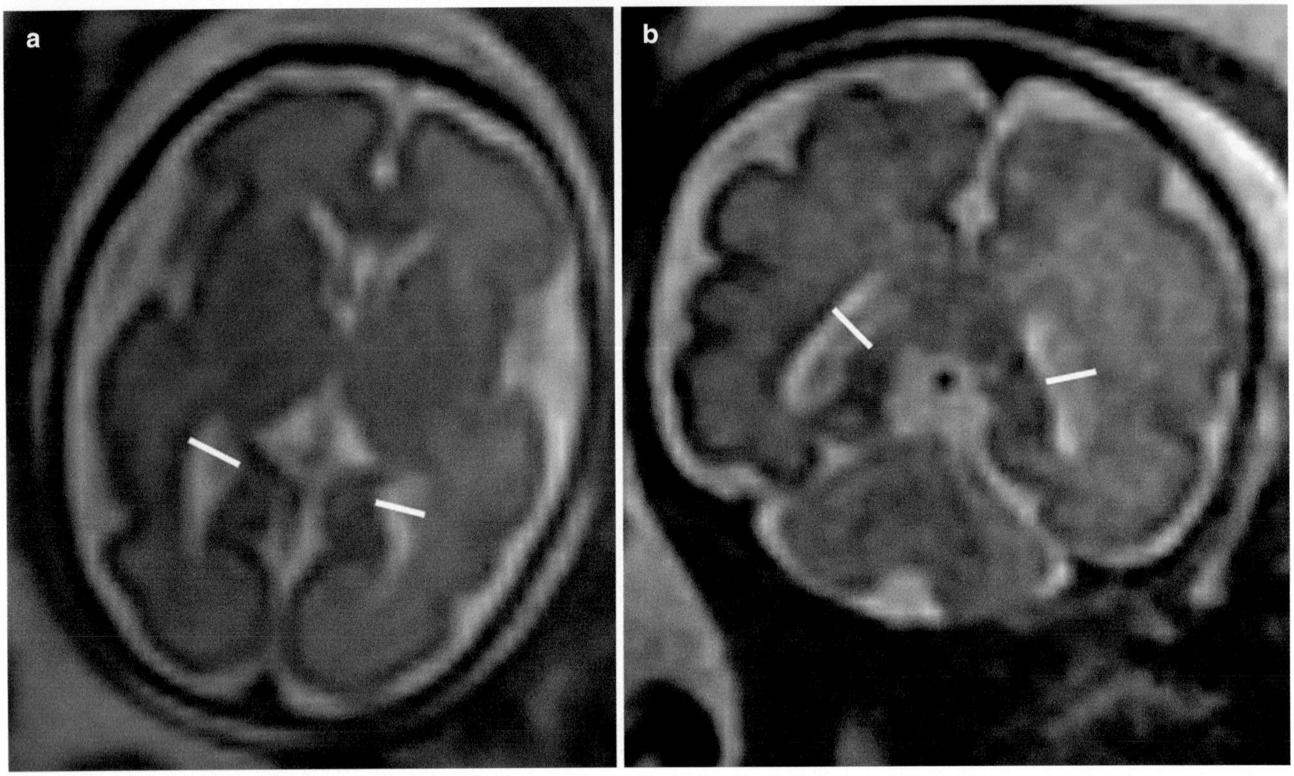

Fig. 7.1 Axial (**a**) and coronal (**b**) T2W Image of a normal 31-week fetal brain. The method of measuring the lateral ventricular width is demonstrated

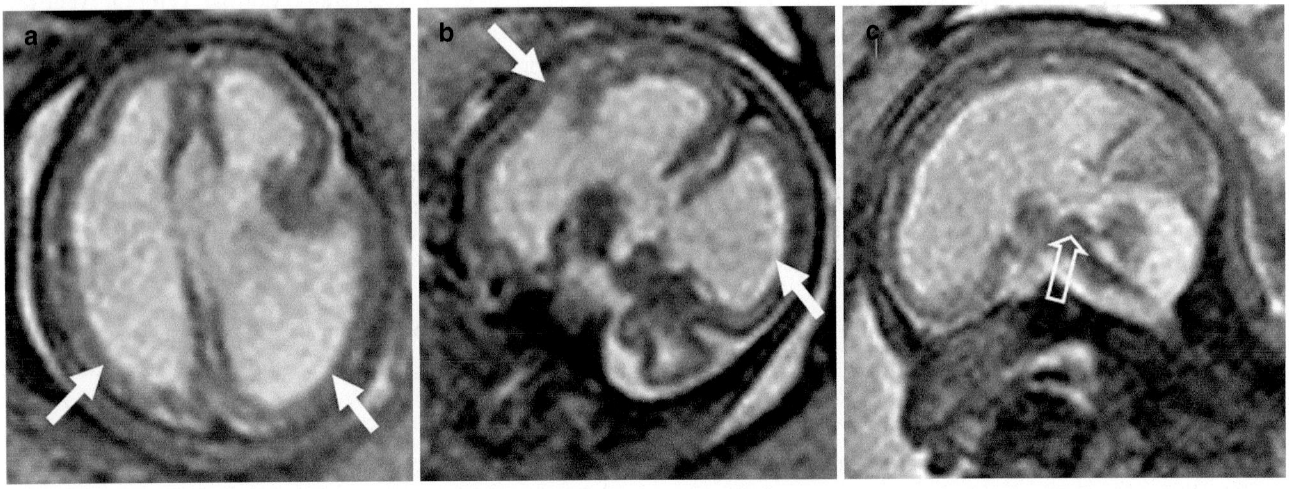

Fig. 7.2 Axial (**a**), coronal (**b**) and sagittal (**c**) T2W images showing ventriculomegaly (arrows) due to aqueduct stenosis (open arrows)

appear smooth in periventricular leukomalacia (Fig. 7.4a, b) Patchy thinning of cerebral cortex.

- Midline structures are normal.
- Posterior fossa structures are normal.
- *Intracranial hemorrhage*—There may be germinal matrix hemorrhage/Hemorrhage along the walls of the ventricles.

7.2 Aqueductal Stenosis

Can be primary or may be associated with malformations like Dandy–Walker, Chiari

- III and lateral ventricles are dilated. IV ventricle is normal (Fig. 7.2a–c).

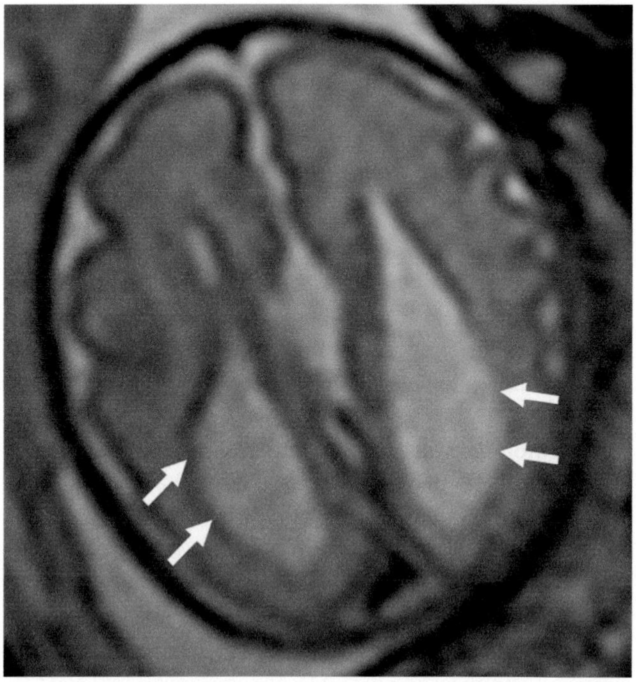

Fig. 7.3 Axial image shows moderate ventriculomegaly and colpocephaly due to agenesis of corpus callosum

- Head size may be increased.
- Thinning of corpus callosum may be seen.

Prognosis May be associated with developmental delay. May require ventricular shunting/endoscopic ventriculostomy postnatally.

7.3 Ventriculomegaly Due to Infection

Infection is an important cause of ventriculomegaly, especially CMV (Fig. 7.5) and toxoplasmosis [6].

Imaging features
- Irregular ventricular wall.
- Subependymal cystic lesions.
- Periventricular calcifications.
- Abnormal signal intensity in the white matter.
- Cortical abnormalities.
- Microcephaly.
- Fetal growth retardation.
- Hepatic calcifications.
- Placentomegaly.

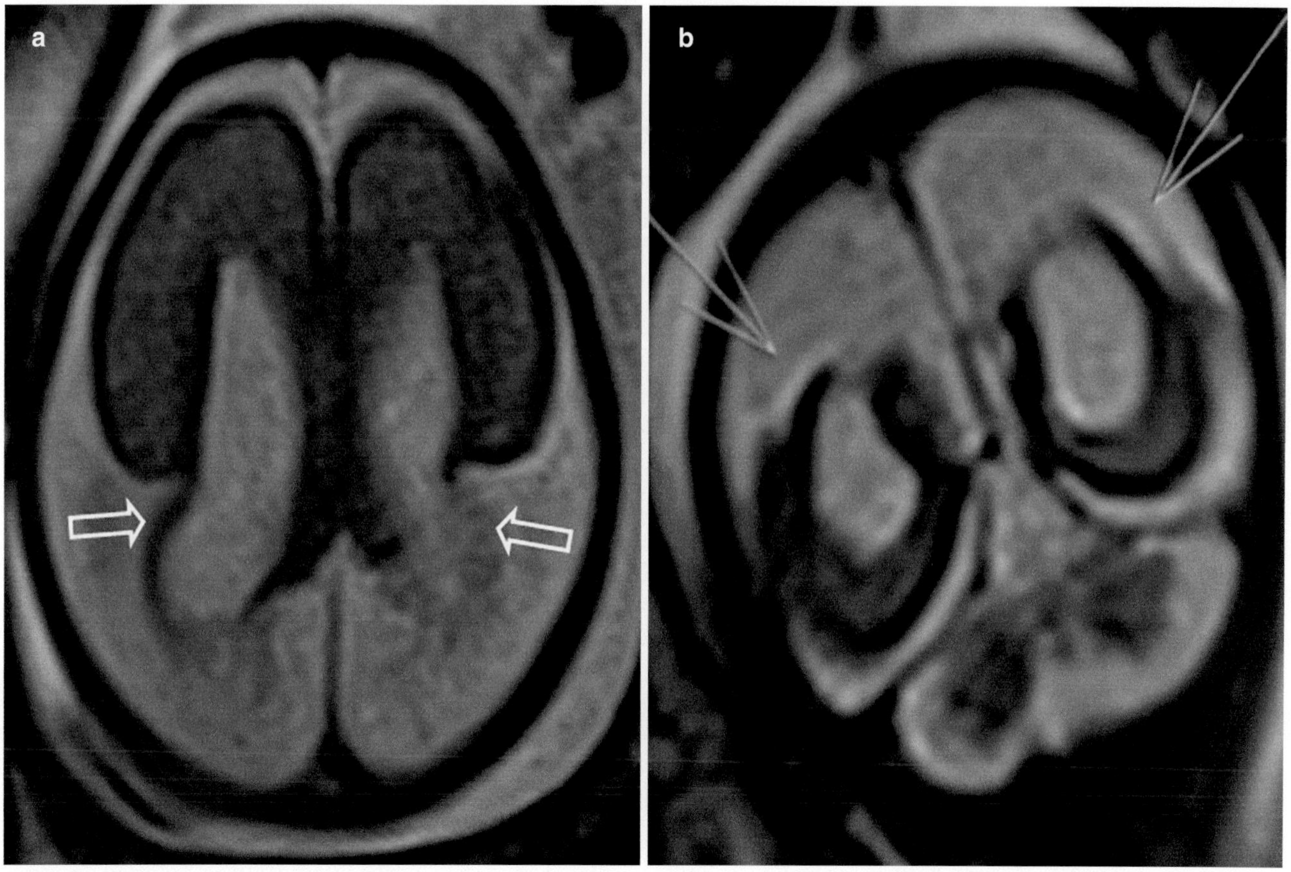

Fig. 7.4 Axial (**a**) and coronal T2W (**b**) images of a 26-week fetus show moderate ventriculomegaly (open arrows) due to encephalomalacic changes in bilateral parieto-occipital lobes (arrow)

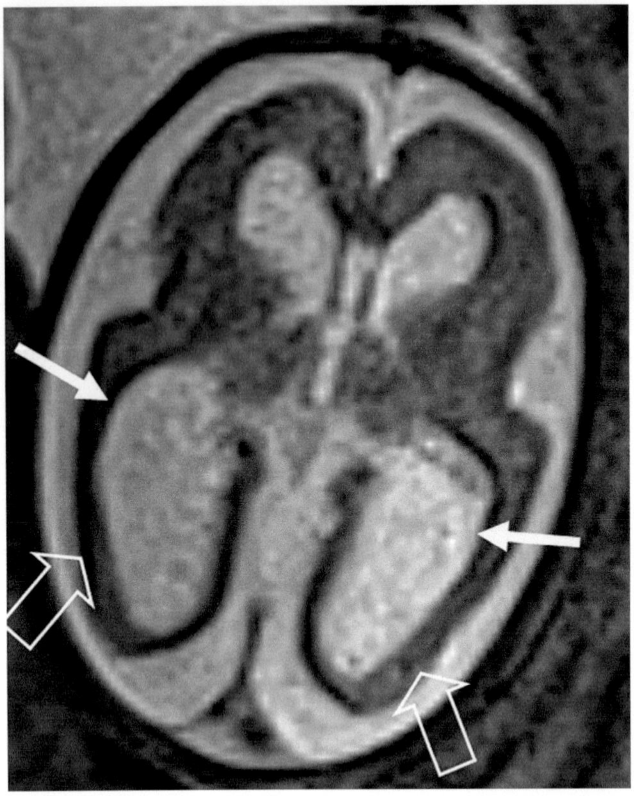

Fig. 7.5 Axial T2W image of a 31-week CMV infected fetus shows ventriculomegaly, diffuse cerebral cortical thinning with generalized reduced sulcation (arrowheads)

- Hepatosplenomegaly.
- Ascites.
- Meconium peritonitis.
- Polyhydramnios.

Differential diagnosis

- Hydranencephaly—The cranial cavity is fluid filled and cortex cannot be identified.
- Holoprosencephaly—there is varying degrees of cleavage abnormality of the structures of prosencephalon.
- Large choroid plexus cyst—Sometimes a large choroid plexus cyst may simulate ventriculomegaly. However, a close examination may show the wall of the cyst and also cause a focal dilatation within the affected ventricle.

7.4 Approach to Mild and Moderate Ventriculomegaly

In fetuses with mild or moderate ventriculomegaly (lateral ventricle measure 10–15 mm), further evaluation is indicated. Such evaluation is done to assess the presence of additional anomalies, genetic abnormalities, or congenital infection because isolated ventriculomegaly shows a good prognosis (Fig. 7.6a, b).

Presence of additional anomalies—are assessed by dedicated sonography and fetal MRI is complementary. Cortical malformations and migrational abnormalities are rarely detected by ultrasound but can be associated with ventriculomegaly and identified by MRI (Fig. 7.7a, b) [7]. MRI is able to demonstrate important additional, 1–14% anomalies as compared to USG in fetuses with mild or moderate ventriculomegaly [8–12].

Amniocentesis with chromosomal microarray analysis may be offered to the affected mothers.

Ventriculomegaly associated with congenital infection

For women who undergo amniocentesis, the amniotic fluid should also be tested by PCR for CMV and toxoplasmosis. Amniocentesis with PCR performed >6 weeks from maternal primary infection has a higher sensitivity and specificity between 97 and 100%.

For the women, where amniocentesis could not be performed—Serum testing for CMV/toxoplasmosis IgG and IgM may be offered. In women with a positive IgM result, IgG avidity testing is recommended; a low avidity IgG and positive IgM indicate infection within the previous 3 months [13, 14].

Follow-up ultrasound after initial detection of fetal ventriculomegaly is helpful to assess resolution, stability, or progression. If the ventriculomegaly resolves or remains stable, the prognosis is generally better [15]. Progression of ventricular dilatation can occur in upto 16% of cases. This can change the diagnosis and prognosis [16, 17].

Prognosis and counseling

Measurements that are around 10 mm are very likely to represent a normal variant, particularly when isolated. In *isolated mild ventriculomegaly*, the outcome is favorable, and the infant is likely to be normal. About 7–10% of fetuses with isolated mild ventriculomegaly can have other structural abnormalities on examination after birth.

The survival rate of infants with isolated mild ventriculomegaly is high (~93–98%) [15, 17, 18]. The likelihood of having normal neurodevelopmental outcomes is greater than 90% [15, 17, 18]. In isolated mild ventriculomegaly, neurodevelopmental delay can be present in 7.9% of children, which is similar to the background rate [18].

In isolated moderate ventriculomegaly (13–15 mm), the outcome is less favorable, and the infant having normal neurodevelopmental outcomes is reported to range from 75 to 93% [15, 19, 20]. The survival rate of infants with isolated moderate ventriculomegaly is reported to range from 80 to 97%. In cases of progressive ventriculomegaly, ventriculoperitoneal shunting may be needed postnatally.

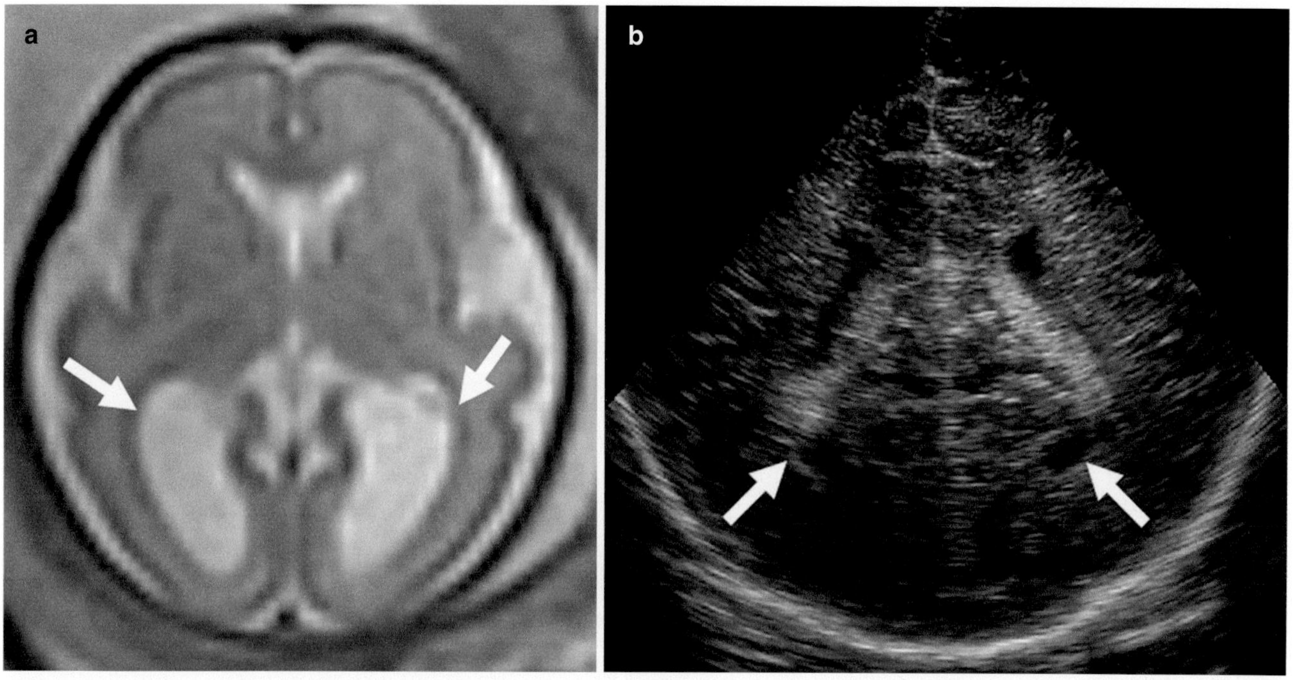

Fig. 7.6 Axial T2W (**a**) image of a 28-week fetus shows mild ventriculomegaly with ventricular diameter of 11 mm. Postnatal neurosonogram (**b**) shows resolution with ventricular diameter of 8 mm

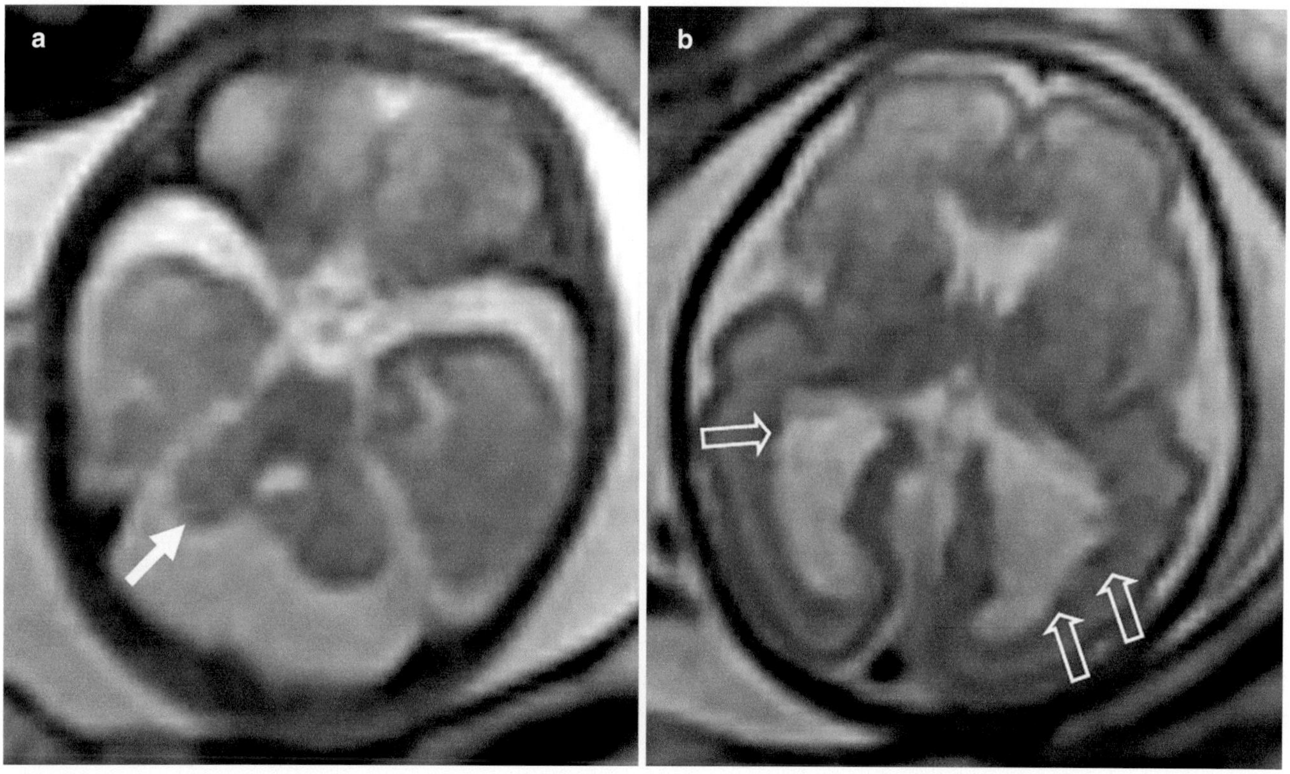

Fig. 7.7 Axial T2W (**a**, **b**) images show mild ventriculomegaly with ventricular diameter of 12 mm. There is associated periventricular nodular heterotopia (open arrows) and hypoplasia of right cerebellar hemisphere (arrow)

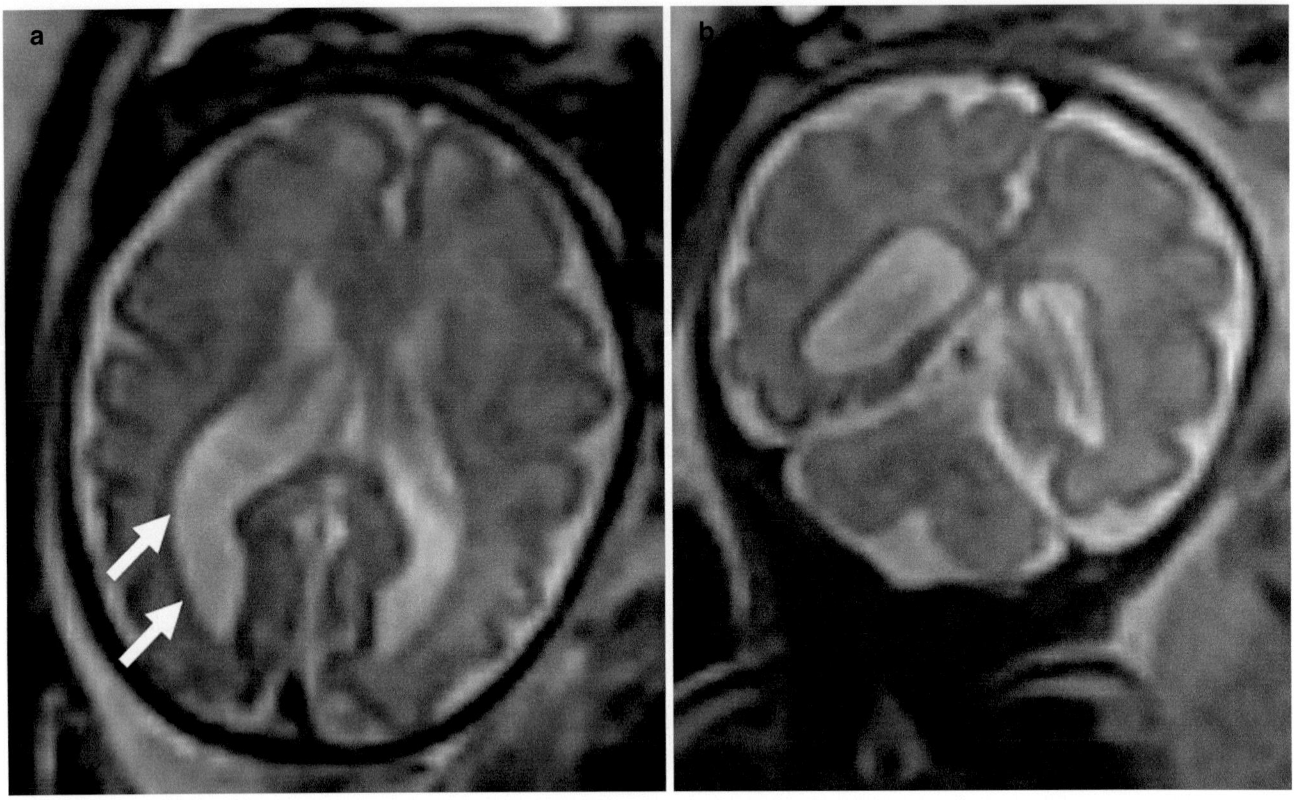

Fig. 7.8 Axial (**a**) and coronal T2W (**b**) images show unilateral ventriculomegaly involving the right lateral ventricle

7.5 Unilateral Ventriculomegaly

There is dilatation of only one lateral ventricle (10 mm or more). Many authors did not differentiate unilateral ventriculomegaly from bilateral ventriculomegaly [21, 22].

In a meta-analysis, infection (8.2%) was the commonest cause and there were no associated chromosomal abnormalities in the affected fetuses [23]. Unilateral mild ventriculomegaly could also represent a normal variant (Fig. 7.8a, b) [24, 25]. There was a progression of ventriculomegaly in 5% of fetuses but was less than that of bilateral ventriculomegaly. MR imaging diagnosed additional brain abnormalities in 5% of cases antenatally but was less than that of bilateral ventriculomegaly [26]. Postnatal follow-up MR imaging diagnosed additional brain abnormalities in 6% of cases. The prevalence of neurodevelopmental delay in isolated unilateral mild/moderate ventriculomegaly was 6% (similar to that in the general population).

Prognosis

Isolated mild/moderate unilateral ventriculomegaly carry a good prognosis.

Unilateral ventriculomegaly with associated anomalies and severe unilateral ventriculomegaly may have an unfavorable prognosis. Antenatal imaging by MRI and infection workup needs to be carried out to confirm that the unilateral ventriculomegaly is truly isolated.

References

1. Salomon LJ, Bernard JP, Ville Y. Reference ranges for fetal ventricular width: a non-normal approach. Ultrasound Obstet Gynecol. 2007;30(1):61–6. https://doi.org/10.1002/uog.4026.
2. Levine D, Barnes PD, Madsen JR, et al. Central nervous system abnormalities assessed with prenatal magnetic resonance imaging. Obstet Gynecol. 1999;94:1011–9.
3. Zimmerman RA, Bilaniuk LT. Magnetic resonance evaluation of fetal ventriculomegaly-associated congenital malformations and lesions. Semin Fetal Neonatal Med. 2005;10(5):429–43.
4. Ritner JA, Frates MC. Fetal CNS: a systematic approach. Radiol Clin N Am. 2014;52(6):1253–64. https://doi.org/10.1016/j.rcl.2014.07.012.
5. Morris JE, Rickard S, Paley MN, et-al. The value of in-utero magnetic resonance imaging in ultrasound diagnosed foetal isolated cerebral ventriculomegaly. Clin Radiol. 2007;62(2):140–4.
6. Malinger G, Lev D, Zahalka N, et-al. Fetal cytomegalovirus infection of the brain: the spectrum of sonographic findings. AJNR Am J Neuroradiol. 2003;24(1):28–32.
7. Rossi AC, Prefumo F. Additional value of fetal magnetic resonance imaging in the prenatal diagnosis of central nervous system anomalies: a systematic review of the literature. Ultrasound Obstet Gynecol. 2014;44:388–93.

8. Parazzini C, Righini A, Doneda C, et al. Is fetal magnetic resonance imaging indicated when ultrasound isolated mild ventriculomegaly is present in pregnancies with no risk factors? Prenat Diagn. 2012;32:752–7.
9. Salomon LJ, Ouahba J, Delezoide AL, et al. Third-trimester fetal MRI in isolated 10- to 12-mm ventriculomegaly: is it worth it? BJOG. 2006;113:942–7.
10. Griffiths PD, Bradburn M, Campbell MJ, et al. MERIDIAN Collaborative Group. Use of MRI in the diagnosis of fetal brain abnormalities in utero (MERIDIAN): a multicenter, prospective cohort study. Lancet. 2017;389:538–46.
11. Whitby EH, Paley MN, Sprigg A, et al. Comparison of ultrasound and magnetic resonance imaging in 100 singleton pregnancies with suspected brain abnormalities. BJOG. 2004;111:784–92.
12. Benacerraf BR, Shipp TD, Bromley B, Levine D. What does magnetic resonance imaging add to the prenatal sonographic diagnosis of ventriculomegaly? J Ultrasound Med. 2007;26:1513–22.
13. Hughes BL, Gyamfi BC. Society for Maternal-Fetal Medicine (SMFM), diagnosis and antenatal management of congenital cytomegalovirus infection. Am J Obstet Gynecol. 2016;214:B5–11. 30.
14. American College of Obstetricians and Gynecologists. Cytomegalovirus, parvovirus B19, varicella zoster, and toxoplasmosis in pregnancy. Practice bulletin no. 151. Obstet Gynecol. 2015;125:1510–25.
15. Gaglioti P, Oberto M, Todros T. The significance of fetal ventriculomegaly: etiology, short- and long-term outcomes. Prenat Diagn. 2009;29:381–8.
16. Fox NS, Monteagudo A, Kuller JA, Craigo S, Norton ME. Mild fetal ventriculomegaly: diagnosis, evaluation, and management. Am J Obstet Gynecol. 2018;219(1):B2–9.
17. Melchiorre K, Bhide A, Gika AD, Pilu G, Papageorghiou AT. Counseling in isolated mild fetal ventriculomegaly. Ultrasound Obstet Gynecol. 2009;34:212–24.
18. Pagani G, Thilaganathan B, Prefumo F. Neurodevelopmental outcome in isolated mild fetal ventriculomegaly: systematic review and metaanalysis. Ultrasound Obstet Gynecol. 2014;44:25.
19. Sethna F, Tennant PW, Rankin J, Robson C, S. Prevalence, natural history, and clinical outcome of mild to moderate ventriculomegaly. Obstet Gynecol. 2011;117:867–76.
20. Beeghly M, Ware J, Soul J, et al. Neurodevelopmental outcome of fetuses referred for ventriculomegaly. Ultrasound Obstet Gynecol. 2010;35:405–16.
21. Tugcu AU, Gulumser C, Ecevit A, Abbasoglu A, Uysal NS, Kupana ES, Yanik FF, Tarcan A. Prenatal evaluation and postnatal early outcomes of fetal ventriculomegaly. Eur J Paediatr Neurol. 2014;18:736–40.
22. Hidaka N, Ishii K, Kanazawa R, Miyagi A, Irie A, Hayashi S, Mitsuda N. Perinatal characteristics of fetuses with borderline ventriculomegaly detected by routine ultrasonographic screening of low-risk populations. J Obstet Gynaecol Res. 2014;40:1030–6.
23. Scala C, Familiari A, Pinas A, Papageorghiou AT, Bhide A, Thilaganathan B, Khalil A. Perinatal and long-term outcomes in fetuses diagnosed with isolated unilateral ventriculomegaly: systematic review and meta-analysis. Ultrasound Obstet Gynecol. 2017;49:450–9.
24. Vergani P, Locatelli A, Strobelt N, Cavallone M, Ceruti P, Paterlini G, Ghidini A. Clinical outcome of mild fetal ventriculomegaly. Am J Obstet Gynecol. 1998;178:218–22.
25. Laskin MD, Kingdom J, Toi A, Chitayat D, Ohlsson A. Perinatal and neurodevelopmental outcome with isolated fetal ventriculomegaly: a systematic review. J Matern Fetal Neonatal Med. 2005;18:289–98.
26. Devaseelan P, Cardwell C, Bell B, Ong S. Prognosis of isolated mild to moderate fetal cerebral ventriculomegaly: a systematic review. J Perinat Med. 2010;38:401–9.

Posterior Fossa Anomalies

8

8.1 Embryology

The fetal posterior fossa comprises of the following structures: the brainstem (pons and bulb), cerebellum (cerebellar hemispheres and vermis), cerebral peduncles, cisterna magna, fourth ventricle, and the tentorium. The structures of the posterior fossa develop from the rhombencephalon (hindbrain), which differentiates into the myelencephalon and metencephalon.

The cerebellum, pons, and upper part of the IV ventricle develop from the metencephalon. The bulb and lower part of the IV ventricle develop from the myelencephalon. In the sixth week of gestation, the pontine flexure develops, with further formation of the anterior and posterior membranous areas. The cerebellar vermis develops from the anterior membranous area. The cisterna magna and a recess known as Blake's pouch develop from the posterior membranous area. Blake's pouch disappears by weeks 16–18 with the fenestration of the IV ventricle (formation of the foramen-Luschka and Magendie) and its closure [1–3]. However, communication between the IV ventricle and the cisterna magna can be present up to 20 weeks of gestation. Cerebellar foliations and verman fissures form from the fifth month of gestation, the primary fissure of the vermis being identified only after 22 week of gestation [4].

Posterior fossa abnormalities can occur due to malformations and disruptions. Malformations are morphological abnormalities resulting from an intrinsically abnormal developmental process. Disruptions are abnormalities that occur due to extraneous interference in an originally normal developmental process [5].

8.2 The MR Imaging Checklist While Examining the Posterior Fossa [6, 7]

- *AP length of cisterna magna* on axial images (Normal <10 mm).
- *Insertion angle of the tentorium*—The tentorium inserts at the level of the torcula and is perpendicular to the occiput.
- *Transcerebellar diameter (TCD)*—It is the widest dimension of cerebellum measured on axial or coronal image (Fig. 8.1a). During 19–25 weeks, the gestational age is equivalent to the TCD expressed in mm.
- *Vermian craniocaudal, anteroposterior dimensions and morphology*—Vermian dimensions on a midsagittal image (Fig. 8.1b) are to be correlated with a normative data. The primary fissure and fastigial point of the vermis (Fig. 8.2) can be demonstrated by 18 weeks on MRI but there can be a physiologic delay up to 24 weeks. An approximately equal length of vermian tissue is normally seen above (47%) and below (53%) the fastigium-declive line. This shows a linear growth with increasing gestation. With increasing gestational age, the vermian foliation also increases [6].
- *Brainstem-vermian angle (BV)*—It is the angle between a line along the posterior surface of the brainstem and a line along the anterior surface of vermis (Fig. 8.1c). Angles between 4° and 17° can be normal, Blake's pouch cyst and vermian hypoplasia are associated with angles of 19–26° and 24–40°, respectively. Dandy–Walker malformation shows an angle of 45–112° [8, 9].
- The normal fourth ventricle shows a triangular shape in the sagittal plane (Fig. 8.2).

Classification of posterior fossa malformations [4]
Cystic Malformations

- Mega cisterna magna
- Blake's pouch cyst
- Vermian hypoplasia
- Dandy–Walker malformation
- Arachnoid cyst

R. Rajeswaran, *MR Imaging of the Fetus*, https://doi.org/10.1007/978-981-16-9209-3_8

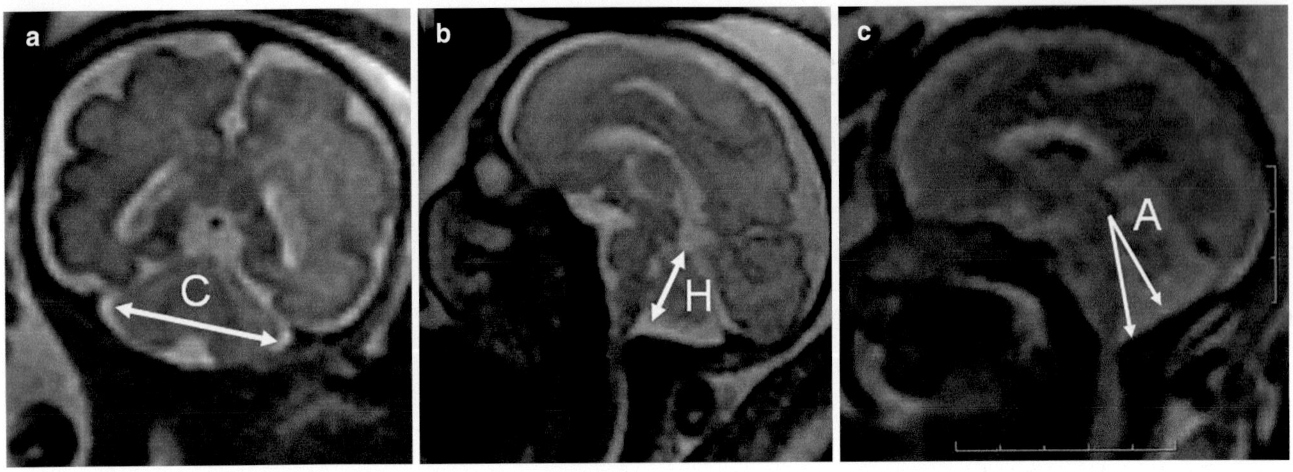

Fig. 8.1 Coronal (**a**) and sagittal (**b**) T2W Image of a normal 31-week fetal brain. The method of measuring the trans-cerebellar diameter (C) and vermian height (H) are shown. Sagittal (**c**) T2W Image of a 21-week fetal brain with blake pouch cyst—the method of measuring the Brainstem Vermian angle (A) is shown

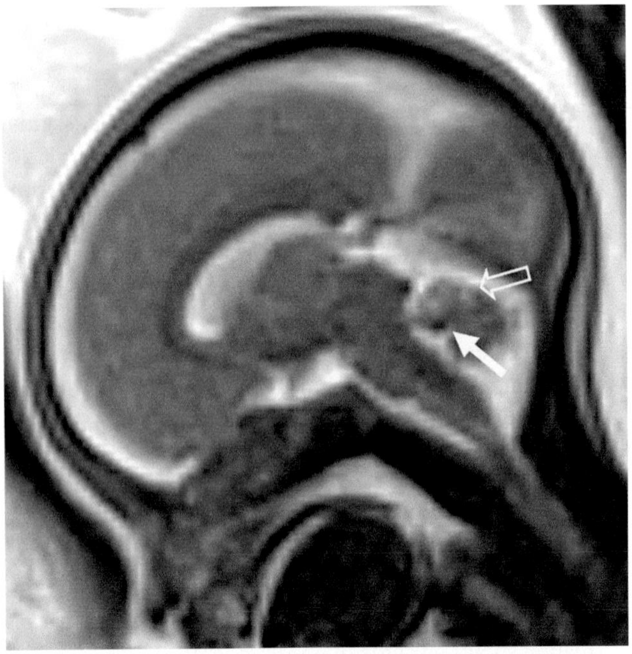

Fig. 8.2 Sagittal T2W Image of a normal 24-week fetus showing normal triangular-shaped IV ventricle, fastigial point (arrow) and primary fissure (open arrow)

Hypoplasia

- Global Cerebellar hypoplasia
- Unilateral Cerebellar hypoplasia
- Ponto-cerebellar hypoplasia
- Vermian agenesis

Dysgenesis

- Rhombencepahlosynapsis
- Joubert syndrome and related disorders
- Kinked/z-shaped brainstem
- Lhermitte Duclos disease
- Focal cortical dysplasia
- Pontine tegmental cap dysplasia

Miscellaneous

Neural tube defects like Chiari malformations, Encephalocele.

8.3 Cystic Malformations

8.3.1 Mega Cisterna Magna

Definition

The cisterna magna measures greater than 10 mm in antero-posterior dimension. It is usually an incidental finding and shows association with other anomalies in less than 20% of cases. Associated anomalies commonly seen are ventriculomegaly and those of trisomy 18.

Imaging features

- Increased CSF space (AP $\geq$ 10 mm) posterior to the cerebellum (Figs. 8.3b and 8.4).
- The cerebellar dimensions are within the normal range for the gestational age.
- The vermis is seen covering the IV ventricle on sagittal sections with a normal brain stem vermian angle.
- The configuration of the IV ventricle, cerebellar hemispheres, its foliation are normal and appropriate for the gestational age.
- There may be scalloping of the inner table of the occipital bone due to CSF pulsations.

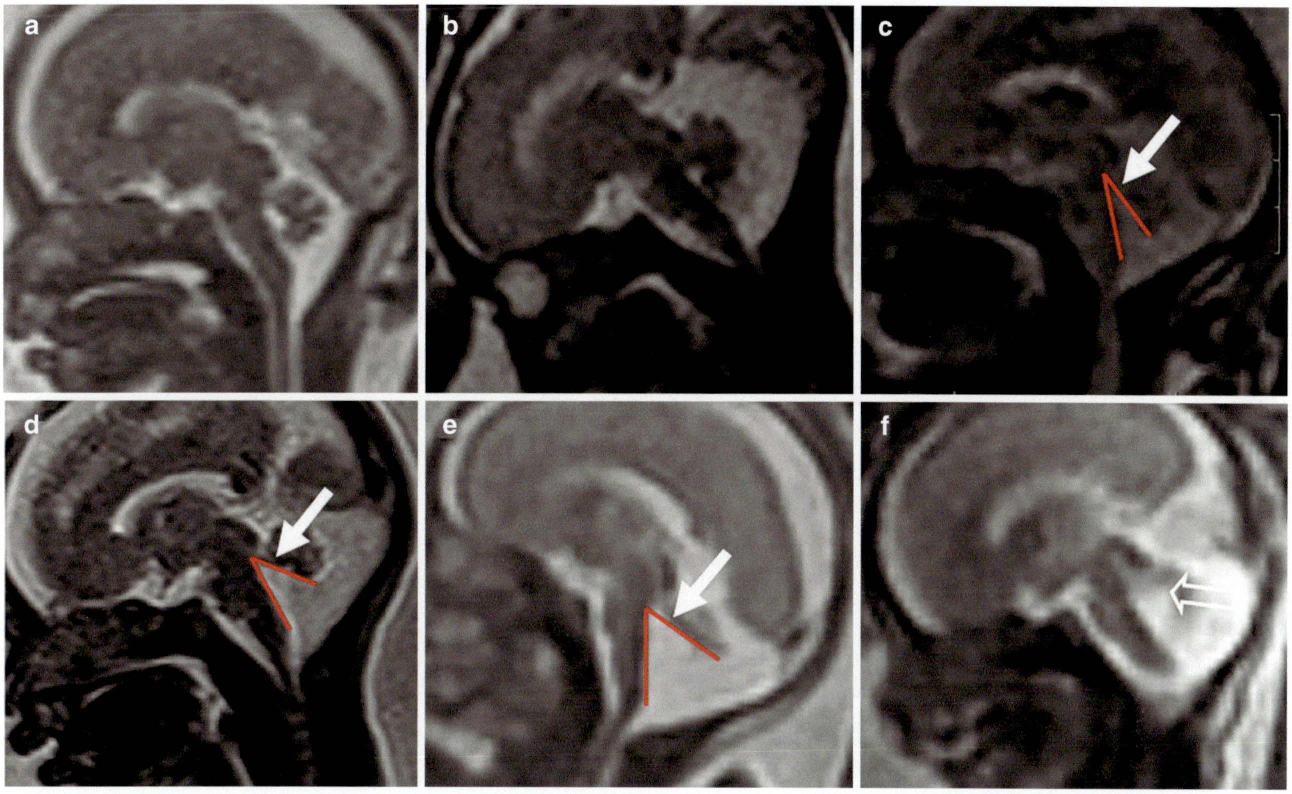

Fig. 8.3 Diagrammatic representation of posterior fossa anomalies with increased retrocerebellar space. (**a**) Normal (**b**) Mega cistern magna—the cerebellum and vermis are adequately developed. (**c**) Blake pouch cyst—the brainstem vermian angle is mildly increased (arrows), the cerebellum and vermis are adequately developed. (**d**) Vermian hypoplasia—the brainstem vermian angle is moderately increased (arrows), the vermis is hypoplastic. (**e**) Dandy–Walker malformation—the brainstem vermian angle is severely increased (arrows), the cerebellum and vermis are poorly developed (**f**) Vermian agenesis—the fastigial point is blunted (open arrows)

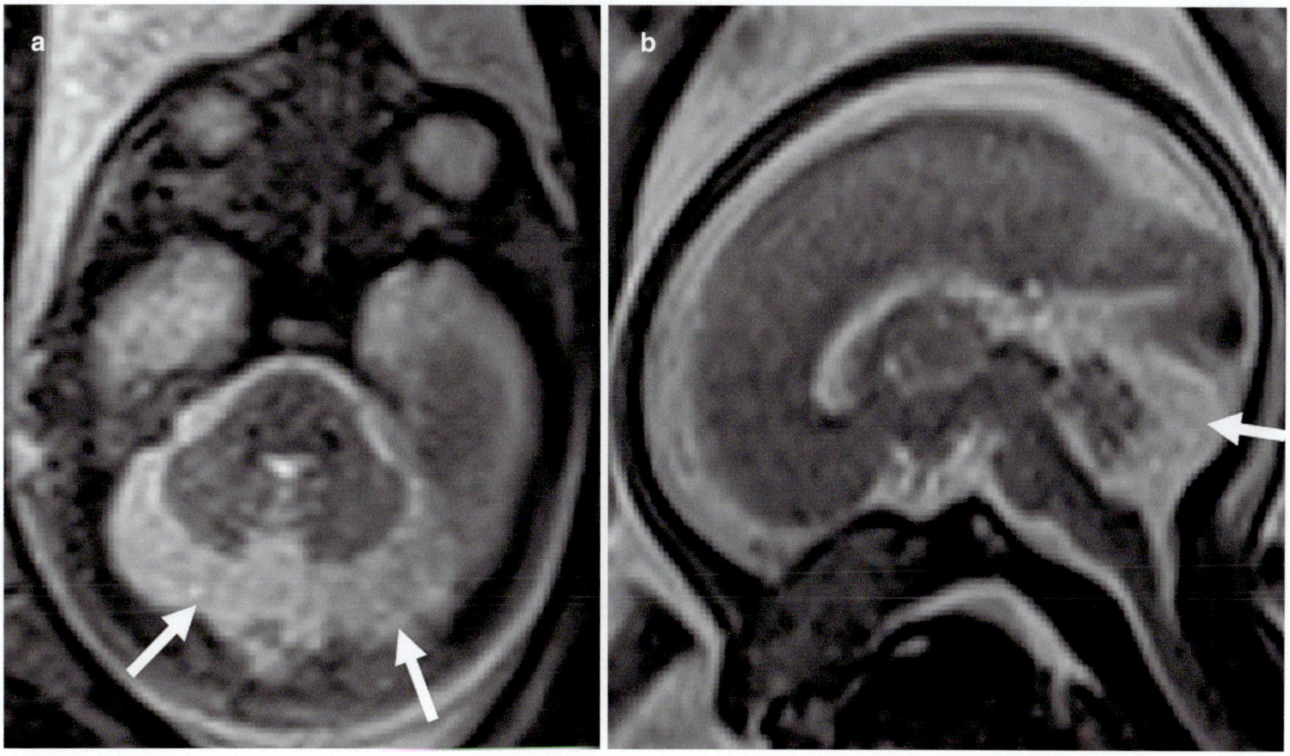

Fig. 8.4 Axial (**a**), sagittal (**b**) T2W images of a 26-week fetus showing a dilated cisterna magna (AP Diameter of 11 mm) (arrows), with normal cerebellar dimensions suggesting mega cisterna magna

Differential diagnosis

- Cerebellar hypoplasia—The cerebellar dimensions are reduced.
- Blake's pouch cyst—The brain stem vermian angle is increased, as the vermis is rotated.
- Arachnoid cyst—there may be mass effect on the cerebellar hemispheres.
- Vermian hypoplasia—The brain stem vermian angle is increased with decreased dimension of vermis.
- Dandy–Walker malformation—The brain stem vermian angle is increased with grossly decreased dimension of vermis. The IV ventricle is enlarged, cystic and communicates with cisterna magna.

Prognosis Good prognosis if it is an isolated finding [10].

8.3.2 Blake's Pouch Cyst (BPC)

Definition

There is delayed/nonperforation of foramen of Magendie, leading to nonregression of BPC. This leads to posterior ballooning of the superior medullary velum into cisterna magna [9, 11, 12].

Imaging features

- CSF-filled cyst seen inferior to the vermis and communicates with the fourth ventricle. The cisterna magna may appear prominent.
- The vermis is rotated and shows normal dimension. MRI is very useful to delineate the normal-appearing vermis and cerebellar hemispheres (Figs. 8.3c and 8.5), though there may be mass effect.
- The BVA is 15°–30°.
- Mostly it resolves spontaneously and very rarely it is associated with hydrocephalus [9, 11].

Differential diagnosis

- Vermian hypoplasia
- Mega cisterna magna
- Arachnoid cyst
- Dandy–Walker malformation

Prognosis

Most of them resolve spontaneously.

Good prognosis in the majority of cases if isolated [13].

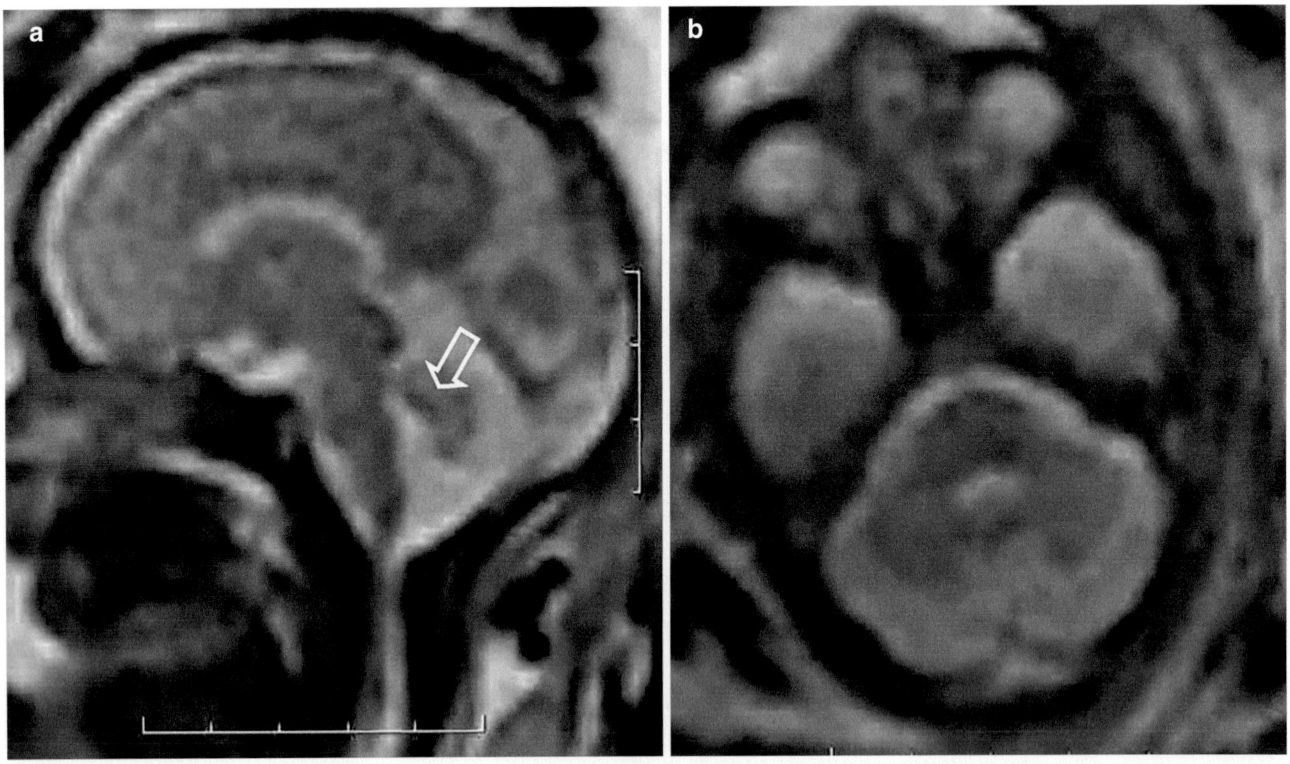

Fig. 8.5 Sagittal (**a**) and axial (**b**) T2W images of a 24-week fetus showing increased brain stem vermian angle of 25° (open arrow), with otherwise normal cerebellar dimensions suggesting persistent blake pouch cyst. However, it regressed on follow-up studies

8.3.3 Vermian Hypoplasia

Definition and Pathology
The cerebellar vermian dimensions are reduced due to faulty development of the superior part of anterior area membranacea in rhombencephalic roof. Mostly it occurs sporadically and sometimes (30% of cases) it is seen with abnormal karyotype.

Imaging features
- Hypoplasia is imaged as "absence of inferior part of vermis." There is communication of the IV ventricle with the cisterna magna in the inferior aspect (Figs. 8.3d and 8.6a, b) [14, 15].
- MRI is useful to identify a small vermis with or without abnormal foliation [16].
- Can be picked up as reduced craniocaudal dimension of vermis on biometry.
- The BVA is 30°–45° (Fig. 8.6c).
- Evaluation of the vermis in all the three planes is important. The sagittal plane can overestimate the amount of vermian tissue due to overlap from the cerebellum.
- Posterior fossa is normal-sized and there is normal insertion of the tentorium.

Differential diagnosis Blake's pouch cyst, Dandy–Walker malformation.

Prognosis Favorable neurologic outcome is seen in up to 77% of patients if it is an isolated anomaly [17]. Delayed motor, mental development, and ataxia can occur in some patients.

8.3.4 Dandy–Walker Malformation

Definition and pathology
It is due to the failure of fenestration fourth ventricle foraminal outlets [15]. There is cystic dilatation of IV ventricle with enlarged posterior fossa and tentorial elevation. There is associated partial or complete agenesis of the cerebellar vermis.

Majority present sporadically. Sometimes they are associated with syndromes (Meckel–Gruber, PHACES syndrome, Walker–Warburg) and chromosomal abnormalities (Trisomy 9, 13, 18, Turner syndrome).

Imaging features
- Sagittal MRI is most important.
- Dilated IV ventricle and is seen continuous with the posterior fossa cyst. There is lack of normal fastigial point.
- Absent or small vermis that is rotated upwards (Figs. 8.3e and 8.7a, c).
- Small cerebellar hemispheres (Fig. 8.7a).
- Superiorly displaced tentorium.
- Increased BVA, >45°.
- Hydrocephalus may be present (Fig. 8.7b).
- Fetal MR is also useful to detect associated CNS anomalies and to evaluate vermis, brainstem.
- Brainstem—may be kinked, thinned, or Z-shaped and may carry worse prognosis.

Differential diagnosis
- Blake Pouch Cyst
- Vermian hypoplasia
- Mega cisterna magna
- Arachnoid cyst

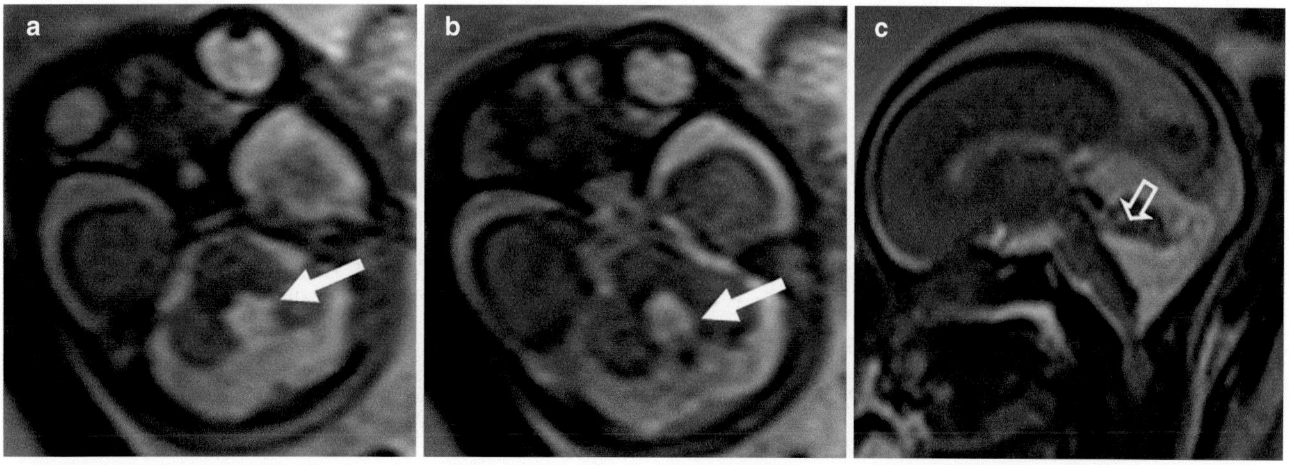

Fig. 8.6 Axial (**a**, **b**), sagittal (**c**) T2W images of a 24-week fetus show prominent IV ventricle (arrows), increased brainstem vermian angle of 40° (open arrows), with reduced cerebellar vermian dimensions suggesting vermian hypoplasia

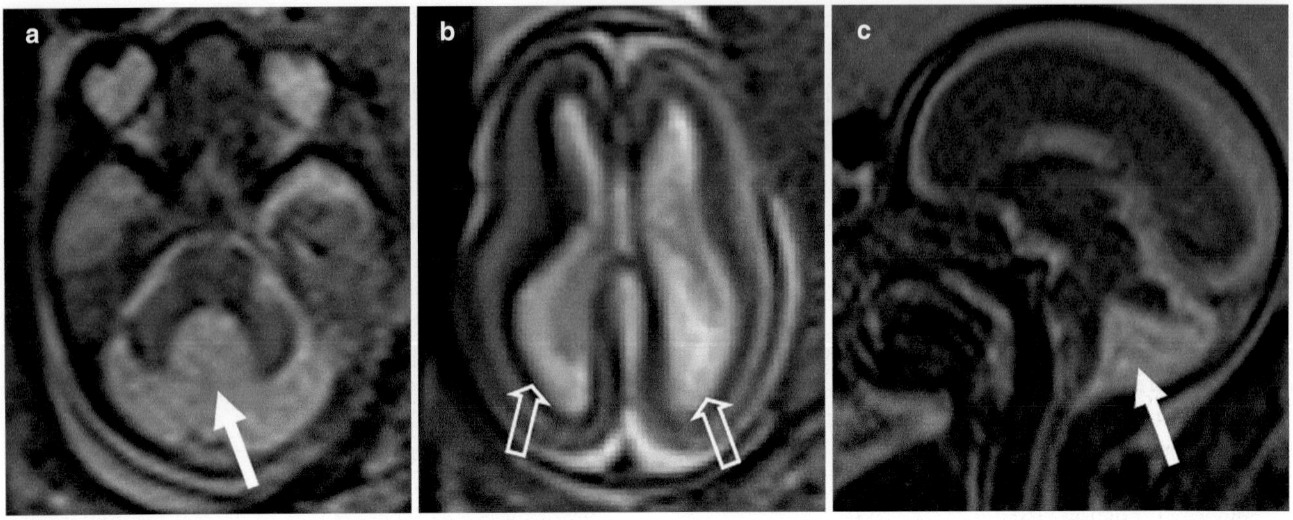

Fig. 8.7 Axial (**a**, **b**), sagittal (**c**) T2W images of a 20-week fetus show a dilated fourth ventricle, which is seen to be continuous with a cystic area posterior to cerebellum. Bilateral cerebellar hemispheres appear separated and ventriculomegaly (open arrows) is visualized. The brainstem vermian angle measures 65° suggesting Dandy–Walker malformation

Prognosis Very likely to have delayed motor/Intellectual development, ataxia, hypotonia, seizures. There is about 40% mortality during infancy and early childhood.

Intelligence is normal in 35% of cases who survive [13].

8.3.5 Posterior Fossa Arachnoid Cyst

- Retrocerebellar extra-axial cystic lesion and not communicating with the fourth ventricle (Fig. 8.8a, b).
- Mass effect may be present on the cerebellum/posterior fossa structures (Fig. 8.8a, b).
- The dimensions of the cerebellum are within normal limits.
- BVA is not increased.

Differential diagnosis
- Blake Pouch Cyst
- Vermian hypoplasia
- Mega cisterna magna

Prognosis Carries a good prognosis.

8.4 Hypoplasia

8.4.1 Global Cerebellar Hypoplasia

Definition and pathology
The cerebellar hemispheres and vermis appear small for the gestational age and show preserved morphology. It is seen sporadically or in association with some chromosomal (Trisomies 9, 13, 18) and complex syndromes (Goldenhar, Moebius). It can result from both disruptions and malformations.

Imaging features
The transverse cerebellar diameter and vermian dimensions are smaller than expected for gestational age and there is prominent subarachnoid spaces (Fig. 8.9a, b). It is important to rule out ponto-cerebellar hypoplasia/associated brain stem abnormalities as they carry worse prognosis.

Differential diagnosis
Mega cisterna magna—The cerebellar dimensions are within the normal range and carries a good prognosis.

8.4.2 Unilateral Cerebellar Hypoplasia

Definition and pathology
One of the cerebellar hemispheres appears smaller. It is usually secondary to disruptions such as infections, cerebellar hemorrhage, other insults. Can sometimes occur with syndromes (e.g., PHACES).

Imaging features
There is asymmetry of the cerebellar hemispheres with one hemisphere appearing smaller than the other (Fig. 8.10a, b). Morphological abnormalities may be identified in the involved hemisphere with or without associated involvement of the adjacent vermis. Gradient echo images may be useful to demonstrate products of hemorrhage.

Prognosis
The prognosis is good if the vermis is not involved and the rest of the brain is normal.

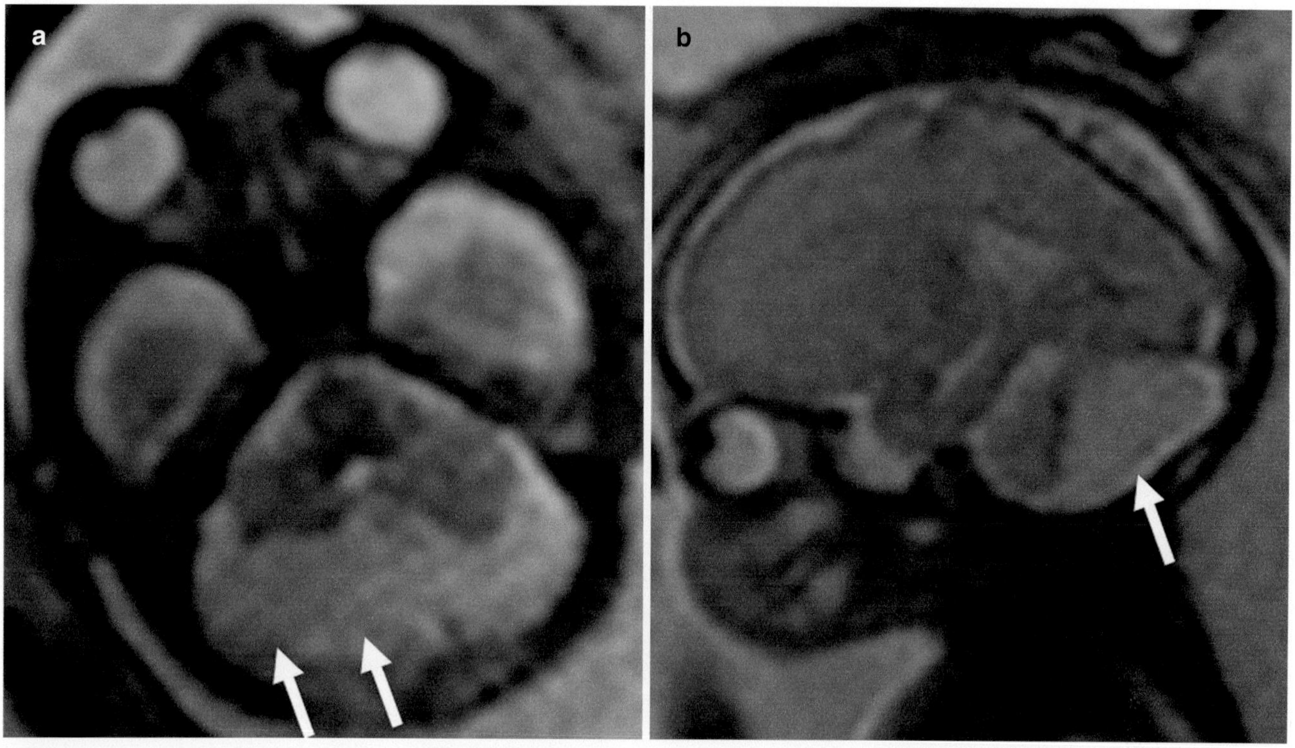

Fig. 8.8 Axial (**a**) sagittal (**b**) T2W images of a 20-week fetus show a retrocerebellar arachnoid cyst (arrow) causing mass effect on the vermis and right cerebellar hemisphere

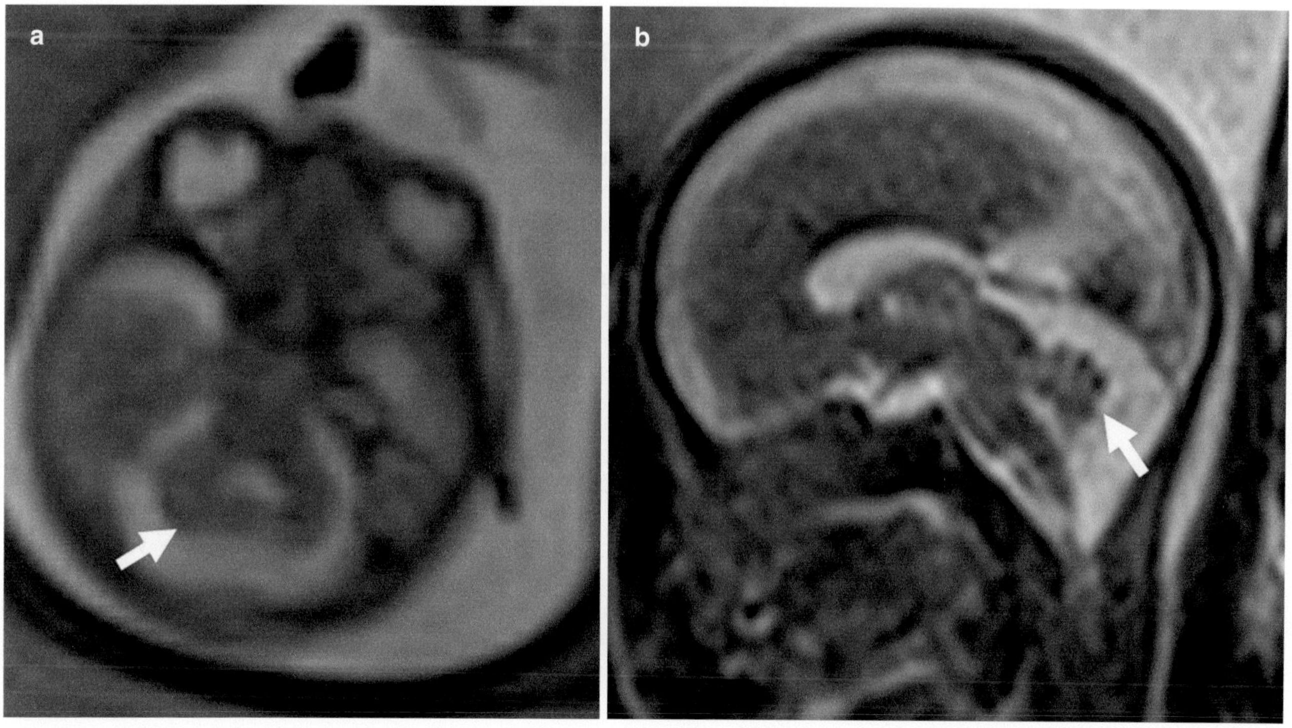

Fig. 8.9 Axial (**a**) and sagittal (**b**) T2W images of a 22-week fetus show reduced cerebellar diameter (18 mm) and vermian height (7.5 mm) suggesting cerebellar hypoplasia

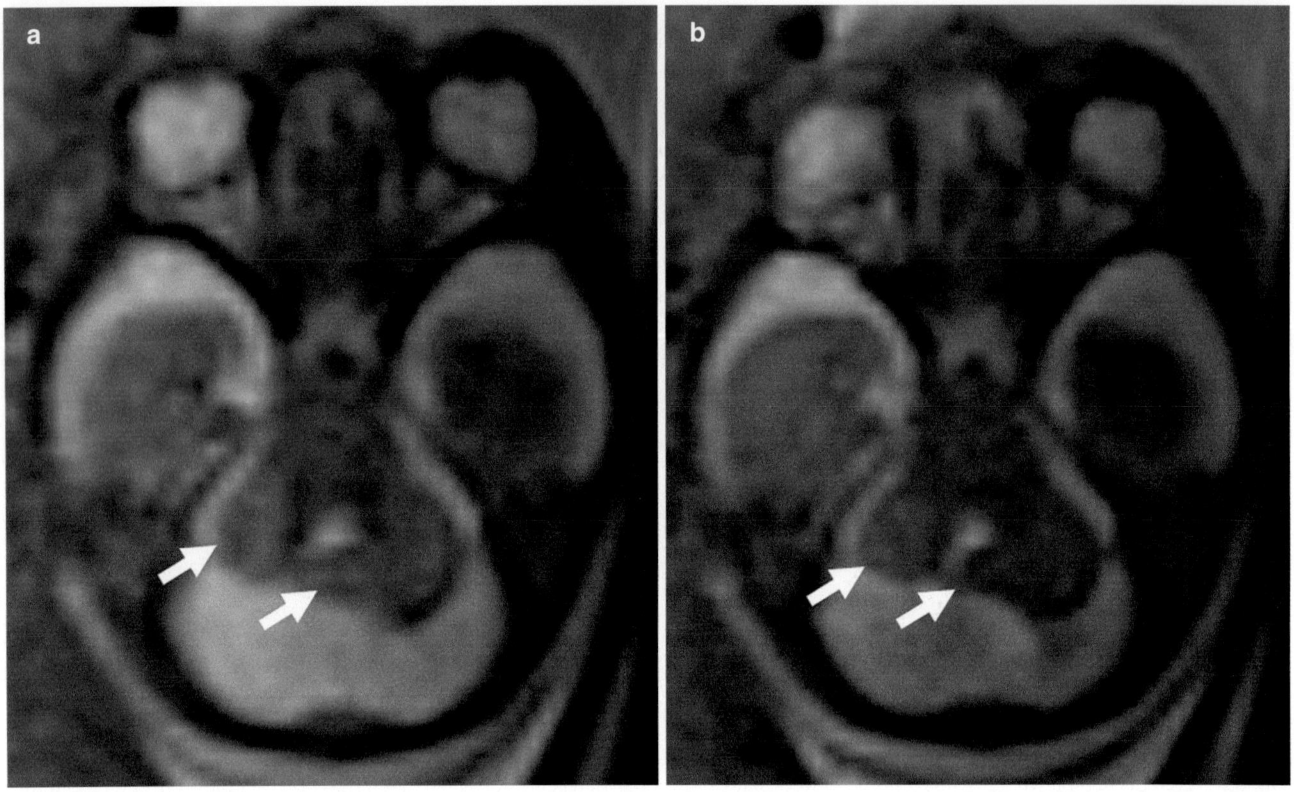

Fig. 8.10 Axial (**a**, **b**) T2W images of a 21-week fetus shows a smaller right cerebellar hemisphere and the adjacent vermis—unilateral hypoplasia of the right cerebellar hemisphere

8.4.3 Ponto-Cerebellar Hypoplasia

Definition and pathology
There is hypoplasia of the cerebellum and pons and the majority of cases are due to mutations in tRNA splicing endonuclease. Atrophy of supratentorial structures can present postnatally. The transmission is autosomal recessive.

Imaging features
The ventral pontine bulge is small or absent. The cerebellum is also small (Fig. 8.11a, b) [4].

Prognosis
It is a progressive condition and shows poor outcome. Genetic counseling is recommended for the parents as there is a 25% recurrence risk of having the next child being affected.

Differential diagnosis
Global cerebellar hypoplasia
Congenital muscular dystrophy

Prognosis
The affected child can have delayed motor/intellectual development with associated hypotonia, ataxia, tremor, Cognitive and speech impairment.

8.4.4 Vermian Agenesis

Definition and pathology
The vermis is absent. It may be isolated or may be an associated finding in conditions like Dandy–Walker malformation, Joubert syndrome, and rhombencephalosynapsis.

Imaging features
- The vermis is absent. The cerebellar hemispheres may oppose each other and produce a pseudo appearance of vermis. However, an abnormal cleft between the opposing cerebellar hemispheres is a clue to diagnosis (Figs. 8.3f and 8.12a, b).
- The fastigial point, primary fissure are not visualized in the midsagittal section (Fig. 8.12c).
- There is an altered configuration of the IV ventricle (Fig. 8.12c).

Prognosis Very likely to have delayed motor/Intellectual development, ataxia.

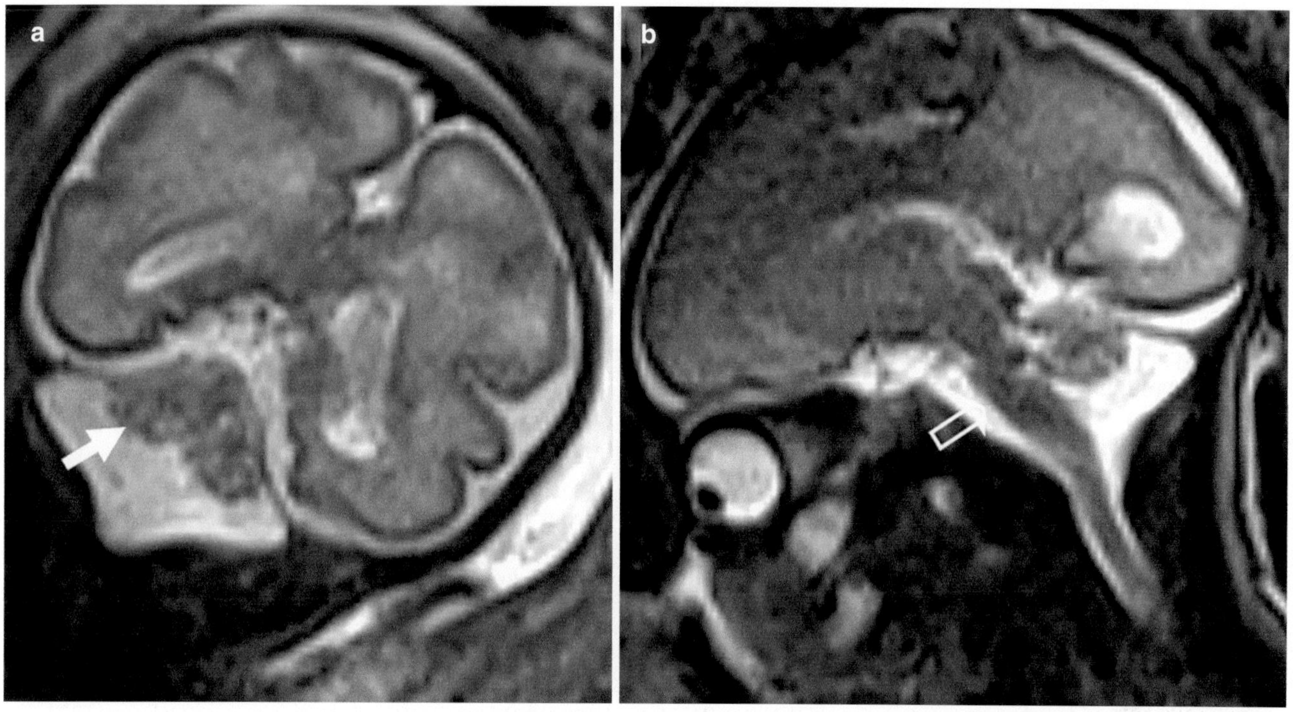

Fig. 8.11 Coronal (**a**) T2W image of a 31-week fetus shows reduced cerebellar diameter (arrow). Sagittal image (**b**) shows flattening of the ventral surface of pons (open arrow) suggesting ponto-cerebellar hypoplasia

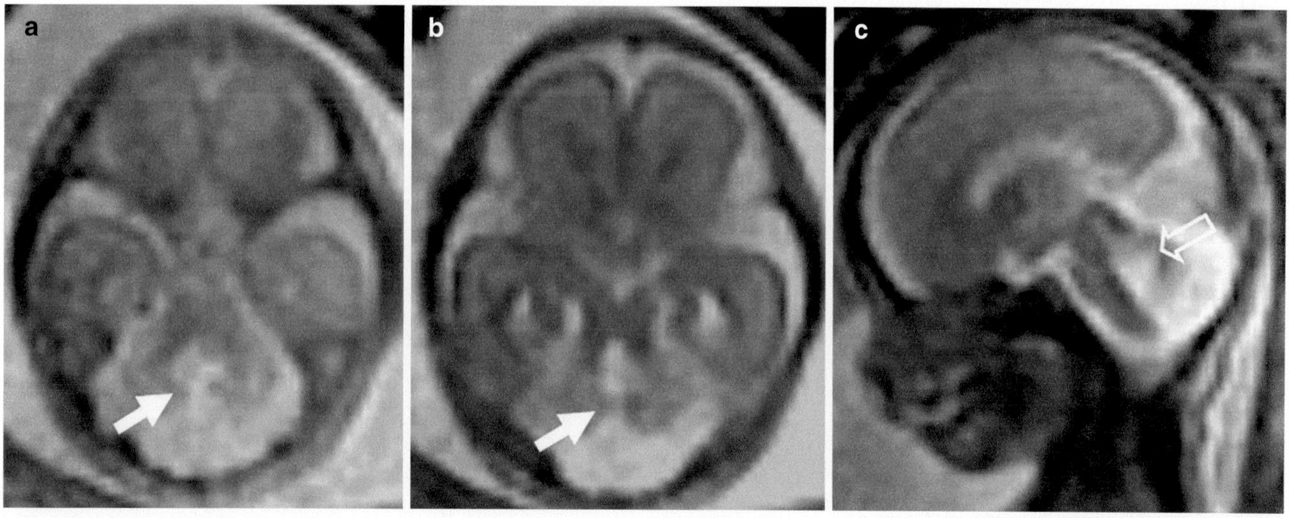

Fig. 8.12 Axial (**a**, **b**) T2W images of a 21-week fetus shows absence of vermis with a cleft separating the cerebellar hemispheres (arrows). Sagittal (**c**) image shows absence of fastigial point (open arrows)—vermian agenesis

8.5 Dysgenesis

8.5.1 Rhombencephalosynapsis

Definition and pathology

- Rare anomaly.
- There is fusion of the cerebellar hemispheres with associated vermian agenesis.
- It is due to a failure vermian differentiation occurring very early in gestation at 5–6 weeks of gestational age [18].
- Can occur in diabetic mothers or due to genetic causes or as a part of multiple anomalies.

Imaging features

- The cerebellar hemispheres appear fused with associated vermian agenesis. The folia are seen traversing horizontally (Fig. 8.13a).
- Reduced trans cerebellar diameter and cerebellar volume.
- The midline sagittal section of cerebellum shows absent fastigial point and primary vermian fissure (Fig. 8.13b).
- Can be associated with hydrocephalus, septal and callosal abnormalities, holoprosencephaly [19–21].

Prognosis

Very likely to have delayed motor/Intellectual development, ataxia, hypotonia, seizures and psychiatry disorders [22]. The prognosis is worse if there is associated ventriculomegaly.

8.5.2 Joubert Syndrome and Molar Tooth Sign Related Disorders

Definition and pathology

This group of autosomal recessive genetic disorders of which Joubert syndrome is the classical example is characterized by impaired ciliary function. There are six subtypes and all of them show molar tooth sign on imaging. Multiple organs like liver, kidneys may also be affected.

Imaging features

- There is lack of decussation of corticospinal tracts, superior cerebellar peduncles, and central pontine tracts.
- Hypoplastic or absent vermis (Fig. 8.14a).
- Axial images at the midbrain level show "molar tooth" appearance due to thickened superior cerebellar peduncles with deep interpeduncular fossa (Fig. 8.14b, c).
- Deformed fourth ventricle giving a bat wing appearance.
- Sometimes associated anomalies like ventriculomegaly, encephalocele, callosal dysgenesis, are present [23].
- Findings are better demonstrated on MRI, though they can be suspected on sonography.

Differential diagnosis

Isolated vermian agenesis.

Dandy–Walker malformation.

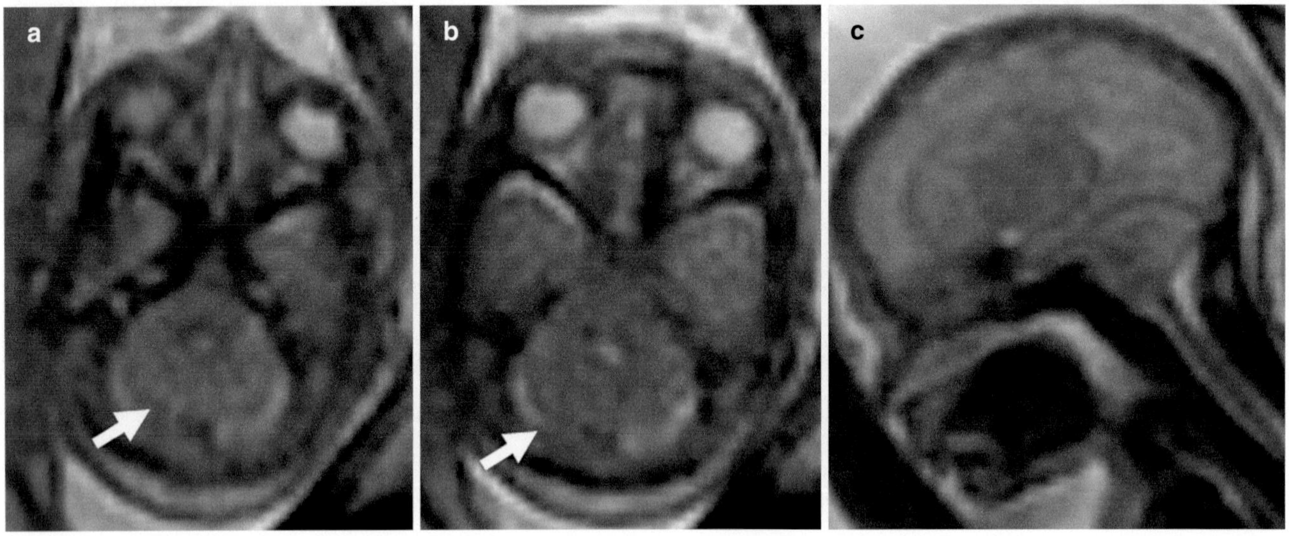

Fig. 8.13 Axial (**a**, **b**) and sagittal (**c**) T2W images of a 21-week fetus show rounded configuration of cerebellum (arrows) with absence of vermis-Rhombencephansynapsis

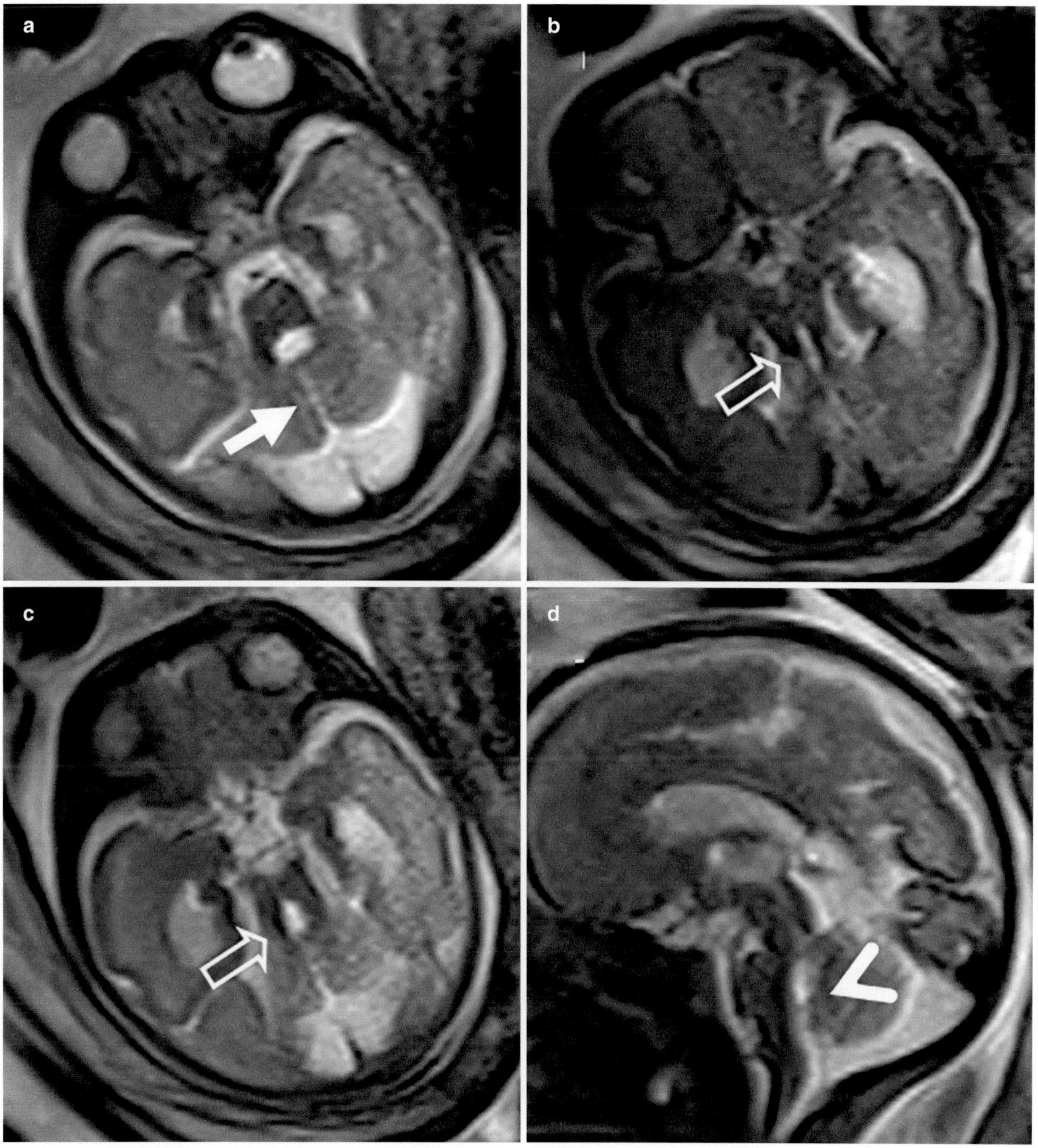

Fig. 8.14 Axial (**a**, **b**, **c**) T2W images of a 30-week fetus show the absence of the vermis (arrow). Bilateral superior cerebellar peduncles are elongated (open arrows) giving a molar tooth appearance to mid-brain. Associated mild dilatation of bilateral lateral ventricles is seen. Sagittal (**d**) image shows absence of fastigial point (arrowhead)

Prognosis

Post-natal outcome is poor with the majority children having severe disability [24], hence, termination of pregnancy is an option. Prenatal diagnosis by DNA testing can be performed if disease-causing mutation is known.

Future pregnancies—The couple to be advised to get an early ultrasound at 20–22 weeks. It can be followed up with MR if necessary.

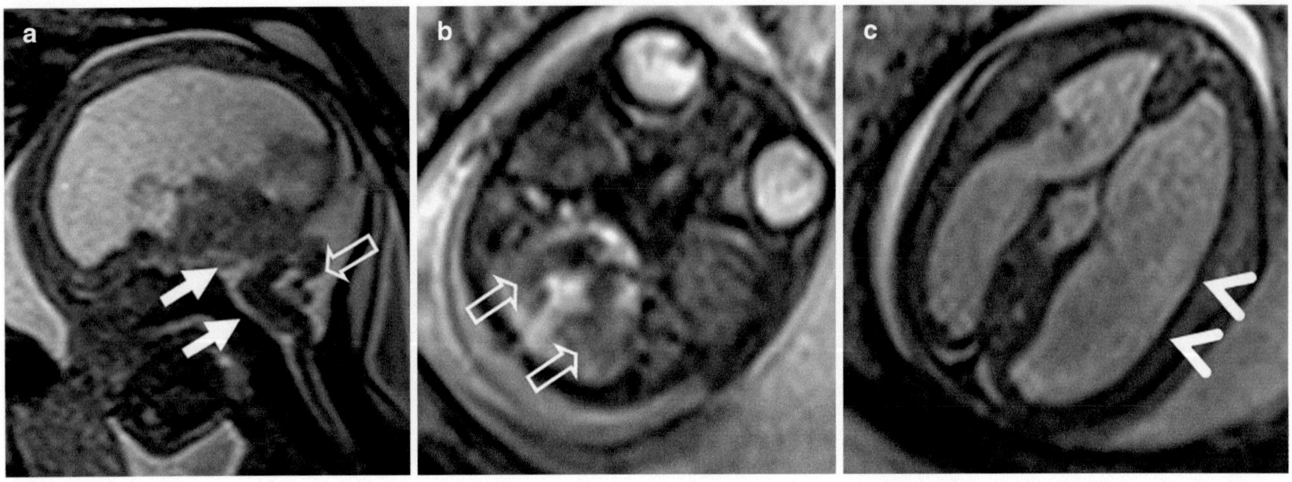

Fig. 8.15 Sagittal (**a**), Axial (**b**) T2W images of a 22-week fetus show an abnormal Z-shaped brainstem (arrow) and a small dysplastic cerebellum-vermis (open arrows). (**c**) Axial T2w image also shows ventriculomegaly–congenital muscular dystrophy

8.5.3 Kinked/z-Shaped Brainstem

Definition and pathology
It is a very rare anomaly caused due to arrested brainstem development at around 7 weeks of gestational age resulting in abnormal brainstem flexures. It can be seen in congenital muscular dystrophies, X-linked hydrocephalus, and tubulinopathies [25].

Imaging features
There is pontomesencephalic kinking or Z-shaped brainstem (Fig. 8.15a), the pons and medulla oblongata may appear bifid. The brainstem shows reduced dimensions. They are always accompanied by other anomalies like cerebellar hypoplasia (Fig. 8.15b), ventriculomegaly (Fig. 8.15c), corpus callosal dysgenesis or neuronal migration disorders.

Prognosis
This condition carries a poor prognosis [26].

8.5.4 Cerebellar Cortical Dysplasia

Definition and pathology
Cerebellar cortical abnormality can be focal or diffuse. They can occur sporadically or be associated with malformations/genetic disorders. Diffuse dysplasia is associated with various genetic disorders, congenital muscular dystrophy syndromes, and congenital cytomegalovirus (CMV) infection [27, 28].

Imaging findings
- Absence of horizontal foliation, disorganized fissures, irregularity of the cerebellar hemispheric surface, hemispheric hypertrophy, heterotopias, and intracerebellar cysts.

8.5.5 Ponto Tegmental Cap Dysplasia

Ponto Tegmental Cap Dysplasia is a very rare condition characterized by flattened ventral pons and a shelf-like protuberance on the dorsal surface of the pons.

8.6 Chiari Malformations (Fig. 8.16)

Have been discussed in the chapter on Neural tube defects.

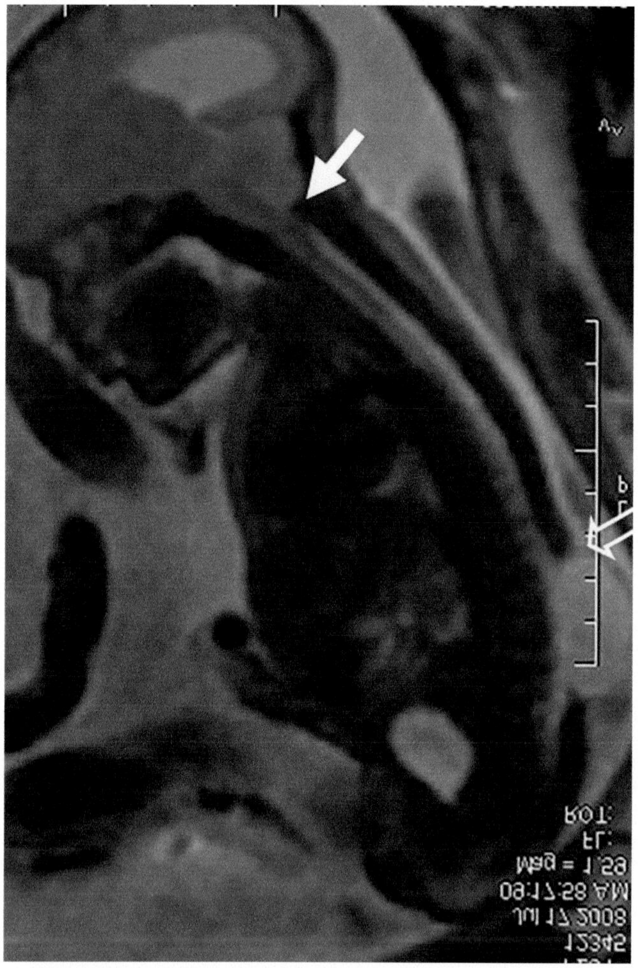

Fig. 8.16 Sagittal T2W images of a 20-week fetus show tonsillar herniation (arrow) and a lumbar meningomyelocele (open arrows)—Chiari 2 malformation

References

1. Gandolfi Colleoni G, Contro E, Carletti A, et al. Prenatal diagnosis and outcome of fetal posterior fossa fluid collections. Ultrasound Obstet Gynecol. 2012;39:625–31.
2. Shekdar K. Posterior fossa malformations. Semin Ultrasound CT MR. 2011;32:228–41.
3. Kollias SS, Ball WS Jr, Prenger EC. Cystic malformation of the posterior fossa: differential diagnosis clarified through embryologic analysis. Radiographics. 1993;13:1221–31.
4. Mahalingam HV, Rangasami R, Seshadri S, Suresh I. Imaging spectrum of posterior fossa anomalies on foetal magnetic resonance imaging with an algorithmic approach to diagnosis. Pol J Radiol. 2021;86:e183–94. https://doi.org/10.5114/pjr.2021.105014.
5. Hennekam RC, Biesecker LG, Allanson JE, Hall JG, Opitz JM, Temple IK, et al. Elements of morphology: general terms for congenital anomalies. Am J Med Genet A. 2013;161A(11):2726–33.
6. Adamsbaum C, Moutard M, Andre C, et al. MRI of the fetal posterior fossa. Pediatr Radiol. 2005;35:124–40.
7. Sreedher G, Mancuso M, Janitz E. Spectrum of fetal brain anomalies depicted on fetal MRI. DO J Am Osteopath Coll Radiol. 2016;5(1):15–22.
8. Volpe P, Contro E, De Musso F, Ghi T, Farina A, Tempesta A, Volpe G, Rizzo N, Pilu G. Brainstem-vermis and brainstemtentorium angles allow accurate categorization of fetal upward rotation of cerebellar vermis. Ultrasound Obstet Gynecol. 2012;39:632–5.
9. Vakakmudi UB, Rangasami R, Gopinath VN. Prenatal Blake pouch cyst with hydrocephalus. Neurol India. 2016;64:830–1.
10. Bolduc M-E, Limperopoulos C. Neurodevelopmental outcomes in children with cerebellar malformations: a systematic review. Dev Med Child Neurol. 2009;51(4):256–67.
11. Ramaswamy S, Rangasami R, Suresh S, Suresh I. Spontaneous resolution of Blake's pouch cyst. Radiol Case Rep. 2015;8(04):877.
12. Robinson AJ, Goldstein R. The cisterna magna septa: vestigial remnants of Blake's pouch and a potential new marker for normal development of the rhombencephalon. J Ultrasound Med. 2007;26:83–95.
13. Ghali R, et al. Perinatal and short-term neonatal outcomes of posterior fossa anomalies. Fetal Diagn Ther. 2014;35(2):108–17.
14. Robinson AJ. Inferior vermian hypoplasia—preconception, misconception. Ultrasound Obstet Gynecol. 2014;43(2):123–36.
15. Robinson AJ, et al. The fetal cerebellar vermis: assessment for abnormal development by ultrasonography and magnetic resonance imaging. Ultrasound Q. 2007;23(3):211–23.
16. Patek KJ, et al. Posterior fossa anomalies diagnosed with fetal MRI: associated anomalies and neurodevelopmental outcomes. Prenat Diagn. 2012;32(1):75–82.
17. Limperopoulos C, Robertson R, Estroff J, et al. Diagnosis of inferior vermian hypoplasia by fetal MRI: potential pitfalls and neurodevelopmental outcome. Am J Obstet Gynecol. 2006;194(4):1070–6.
18. Passi GR, et al. Rhombencephalosynapsis. Pediatr Neurol. 2015;52(6):651–2.
19. Whitehead MT, et al. Rhombencephalosynapsis as a cause of aqueductal stenosis: an under-recognized association in hydrocephalic children. Pediatr Radiol. 2014;44(7):849–56.
20. Cagneaux M, et al. Severe second-trimester obstructive ventriculomegaly related to disorders of diencephalic, mesencephalic and rhombencephalic differentiation. Ultrasound Obstet Gynecol. 2013;42(5):596–602.
21. Ishak GE, et al. Rhombencephalosynapsis: a hindbrain malformation associated with incomplete separation of midbrain and forebrain, hydrocephalus and a broad spectrum of severity. Brain. 2012;135(Pt 5):1370–86.
22. Koprivsek KM, et al. Partial rhombencephalosynapsis: prenatal MR imaging diagnosis and postnatal follow up. Acta Neurol Belg. 2011;111(2):157–9 (Pasquier L et al: Rhombencephalosynapsis and related anomalies: a neuropathological study of 40 fetal cases. Acta Neuropathol. 117(2):185–200, 2009)
23. Bosemani T, Orman G, Boltshauser E, Tekes A, Huisman TAGM, Poretti A. Congenital abnormalities of the posterior fossa. Radiographics. 2015;35(1):200–20.
24. Fennell EB, Gitten JC, Dede DE, Maria BL. Cognition, behavior, and development in Joubert syndrome. J Child Neurol. 1999;14(9):592–6.
25. Amir T, Poretti A, Boltshauser E, Huisman TAGM. Differential diagnosis of ventriculomegaly and brainstem kinking on fetal MRI. Brain and Development. 2016;38(1):103–8.
26. Smith AS, Levine D, Barnes PD, Robertson RL. MRI of the kinked fetal brainstem: a sign of severe dysgenesis. J Ultrasound Med Off J Am Inst Ultrasound Med. 2005;24(12):1697–709.
27. Massoud M, Clerc J, Cagneux M, Vasiljevic A, Massardier J, Doret M, et al. Prenatal diagnosis of cerebellar cortical dysplasia associated with abnormalities of foliation. Ultrasound Obstet Gynecol. 2012;40(2):243–4.
28. Severino M, Huisman TAGM. Posterior fossa malformations. Neuroimaging Clin N Am. 2019;29(3):367–83.

9 Abnormalities of Proliferation, Neuronal Migration, and Cortical Organization

Malformations of cortical development (MCD) occur due to various causes like genetic syndromes, infections, vascular, or metabolic disorders [1, 2]. MCD is characterized by cortical abnormalities or the presence of heterotopic gray matter (Fig. 9.1) or abnormal brain size (megalencephaly or microcephaly).

Sonography has limitations in the evaluation of the peripheral brain structures, the sulci, and gyri. MRI allows better visualization of the heterotopic tissues and structures of the brain periphery [3]. However, gestational age at the time of MRI scan can limit the diagnostic accuracy, as some findings may be visualized only in the third trimester [4].

9.1 Embryology

The development of the cerebral cortex occurs in three overlapping phases:

1. Neuronal proliferation and apoptosis
2. Neuronal migration
3. Neuronal organization and maturation.

Neuronal proliferation and apoptosis occur during 4–16 weeks of gestation age in the germinal zones, i.e., along the margins of the lateral ventricles. Neuronal migration occurs during 8–24 weeks, as neurons radially migrate from the germinal zones to the cortex peripherally. The early migrating neurons occupy the deeper aspect of cortex and the later migrating neurons get placed in the superficial aspect of the cortex. Neuronal organization and maturation start by 22–24 weeks of gestation age and progresses until 2 years of postnatal age, as six layers of functional cortex develop with the establishment of interneuron connections. At the end of the proliferation and migration stage, the brain shows most structures but the cortex appears smooth (less sulcation). At the end of organization and maturation, the sulci and gyri are increased as also the cortical thickness [5, 6]. The sulcal development progresses throughout the second and third trimesters (Table 9.1; Fig. 9.1) [7]. Primary sulci are indentations that occur initially on the brain surface. The secondary and tertiary sulci develop as ramifications of the primary sulci at a later stage.

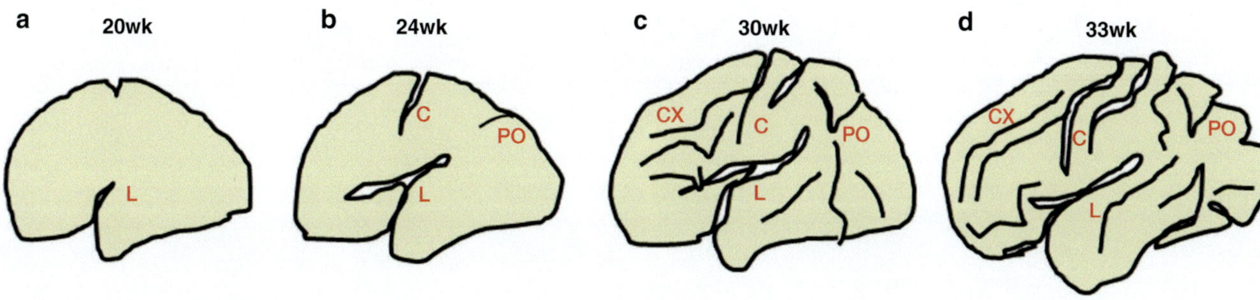

Fig. 9.1 (**a–d**) Schematic diagram showing the development of sulcal spaces on the lateral cerebral surface. *L* lateral sulcus, *C* central sulcus, *PO* Parieto-occipital sulcus, *CX* convexity sulci

R. Rajeswaran, *MR Imaging of the Fetus*, https://doi.org/10.1007/978-981-16-9209-3_9

Sylvian Fissure
The Sylvian fissure is first seen by 18 weeks on MRI (Fig. 9.2a), shows an obtuse angle and progresses to show acute angulation by 25 weeks (Fig. 9.2d). The development stages are shown in Figs. 9.2a–i and 9.4a–i.

Parieto-Occipital Fissure
The parieto-occipital fissure separates the parietal lobe from the occipital lobe and is seen as a cleft on the medial surface of the brain (Fig. 9.2a–i). On MR imaging, it is well demonstrated on the axial (Fig. 9.2a–i) and sagittal sections (Fig. 9.3a–i).

Cingulate Sulcus
This sulcus is seen on the medial surface of the brain. It is seen running parallel to the rostrum, body, and splenium of the corpus callosum. Because of its curved course, on MR imaging, the anterior part is well demonstrated on axial images, and the middle part is well depicted on the coronal images (Fig. 9.4a–i).

Table 9.1 Gestational age when fissures and primary sulci become visible on MR Imaging

Gestational age	Sulcation
18–22 weeks	Sylvian fissure
19–23 weeks	Parieto-occipital fissure
19–23 weeks	Calcarine fissure
26–27 weeks	Central sulcus
25–29 weeks	Cingulate sulcus
27–29 weeks	Convexity sulci
>33 weeks	Extensive sulcation

Central (Rolandic) Sulcus
The central sulcus is demonstrated on MR images by 26–27 weeks of gestation. It is well seen on the axial (Fig. 9.5a–i) and sagittal sections (Fig. 9.3a–i).

Calcarine Fissure
The calcarine fissure is visualized on the medial surface of the occipital lobe. It starts from the medial aspect of the parieto-occipital fissure and proceeds posteriorly to the occipital pole. On MR imaging, it is well demonstrated on the sagittal (Fig. 9.3a–i) and coronal sections (Fig. 9.6a–i).

Convexity Sulci
As the fetal brain matures, these convexity sulci can be visualized on the lateral surfaces of the cerebral hemispheres (Fig. 9.6a–i). These convexity sulci include the central sulcus, superior temporal sulcus, and other sulci on the lateral surface of cerebral hemisphere. MR imaging is superior to sonography in demonstrating sulci of the inferior and lateral surfaces of the cerebral hemispheres [7].

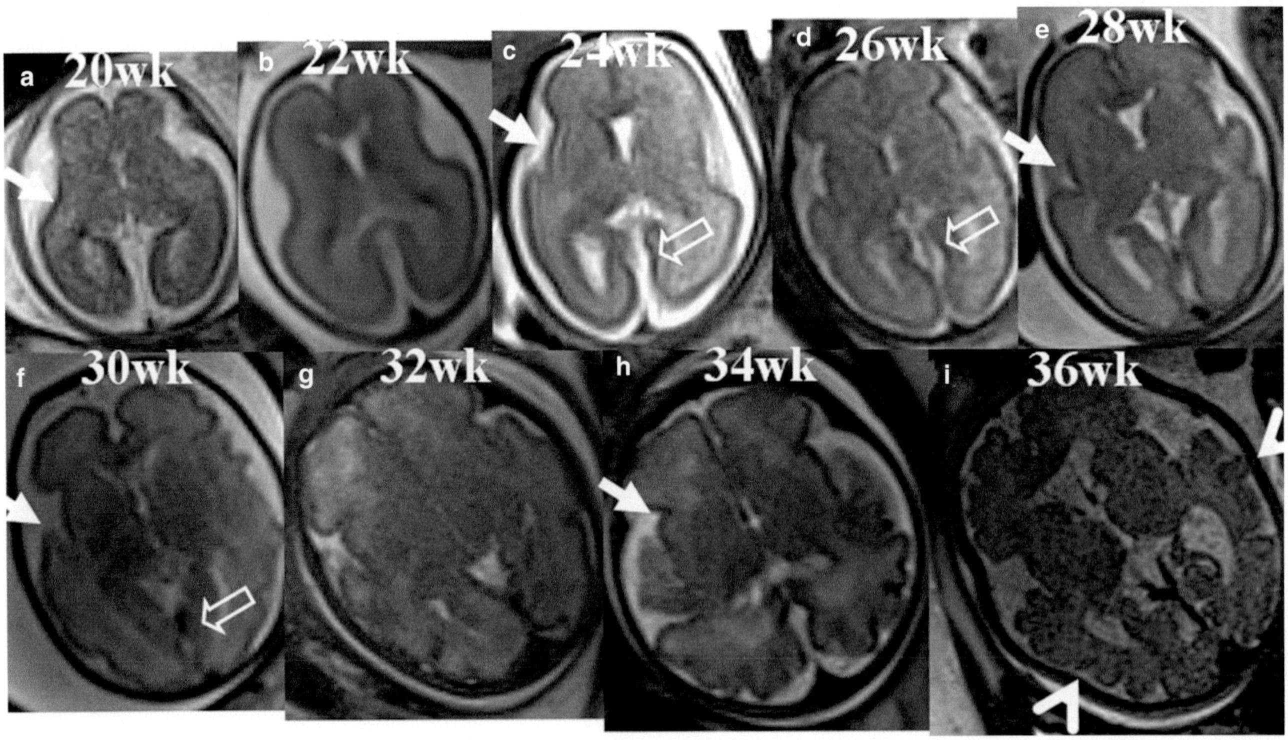

Fig. 9.2 (a–i) Axial T2W images of fetuses at different gestational ages at the level of III ventricle showing the development of Sylvian fissure (arrow), parieto-occipital (open arrows), and cortical sulci (arrowheads)

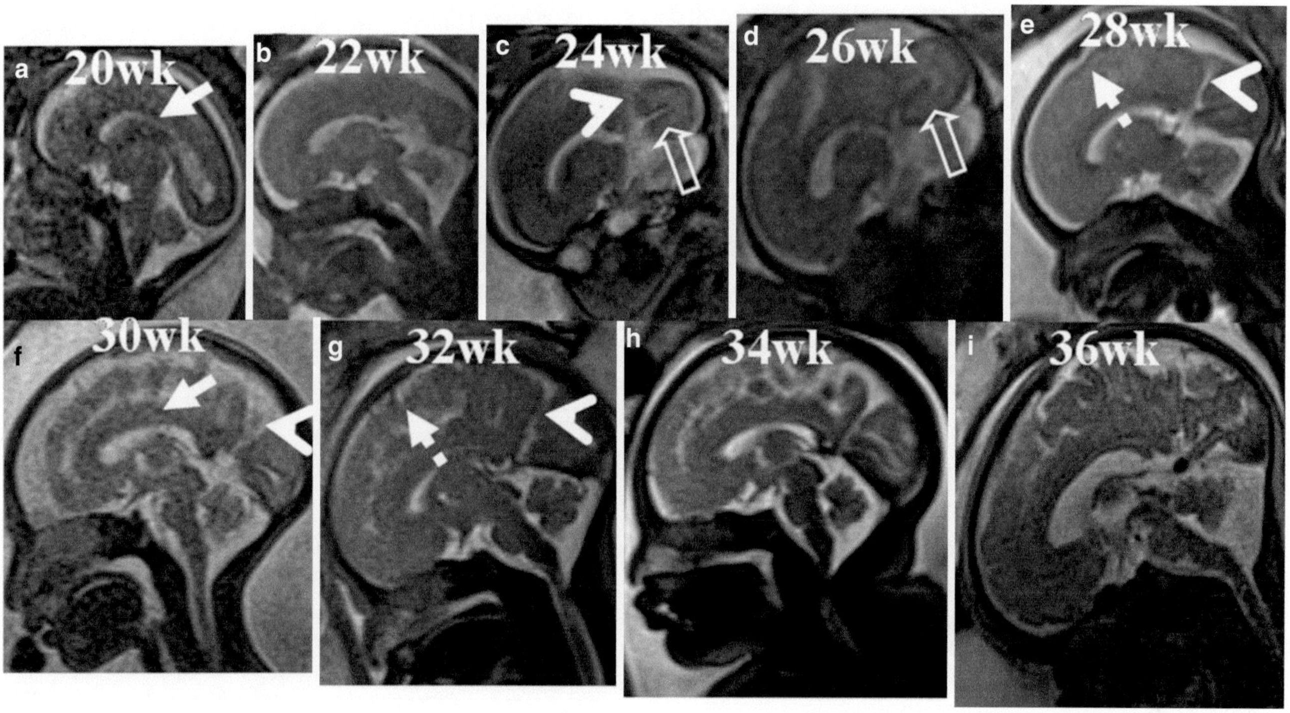

Fig. 9.3 (**a–i**) Mid-sagittal T2W images of fetuses at different gestational ages showing the development of corpus callosum(arrows), parieto-occipital (arrowheads), calcarine (open arrows), and central sulci (broken arrows)

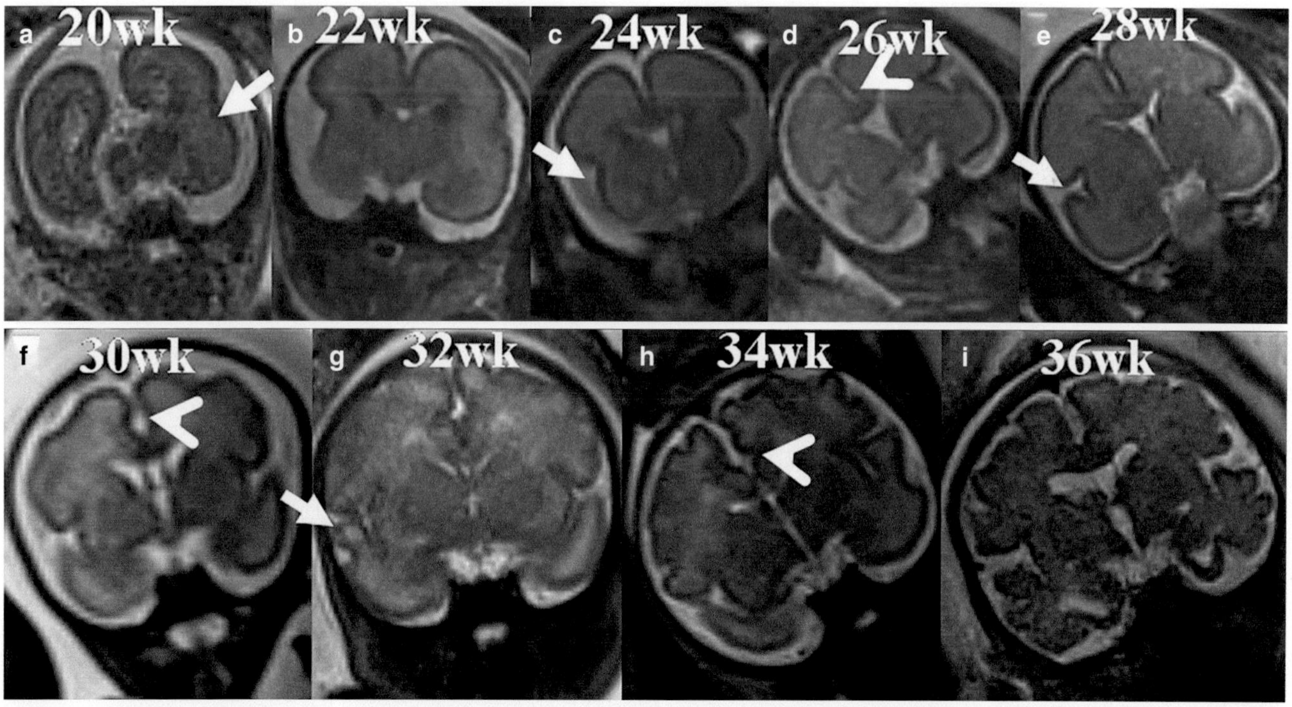

Fig. 9.4 (**a–i**) Coronal T2W images of fetuses at different gestational ages at the level of sella showing the development of Sylvian fissure (arrow), and cingulate sulcus (arrowheads)

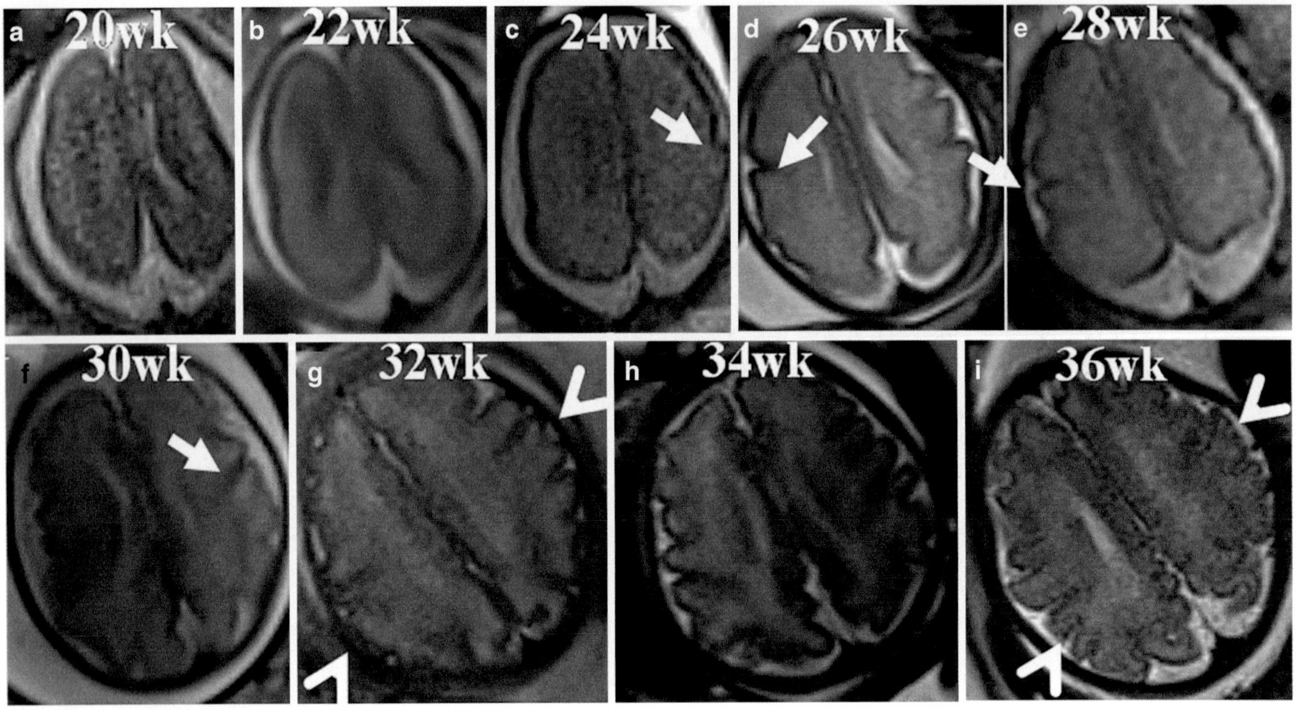

Fig. 9.5 (**a–i**) Axial T2W images of fetuses at different gestational ages at the level of corona radiata showing the development of central (arrow), and cortical sulci (arrowheads)

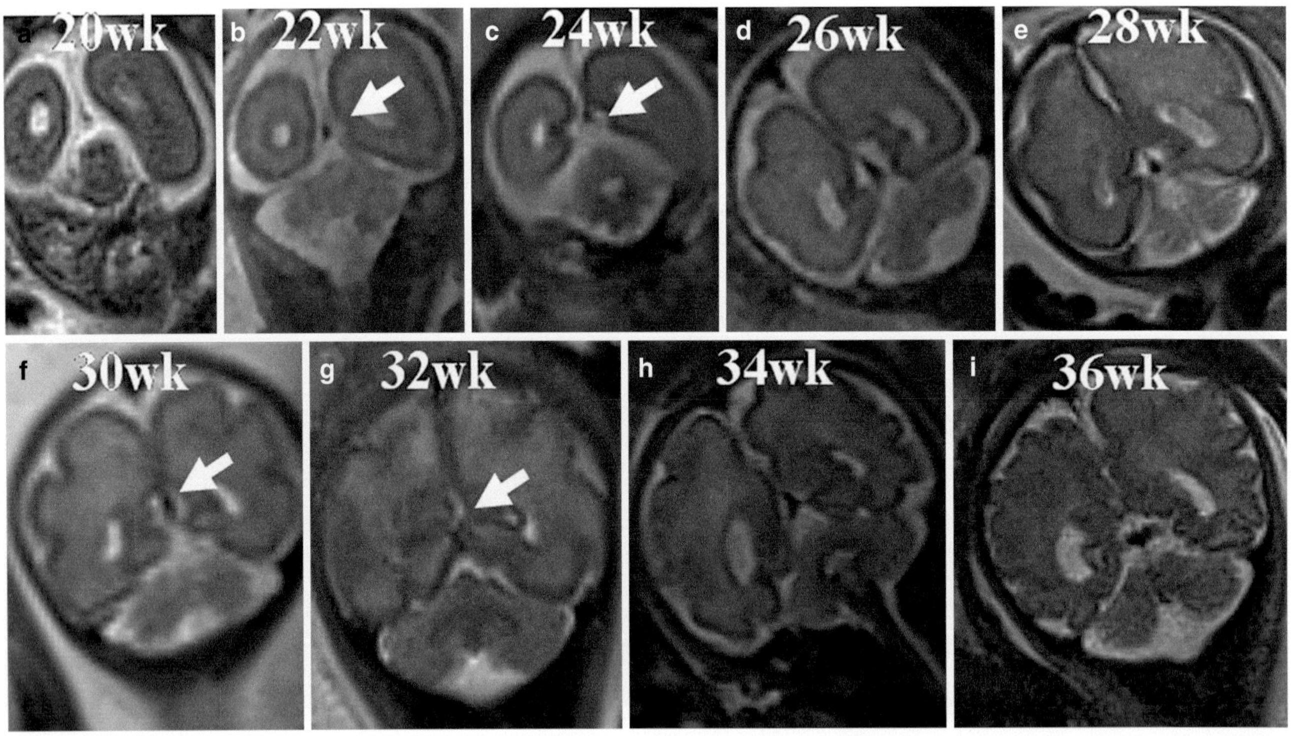

Fig. 9.6 (**a–i**) Coronal T2W images of fetuses at different gestational ages at the level of occipital lobe showing the development of calcarine sulcus (arrows)

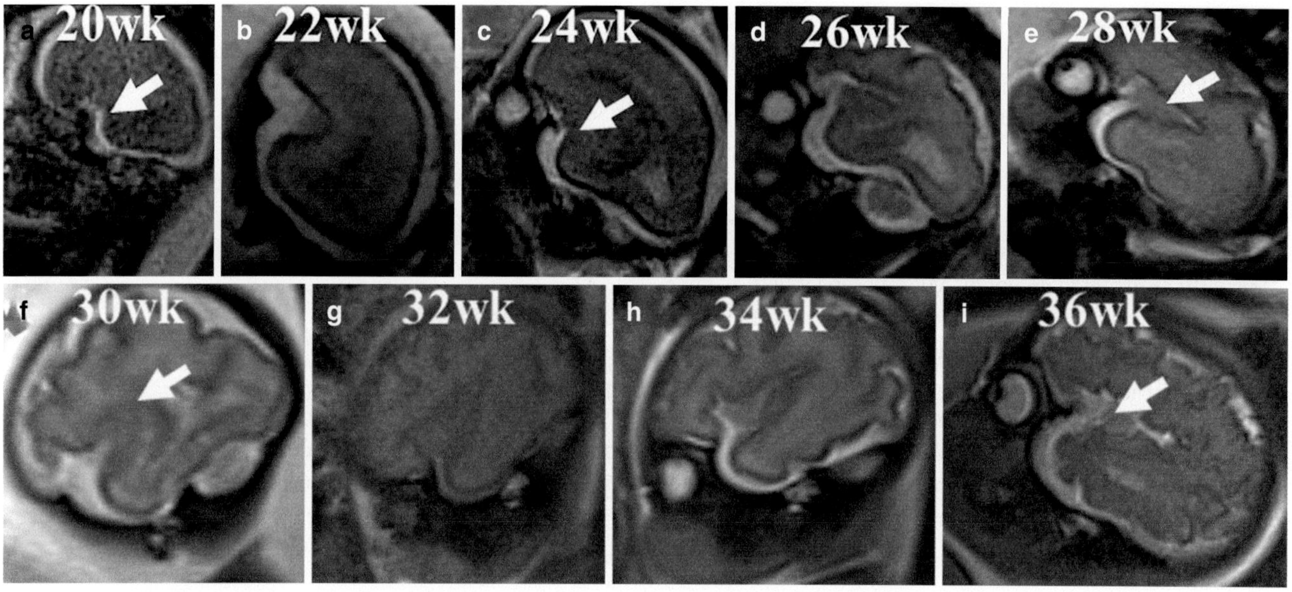

Fig. 9.7 (a–i) Parasagittal T2W images of fetuses at different gestational ages showing the development of lateral sulcus (arrows)

Lateral Sulcus
It is one of the most conspicuous structures separating the temporal from the parietal lobe. It is seen from 18 weeks and well demonstrated on sagittal sections (Fig. 9.7a–i).

The classification for malformations of cortical development organizes many conditions into one of four major groups according to the main underlying mechanism [8–10]:

Classification of the Malformations of Cortical Development

- *Group I: Abnormal cell proliferation or apoptosis*
- *Group II: Abnormal neuronal migration*
- *Group III: Abnormal post migrational development (organization)*
- *Group IV: Malformations secondary to inborn errors of metabolism*

The important disorders within these groups of cortical development are enumerated and discussed.

9.2 Group I: Abnormal Cell Proliferation or Apoptosis [9]

1. *Microcephaly*
   (a) With normal to simplified cortical pattern
   (b) Microcephaly with lissencephaly
   (c) Microcephaly with extensive polymicrogyria
2. *Megalencephaly/macrocephaly*
3. *Abnormal cell proliferation*
   (a) *Non-neoplastic*
      (i) Tuberous sclerosis (Hamartomas)
      (ii) Hemimegalencephaly
      (iii) Focal cortical dysplasia (Types I and IIb)
   (b) *Neoplastic*
      (i) Ganglioglioma, Dysembryoplastic neuroepithelial tumor

Disorders of abnormal cell proliferation can result in the formation of too many neurons or reduced number of neurons or abnormal neurons [10]. Increased proliferation of neurons or decreased apoptosis results in the formation of megalencephaly and hemimegalencephaly. Microlissencephaly results from decreased proliferation of neurons or due to increased apoptosis. Focal cortical dysplasia occurs due to the formation of abnormal cells.

9.2.1 Microcephaly

Definition
The term microcephaly is used when the fetal head measurements fall under the 3rd percentile.

Pathology
Many genetic disorders, syndromes, infection, and several causes have been identified that result in microcephaly It can be primary microcephaly when the brain is abnormal from the early stage. In secondary microcephaly, there is normal brain development and it gets arrested by some insult/event.

Primary microcephaly results from either decreased cell production or due to increased apoptosis. It has two subtypes: (1) Microcephaly with a simplified gyral pattern (mild form) and (2) Microlissencephaly (severe form).

Imaging Features

- Volume of the brain is reduced. The head circumference is below the 3rd percentile (Fig. 9.8a, b)
- Sloping forehead, small frontal lobes (Fig. 9.8c), enlarged subarachnoid spaces and thick placenta (measuring > 5 cm) [11]
- Microcephaly with a simplified gyral pattern shows few shallow sulci, normal cortical thickness (3 mm), and is usually an isolated anomaly. Microlissencephaly is characterized by a thickened cortex (>3 mm), smooth cortical surface and is usually associated with other brain anomalies [12] (Fig. 9.9a–c).
- Those presenting in the II trimester may have associated holoprosencephaly or encephalocele.
- Those presenting in the III trimester may have abnormalities of sulcation or neuronal migration.
- Fetal brain MRI (at or after 32 weeks) is useful to detect abnormalities of neuronal migration, such as lissencephaly and polymicrogyria.

Prognosis

Most cases of microcephaly have intellectual and neurological disabilities.

9.2.2 Megalencephaly

Definition

It is characterized by an abnormally large brain and can be unilateral or bilateral. Megalencephaly can involve the entire cerebral hemisphere or part of the cerebral hemisphere. It can be isolated or be associated with syndromes.

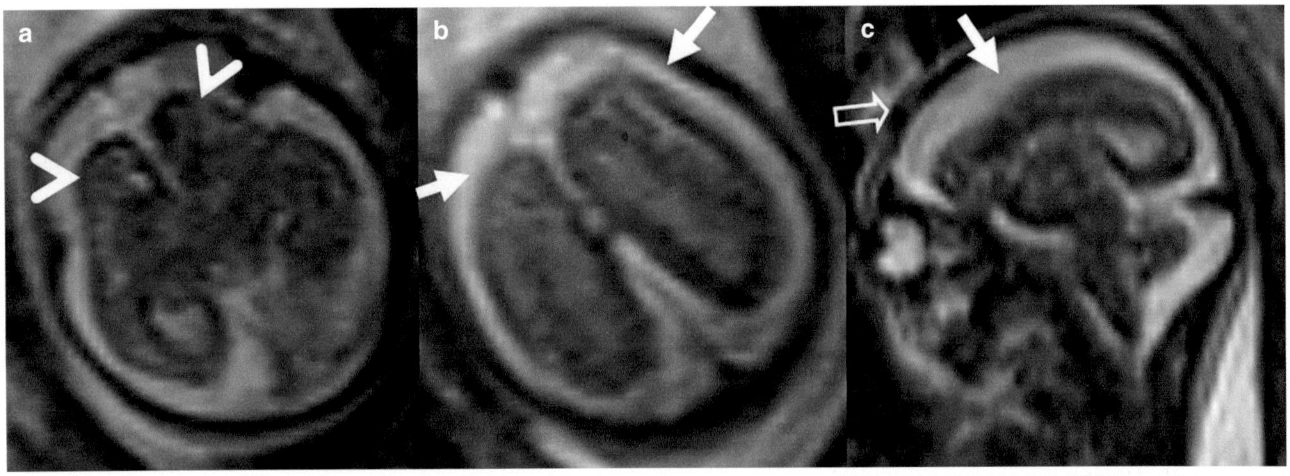

Fig. 9.8 Axial (**a**, **b**), sagittal (**c**) images of a 23-week fetus show reduced volume of bilateral cerebral hemispheres, especially in frontal lobes (arrowhead), enlarged subarachnoid space (arrows), and sloping forehead (open arrows) suggesting microcephaly

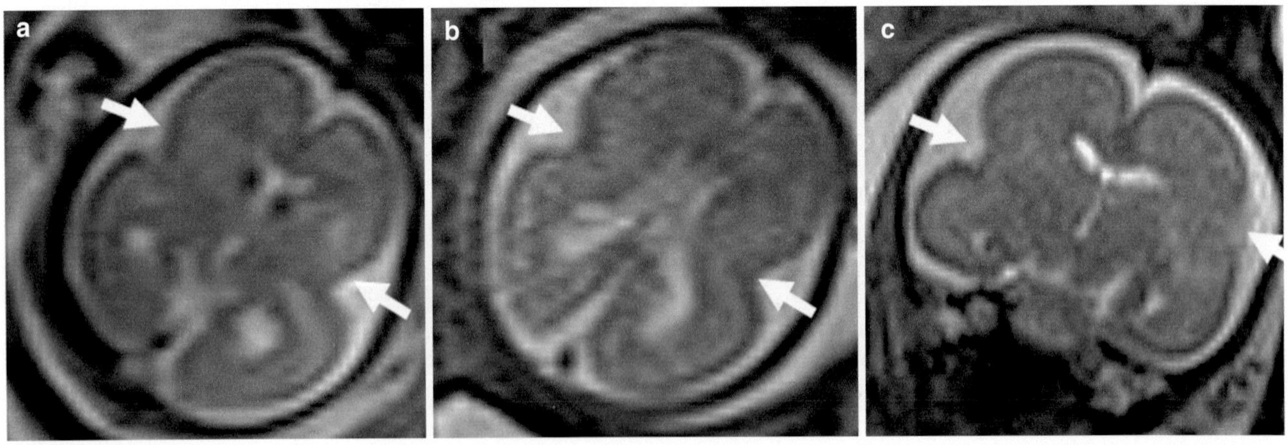

Fig. 9.9 Axial (**a**, **b**), coronal (**c**) images of a 27-week fetus with reduced head dimensions showing generalized reduced sulcal development and shallow lateral sulcus (arrow), suggesting microlissencephaly

Pathology

Megalencephaly is a congenital malformation in which increased cell production or decreased apoptosis results in hamartomatous overgrowth of a hemisphere. Macroscopically the affected hemisphere shows overgrowth, abnormal cortical development with areas of lissencephaly, polymicrogyria, pachygyria and agyria in varying proportions, with intervening normal-appearing brain.

Imaging Features

- The head circumference may be increased.
- Unilateral or bilateral cerebral hemispheres show increased volume.
- Ipsilateral ventricular dilatation with thickened cortex on the side of the megalencephaly, better demonstrated on MRI (Fig. 9.10a, b) [13].
- It is commonly associated with heterotopia, agyria, or polymicrogyria (Fig. 9.10b).

Differential Diagnosis

Macrocephaly is characterized by head circumference > 2 standard deviations above the population mean and has several causes. It commonly shows normal brain anatomy with normal signal intensity.

Prognosis

The affected child can have mental retardation, seizures, and neurological abnormalities.

9.2.3 Abnormal Proliferation: Abnormal Cell Type—Tuberous Sclerosis

Definition and Pathology

It is a neurocutaneous disorder involving multiple organs and characterized by the development of multiple benign tumors/hamartomas.

Spontaneous mutations account for 50–85% of cases. The remainder show inheritance as an autosomal dominant condition.

Prenatal MRI evaluation is usually done in affected families or in fetuses whose sonography show cardiac rhabdomyomas.

Imaging Features

- Can be difficult to identify on USG, hence fetuses with cardiac masses/rhabdomyomas (Fig. 9.11a) need to be further evaluated by MRI.
- Periventricular, cortical, and subcortical tubers may be seen—These lesions appear hypointense on T2 weighted

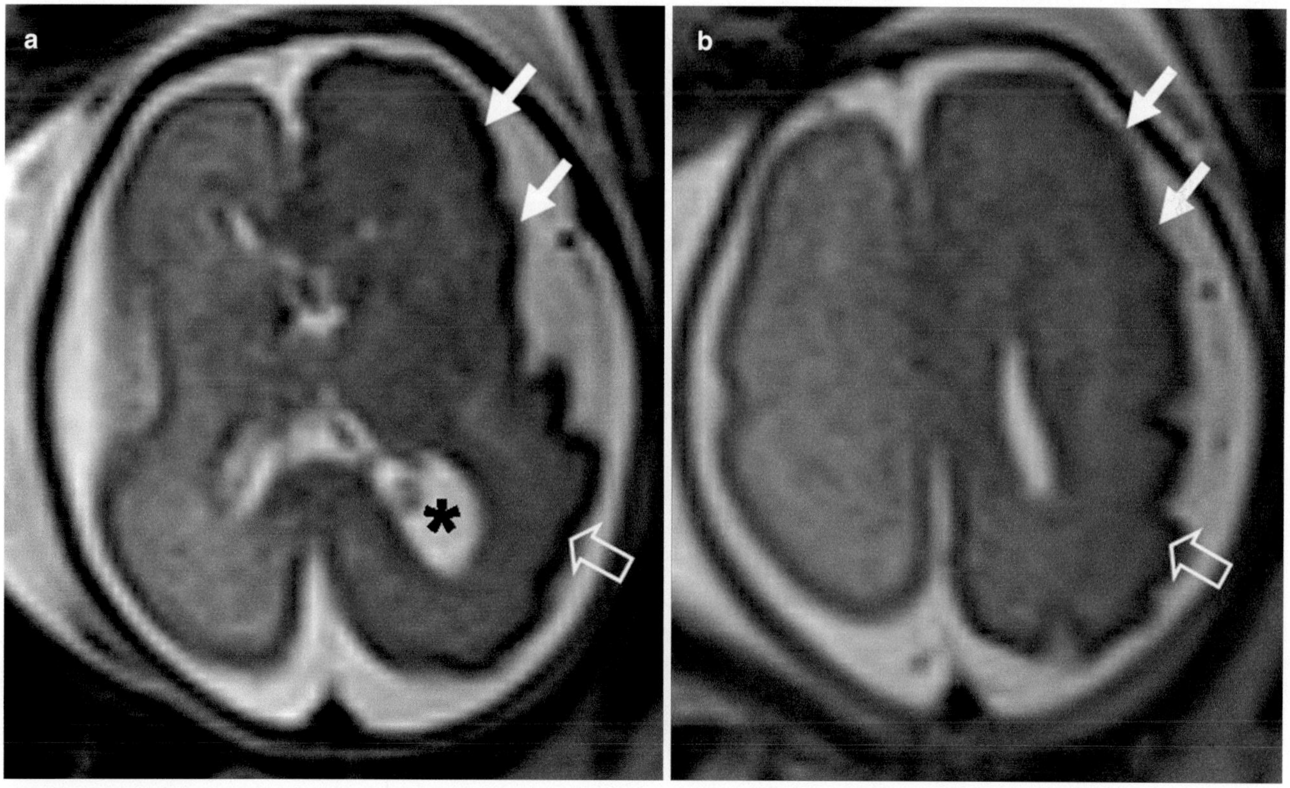

Fig. 9.10 Axial (**a**, **b**) images of a 25-week fetus show enlarged left cerebral hemisphere (arrow) with mild dilatation of ipsilateral lateral ventricle (asterisk). The affected cerebral hemisphere shows advanced myelination and polymicrogyria (open arrows)

images (Fig. 9.11c) and hyperintense on T1 weighted images due to unmyelinated surrounding tissue [14, 15].

- The tubers are irregular in shape with their long axis perpendicular to the ventricular wall.
- Subependymal giant cell astrocytoma—is seen as a mass adjacent to the foramen of Monro (Fig. 9.11b) and may cause hydrocephalus.
- A normal MRI brain does not exclude the diagnosis of tuberous sclerosis.

Prognosis

Multiple organs may be affected. Even if the prenatal scan is normal, Postnatal MRI brain is warranted in high-risk patients.

Rhabdomyomas may resolve spontaneously, remain stable, or may be associated with arrhythmias.

Affected children may have the clinical triad of: Adenoma Sebaceum, intellectual impairment, seizures.

There is a high risk of developing subependymal giant cell astrocytoma in the cerebral tubers.

Differential Diagnosis

Heterotopia: Is isointense with gray matter.

9.3 Group II: Abnormal Neuronal Migration

1. *Lissencephaly*
   (a) Classic Lissencephaly (type I)
   (b) Cobblestone Lissencephaly (type II)
2. Heterotopia
   (a) Subependymal heterotopia
   (b) Subcortical heterotopia
   (c) Marginal glioneuronal heterotopia

Disorders of neuronal migration include classic lissencephaly, which results due to the cessation of neuronal migration; cobblestone lissencephaly, which results from overmigration of the neurons. Heterotopia results due to ectopic neuronal migration (Fig. 9.12).

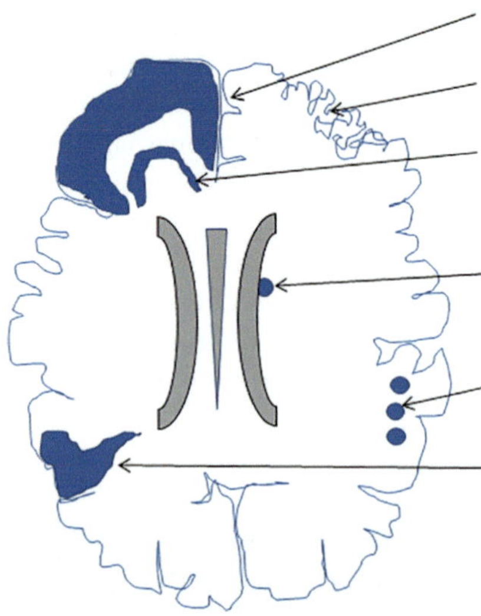

Fig. 9.12 Schematic diagram showing lissencephaly, polymicogyria, heteropias, and focal cortical dysplasia

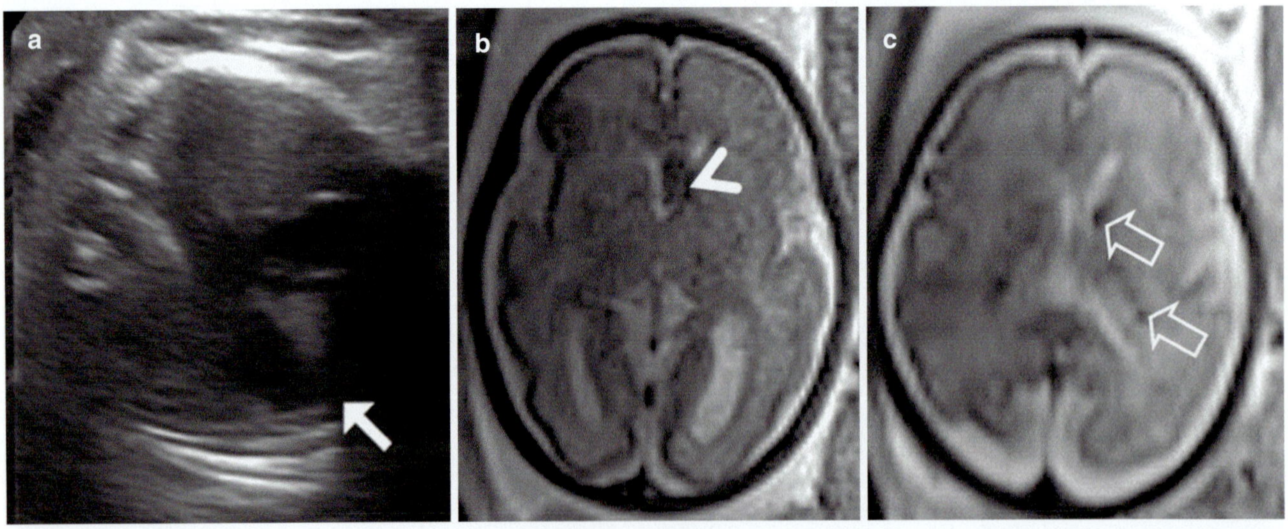

Fig. 9.11 Sonographic image of a 28-week fetus (**a**) shows hyperechoic lesion in the heart—rhabdomyoma (arrow). Axial MR images (**b**, **c**) show subependymal giant cell astrocytoma in Foramino of Monro region (arrowhead) and bilateral periventricular tubers (open arrows) suggesting tuberous sclerosis

9.3.1 Diffuse Neuronal Migration Arrest: Classical Lissencephaly (Type I)

Definition

In lissencephaly, the brain appears smooth with thick featureless cortex and absent sulcation. It can also show associated pachygyria/band heterotopia (Fig. 9.13).

Imaging Features

- Complete form—there is diffusely smooth brain surface (Fig. 9.13).
- Incomplete form—Consists of parieto-occipital agyria with few shallow sulci in the temporal lobe and inferior aspect of the frontal lobe. The cerebral hemispheres may show shallow Sylvian fissures giving a "figure of eight or hourglass" configuration).
- The thickened cortex may show three layers—a thin peripheral T2 hypointense layer, thin T2 hyperintense intermediate cell sparse layer, and a thick inner T2 hypointense layer of gray matter suggesting neuronal arrest. The subcortical white matter appears thin with the absence of the normal interdigitation of white matter into the gyri.
- While interpreting fetal MRI, it is important to know the gestational age before commenting on lissencephaly. A smooth appearance of the brain is normal until 20 weeks gestation. Lissencephaly can be suspected by 24 weeks' gestation on MRI, when the Sylvian and parieto-occipital fissures are absent or appear shallow [16, 17].
- Cystic areas can be seen in the germinal matrix—a sign of halted brain development

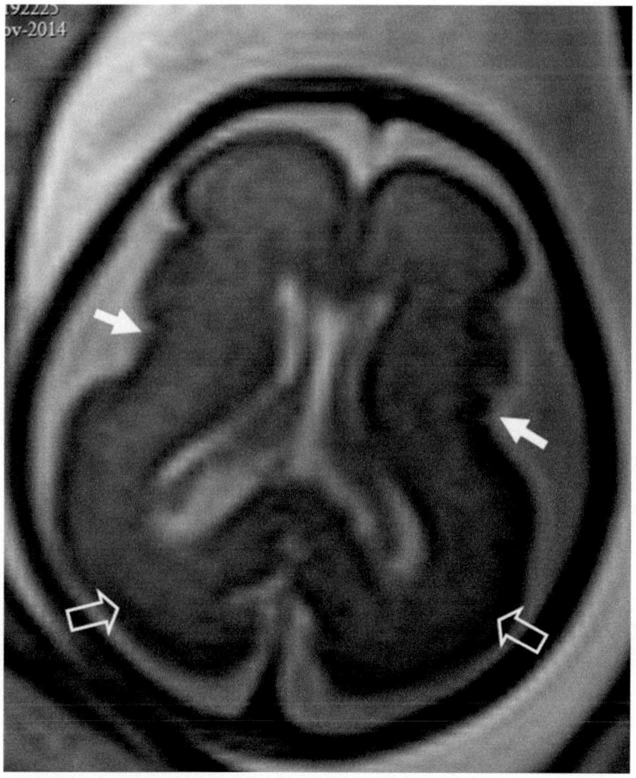

Fig. 9.13 Axial T2W image of a 28-week fetus showing reduced sulcal development (arrows) and band hetertopia in bilateral parieto-occipital regions (open arrows)

9.3.2 Neuronal Overmigration: Cobblestone Lissencephaly (Type 2)

Definition and Pathology

This condition is characterized by nodular cortical surface. It results from over migration of the germinal matrix neurons beyond the gyri.

It may be associated with congenital muscular dystrophy, syndromes, and mutational disorders.

Imaging Features

- There is a deficiency of normal sulcation.
- The cerebral cortical surface appears nodular, being common in the anterior aspect of the brain.
- Associated abnormalities include—ventriculomegaly, callosal dysgenesis, aqueductal stenosis, inferior vermian hypoplasia, and pontomesencephalic kink giving "Z" appearance· [18, 19].

Prognosis

It is associated with severe mental retardation, developmental delay, seizures, and failure to thrive. In severe cases, death occurs in the first few years of life.

If mutation is known, early prenatal diagnosis can be obtained with DNA analysis.

Termination of pregnancy is an option and may be offered to the couple.

9.3.3 Focal Neuronal Migration Arrest: Heterotopia

Definition

Due to arrest of migration, collections of neurons are seen in abnormal locations—anywhere along the course of subependymal region to the subcortical region (Fig. 9.12).

They may occur in isolation or may be associated with other brain anomalies/syndromes. Heterotopias may be either of the nodular type (subependymal or subcortical) or of the band type [20, 21].

Imaging Features

- *Subependymal nodular heterotopia*: Few or multiple oval or round nodules may be seen along the lateral ven-

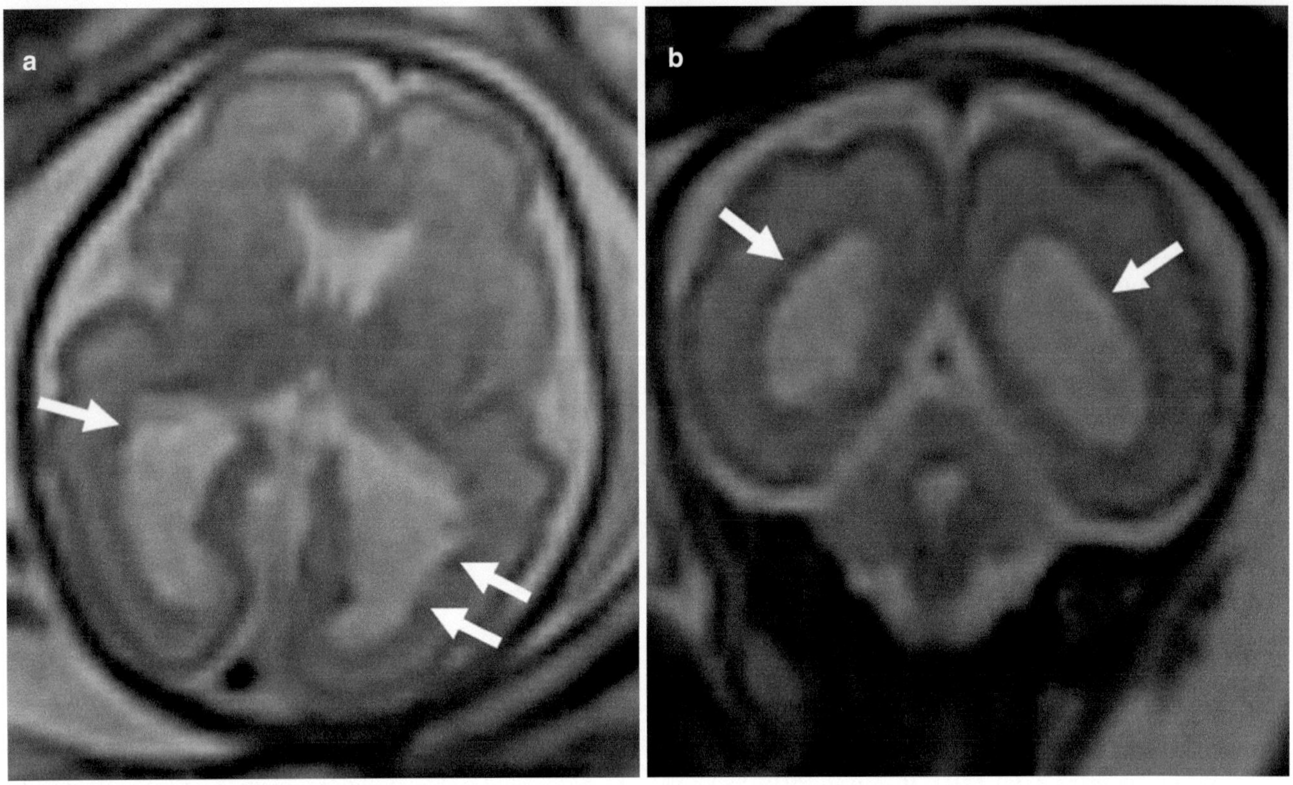

Fig. 9.14 Axial (**a**), coronal (**b**) T2W image of a fetus shows ventriculomegaly with associated bilateral periventricular nodular heterotopia

tricular walls, commonly along the trigonal or occipital horn regions of bilateral lateral ventricles (Figs. 9.12 and 9.14a, b).

- These nodules appear isointense to gray matter on all imaging sequences and are seen with their long axis parallel to the ventricular wall. There is no surrounding edema. They may be associated with malformations like ventriculomegaly.
- *Subcortical nodular heterotopia*: These nodules are seen in the subcortical region, in contiguity with the overlying thin cortex. They may vary in size from subcentimeter lesions to large lesions (Fig. 9.12) that occupy most of the cerebral hemisphere [22].
- *Band heterotopia* ("*Double cortex*"): Band heterotopias are more common in females and may be familial (X-linked dominant). It is seen as a smooth stripe of gray matter located in the subcortical region. Band heterotopias are seen parallel to the overlying cortex (Figs. 9.12 and 9.13). They are also considered as a mild form of lissencephaly and can be partial or complete. The overlying cortex shows shallow sulci with normal thickness or reduced thickness [23].

Differential Diagnosis

Tuberous sclerosis—the tubers appear irregular in shape with the long axis perpendicular to the ventricular wall. Some of the tubers may show surrounding edema.

Intracranial Hemorrhage—May cause nodularity along the ependyma and may be associated with hemorrhage in the caudothalamic groove and ventricles. MRI, especially gradient sequence is diagnostic.

Infection—Especially cytomegalovirus infection may cause abnormal neuronal migration, and may be associated with fetal growth retardation and hydrops.

9.4 Group III: Abnormal Post Migrational Development (Organization)

1. Polymicrogyria and schizencephaly
2. Cortical dysgenesis secondary to inborn errors of metabolism
3. Type I and type III focal cortical dysplasia
4. Post-migrational microcephaly (also in group I)

Prenatal causes like ischemia or infection may lead to disorders of cortical organization. Injury of the superficial part of the brain may result in polymicrogyria, whereas insult of the whole thickness of the brain may result in schizencephaly.

9.4.1 Polymicrogyria (PMG)

Definition
Polymicrogyria refers to increased number of small gyri. It may be associated with pachygyria which means broad flattened gyri. Polymicrogyria can occur as an isolated entity or be associated with syndromes and other brain anomalies.

Imaging Features

- Polymicrogyria can be diffuse or focal and unilateral or bilateral
- There is excessive number of small gyri that produces an "Over-folded cortex" or "fine saw tooth appearance" to the cortex (Figs. 9.12 and 9.15).
- Sometimes there is fusion of the microsulci that may give an appearance of smooth cortical surface [24, 25].
- An abnormal gyral pattern, abnormal gray-white matter junction or asymmetry of cerebral hemispheres may be the clue to conduct a detailed examination.

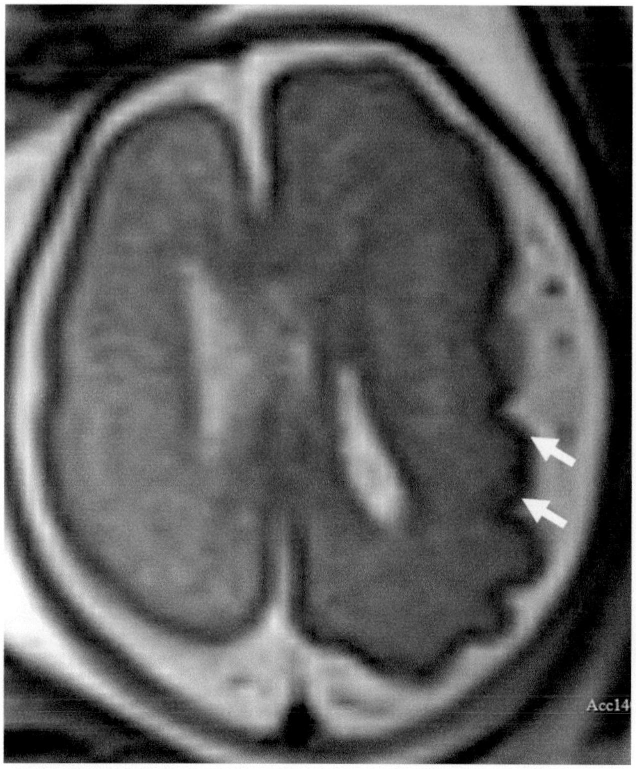

Fig. 9.15 Axial T2W image of a 25-week fetus shows hemimegalencephaly of the left cerebral hemisphere with associated polymicrogyria (arrow)

- Polymicrogyria commonly occurs in the perisylvian location. The Sylvian fissures appear deep and wide due to the malformation.
- The polymicrogyric cortex may be of normal thickness (3 mm) or thickened (4–6 mm). The adjacent white matter may show abnormal T2 hyperintensity.
- It may be associated with brain anomalies like corpus callosal dygenesis, hemimegalencephaly, or microcephaly.

Differential Diagnosis Lissencephaly, Congenital CMV infection.

Prognosis
PMG is a common malformation and affected patients often present with seizures.

Prognosis becomes worse when there is an associated abnormality/syndrome.

9.4.2 Schizencephaly

Definition
It represents a cleft extending from the cortical surface to the ventricle and is lined by gray matter. It can occur sporadically, following prenatal insult or rarely be familial. Schizencephaly can occur unilaterally or bilaterally. There are two types—closed lip and open lip Schizencephaly.

Imaging Features

- Closed lip Schizencephaly (type 1)—The lips of the cleft are in contact with each other and are commonly unilateral (Fig. 9.16).
- Open lip (type 2)—The lips of the cleft are separated from each other by intervening cerebral spinal fluid (CSF) extending from the lateral ventricle. It commonly occurs bilaterally. The cleft is wedge shaped, with the apex toward the ventricles and base toward the brain surface (Fig. 9.17a, b)
- The gray matter lining the clefts may show areas of pachygyria or polymicrogyria. Subependymal heterotopia may occur in the periventricular region [26, 27].
- Though the open lip Schizencephaly can be easily identified on fetal MRI, the closed lip type may be difficult to diagnose, often displaying as a small depression along the ventricular walls.
- Schizencephaly is commonly associated with septal agenesis and septo-optic dysplasia.

Differential Diagnosis
Porencephaly—occurs after a destructive insult and is not lined by gray matter.

Arachnoid Cyst—Seen as extra-axial cyst. The adjacent parenchyma is displaced or remodeled.

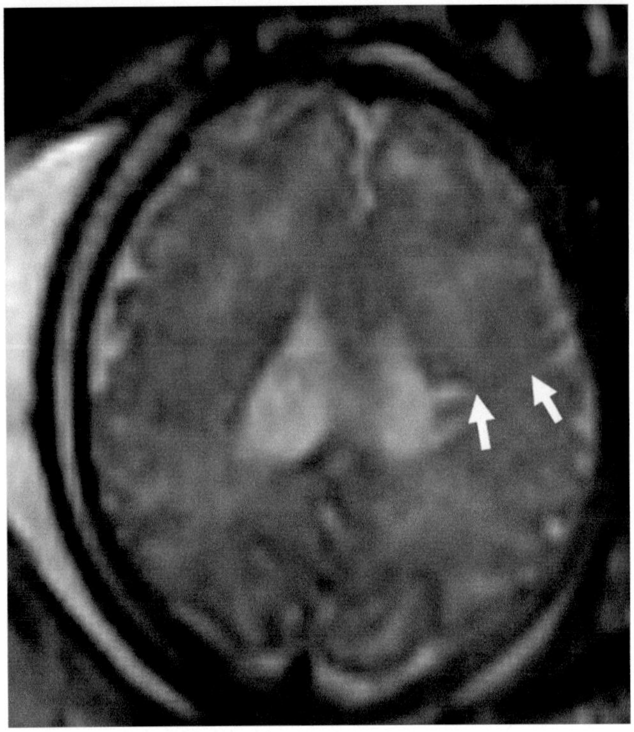

Fig. 9.16 Axial T2W image of a 33-week fetus shows gray matter lined cleft (arrows) in the left frontal region suggesting closed-lip schizencephaly

Prognosis

Can be associated with drug-resistant seizure.

If small or closed lip, neurologic deficit is mild.

When the cleft is large, there may be severe neurological deficit. Termination may be offered.

9.4.3 Cortical Dysplasia

Definition

Represents a heterogeneous group of cortical malformation and is a common cause of epilepsy postnatally.

Imaging Features

- Cortical dysplasia can be difficult to appreciate on fetal MRI and descriptions are based on postnatal high-resolution MR studies
- It is important to check for associated cortical dysplasia in fetuses with brain anomalies, such as corpus callosal dysgenesis.
- There may be focal cortical thickening, abnormal T2 hyperintensities or abnormal sulcal—gyral pattern (Fig. 9.18).
- There may be associated segmental or lobar hypoplasia/atrophy.

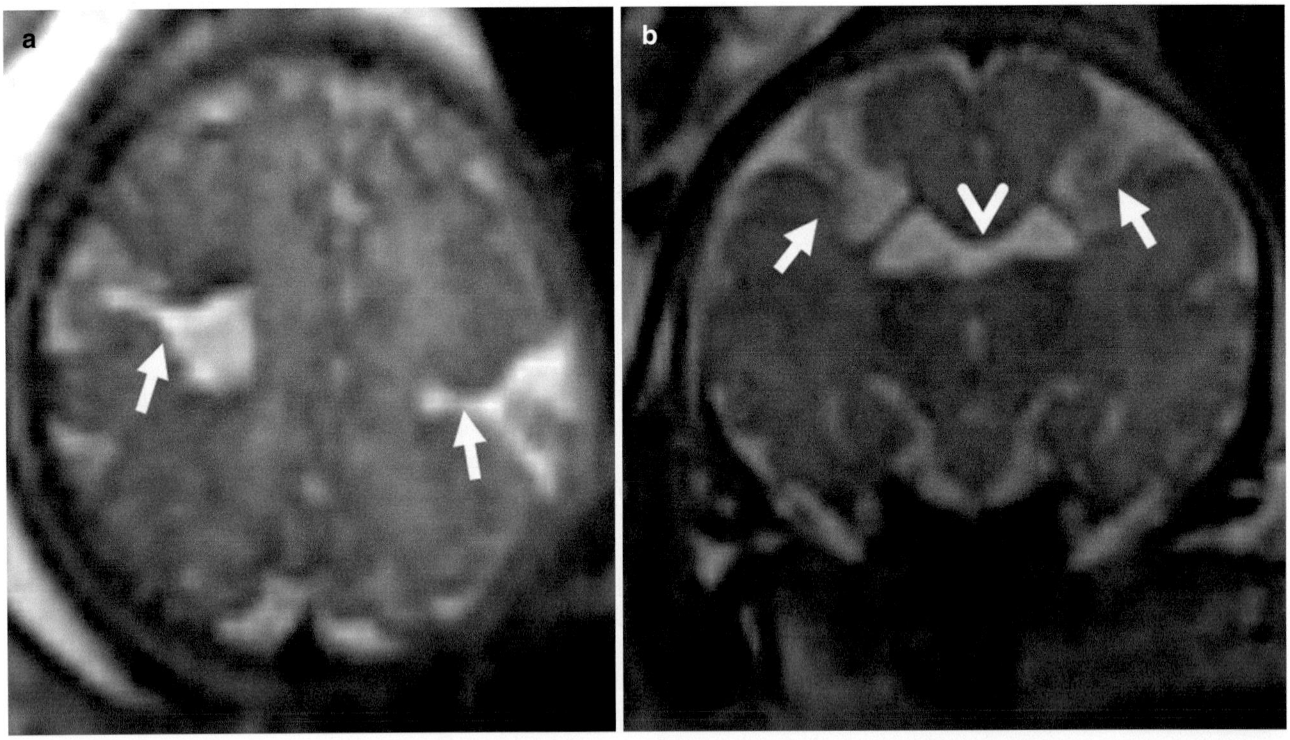

Fig. 9.17 Axial (**a**), coronal (**b**) T2W image of a 34-week fetus shows gray matter lined wide cleft (arrows) in bilateral frontal region suggesting open lip schizencephaly. Associated septal agenesis is also seen (arrowhead)

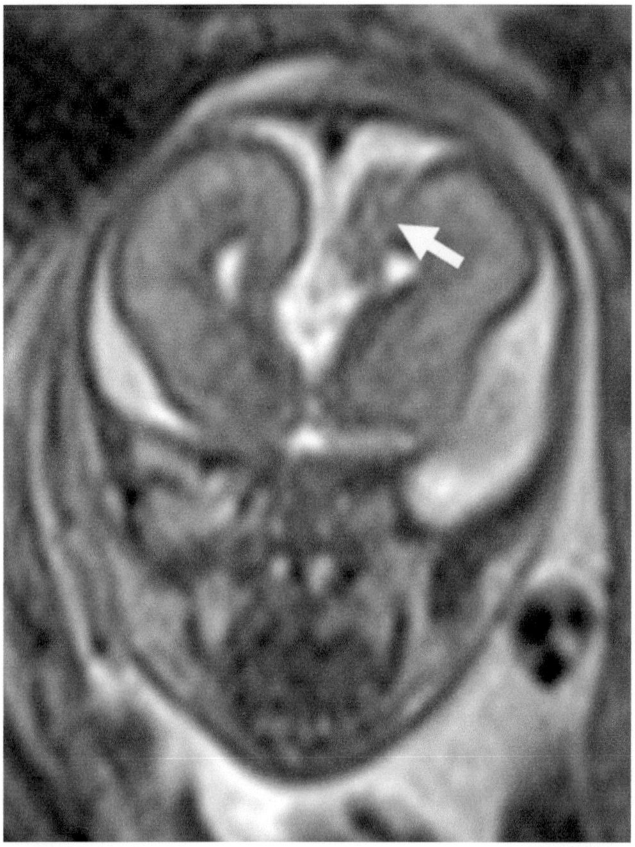

Fig. 9.18 Coronal image of a 27-week fetus shows focal cortical abnormality (dysplasia) (arrow) in the left frontal lobe in a case of agenesis of corpus callosum

Prognosis

It is a common cause of epilepsy postnatally and may require resection. Prognosis also varies depending upon the associated brain anomalies.

9.5 Group IV: Inborn Errors of Metabolism

Sometimes inborn errors of metabolism may manifest with cortical malformations—e.g., Microcephaly, Macrocephaly, heterotopias, and polymicrogyria [28, 29]. Associated findings include prominent subarachnoid spaces, subependymal or subcortical cysts, ventriculomegaly, cerebellar abnormalities, and corpus callosal dysgenesis.

References

1. Barkovich AJ, Guerrini R, Kuzniecky RI, Jackson GD, Dobyns WB. A developmental and genetic classification for malformations of cortical development: update 2012. Brain. 2012;135:1348–69.
2. Raybaud C, Widjaja E. Development and dysgenesis of the cerebral cortex: malformations of cortical development. Neuroimaging Clin N Am. 2011;21(3):483–543.
3. Rajeswaran R, Chandrasekharan A, Joseph S, Venkata Sai PM, Dev B, Reddy S. Ultrasound versus MRI in the diagnosis of fetal head and trunk anomalies. J Matern Fetal Neonatal Med. 2009;22(2):115–23.
4. Mohan A, Rangasami R, Chandrasekharan A, et al. Role of MRI in the diagnosis of fetal anomalies at 18–20 weeks gestational age. J South Asian Feder Obst Gynae. 2019;11(5):292–6.
5. Barkovich J, Gressens P, Evrard P. Formation, maturation and disorders of brain neocortex. AJNR Am J Neuroradiol. 1992;13:423–46.
6. Grissens P. Mechanisms and Disturbances of Neuronal Migration. Pediatr Res. 2000;48(6):725–30.
7. Ghai S, Fong K, Tai A, et al. Prenatal US and MR imaging findings of lissencephaly: review of fetal cerebral sulcal development. Radiographics. 2006;26:389–406.
8. Barkovich AJ, Kuzniecky RI, Jackson GD, et al. A developmental and genetic classification for malformations of cortical development. Neurology. 2005;65(12):1873–87.
9. Barkovich AJ, Guerrini R, Kuzniecky RI, et al. A developmental and genetic classification for malformations of cortical development: update 2012. Brain. 2012;135(5):1348–69.
10. Abdel Razek AA, Kandell AY, Elsorogy LG, et al. Disorders of cortical formation: MR imaging features. AJNR Am J Neuroradiol. 2009;30(1):4.
11. Guibaud L. Contribution of fetal cerebral MRI for diagnosis of structural anomalies. Prenat Diagn. 2009;29:420–33.
12. Sztriha L, Dawodu A, Gururaj A, et al. Microcephaly associated with abnormal gyral pattern. Neuropediatrics. 2004;35:346–52.
13. Vaishnavathy VV, Rangasami R, Suresh S, Suresh I. Fetal hemimegalencephaly. Neurol India. 2015;63:636–7.
14. Sonigo P, Elmaleh A, Fermont L, Delezoide AL, Mirlesse V, Brunelle F. Prenatal MRI diagnosis of fetal cerebral tuberous sclerosis. Pediatr Radiol. 1996;26:1–4.
15. Levine D, Barnes P, Korf B, Edelman R. Tuberous sclerosis in the fetus: second trimester diagnosis of subependymal tubers with ultrafast MR imaging. AJR. 2000;175:1067–9.
16. Okamura K, Murotsuki J, Sakai T, Matsumoto K, Shirane R, Yajima A. Prenatal diagnosis of lissencephaly by magnetic resonance image. Fetal Diagn Ther. 1993;8:56–9.
17. Fogliarini C, Chaumoitre K, Chapon F, Fernandez C, Levrier O, Figarella-Branger D, et al. Assessment of cortical maturation with prenatal MRI. Part I: normal cortical maturation. Eur Radiol. 2005;15:1671–85.
18. Kojima K, Suzuki Y, Seki K, Yamamoto T, Sato T, Tanaka T, Suzumori K. Prenatal diagnosis of lissencephaly (type II) by ultrasound and fast magnetic resonance imaging. Fetal Diagn Ther. 2002;17:34–66.
19. Stroustrup Smith A, et al. MRI of the kinked fetal brainstem: a sign of severe dysgenesis. J Ulrasound Med. 2005;24(12):1697–709.
20. Barkovich J, Kuzniecky R. Grey matter heterotopia. Neurology. 2000;55:1603–8.
21. Blondiaux E, Sileo C, Nahama-Allouche C, et al. Periventricular nodular heterotopia on prenatal ultrasound and magnetic resonance imaging. Ultrasound Obstet Gynecol. 2013;42:149–55.
22. Barkovich J. Morphologic characteristics of subcortical heterotopia: MR imaging study. AJNR Am J Neuroradiol. 2000;21:290–5.
23. DiMario FJ Jr, Cobb RJ, Ramsby GR, Leicher C. Familial band heterotopias simulating tuberous sclerosis. Neurology. 1993;43:1424–6.
24. Righini A, Zirpoli S, Mrakic F, et al. Early prenatal MR imaging diagnosis of polymicrogyria. AJNR Am J Neuroradiol. 2004;25:343–6.
25. Dhombres F, et al. Prenatal ultrasonographic diagnosis of polymicrogyria. Ultrasound Obstet Gynecol. 2008;32:951–4.
26. Denis D, Maugey-Laulom B, Carles D, Pedespan JM, Brun M, Chateil JF. Prenatal diagnosis of schizencephaly by fetal magnetic resonance imaging. Fetal Diagn Ther. 2001;16:354–9.

27. Oh KY, Kennedy AM, Frias AE Jr, Byrne JL. Fetal schizencephaly: pre- and postnatal with a review of the manifestations. Radiographics. 2005;25:647–57.
28. Mellerio C, Marignier S, Roth P, et al. Prenatal cerebral ultrasound and MRI findings in glutaric aciduria Type 1: a de novo case. Ultrasound Obstet Gynecol. 2008;31:712–4.
29. Poll-The BT, Gärtner J. Clinical diagnosis, biochemical findings and MRI spectrum of peroxisomal disorders. Biochim Biophys Acta. 2012;1822:1421–9.

10 Intracranial Cysts, Tumors, and Masses

10.1 Intracranial Cysts

The common intracranial cysts are arachnoid cyst, porencephalic cyst, choroid plexus cyst, and periventricular pseudocysts.

10.1.1 Arachnoid Cyst

Definition

Extra-axial cyst, made up of CSF and contained within the layers of the arachnoid membrane.

Imaging Features

- The role of MRI is to confirm the diagnosis, to differentiate from other cyst, and to rule out any cortical malformation.
- Extra-axial CSF intensity cyst seen [1].
- The common sites are interhemispheric region, collicular region, Sylvian fissure, skull base, and suprasellar regions.
- Can cause mass effect on the adjacent brain (Fig. 10.1)
- The adjacent calvarium may show scalloping.
- Doppler examination is useful to see the vascularity—to rule out vascular malformation resembling cyst.

Prognosis

Arachnoid cysts are associated with good prognosis if it is an isolated finding.

Commonly these cysts may resolve with increasing gestation [2, 3]. The remaining brain parenchyma is normal in most of the cases.

Very rarely when the cyst grows rapidly, they need to be monitored at regular intervals.

These cysts may require resection postnatally when there is a considerable mass effect. Shunting may be required when there is associated hydrocephalus due to the mass effect on the CSF pathway.

Differential Diagnosis

- Porencephalic cyst—Discussed in 10.1.2
- Schizencephaly—Communicate with lateral ventricle and the cleft is lined by grey matter.
- Dandy–Walker malformation—Is associated with enlarged IV ventricle and increased brainstem-vermian angle (>45 degrees). In case of posterior fossa arachnoid cyst, there may be mass effect with compression of cerebellar hemispheres and IV ventricle.
- Interhemispheric cyst associated with corpus callosum dysgenesis (Fig. 10.2a, b)—cyst may show septations, mass effect, and asymmetry of ventricles.

10.1.2 Porencephalic Cyst

Definition and Pathology

There is cyst formation due to infarction or focal destruction of the brain. The common causes are infection, hemorrhage, and ischemia due to placental abruption [4].

Imaging Features

- Smooth walled intraparenchymal cyst, sometimes communicating with the ventricle. There may be associated products of hemorrhage along the cyst. There is no mass effect (Fig. 10.3).
- MRI is useful to assess the associated parenchymal changes/encephalomalacia.

Differential Diagnosis

Arachnoid cyst—extra-axial in nature and may show mass effect.

Schizencephaly—Porencephalic cysts communicating with the lateral ventricles need to be differentiated from schizencephaly, which usually shows gray matter lining the walls.

R. Rajeswaran, *MR Imaging of the Fetus*, https://doi.org/10.1007/978-981-16-9209-3_10

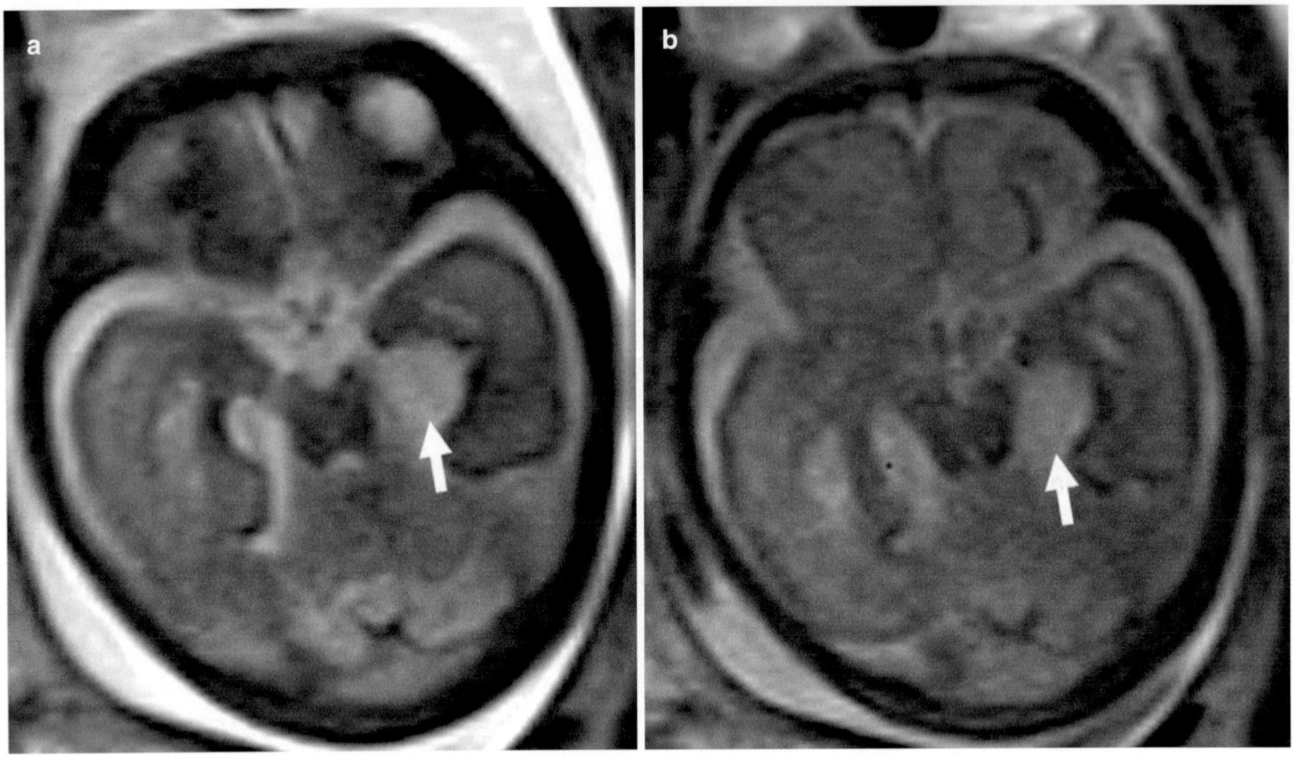

Fig. 10.1 Axial (**a**, **b**) T2W images of a 31-week fetus show an extra-axial cyst (arrows) in left median temporal region—Arachnoid cyst

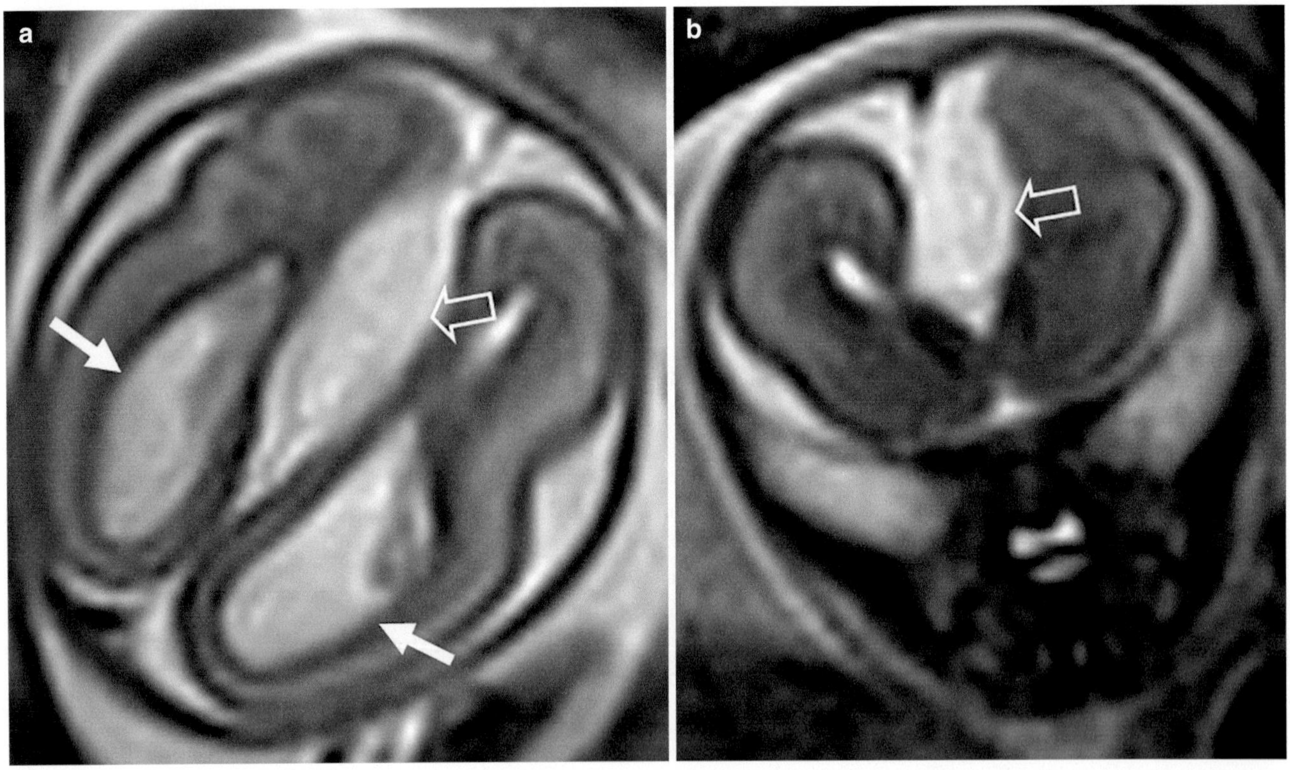

Fig. 10.2 Axial (**a**), coronal (**b**) T2W image of a 26-week fetus shows agenesis of corpus callosum, ventriculomegaly (arrow), and interhemispheric cyst (open arrows)

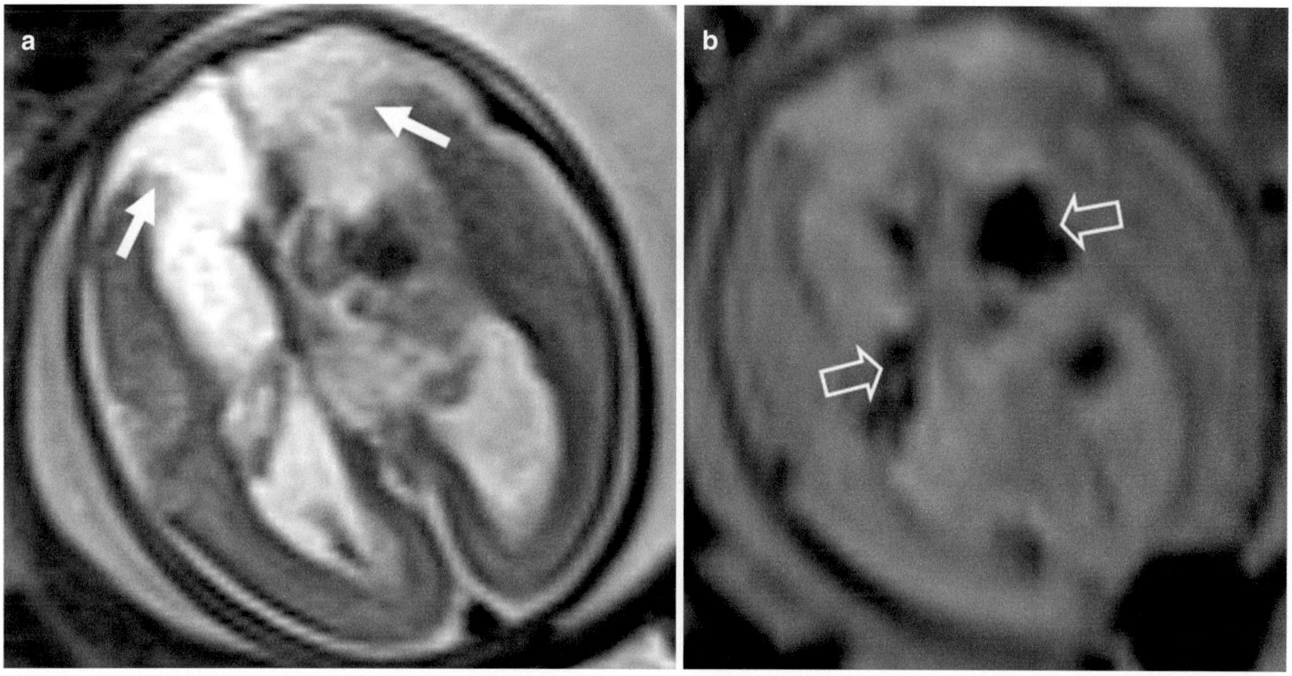

Fig. 10.3 Axial (**a**)-T2 and (**b**)-GRE images of a 25-week fetus show porencephalic cyst (arrows) in bilateral frontal region. Germinal matrix intraventricular hemorrhage is seen bilaterally (open arrows)

Prognosis
Depends on the location, the size, and the associated parenchymal changes. There can be associated seizure [5].

10.1.3 Choroid Plexus Cyst

It is seen along choroid plexus of the lateral ventricle. It may be incidental finding or may be associated with anomalies/trisomy 18 [6, 7].

Prognosis
Isolated choroid plexus cysts have a favorable outcome. Multiple choroid plexus cysts are a marker for Trisomy 18.

10.1.4 Periventricular Pseudocysts

They can occur secondary to infections, metabolic disorders, and chromosomal abnormalities (Fig. 10.4). Caudothalamic groove cysts can occur following a germinal matrix hemorrhage.

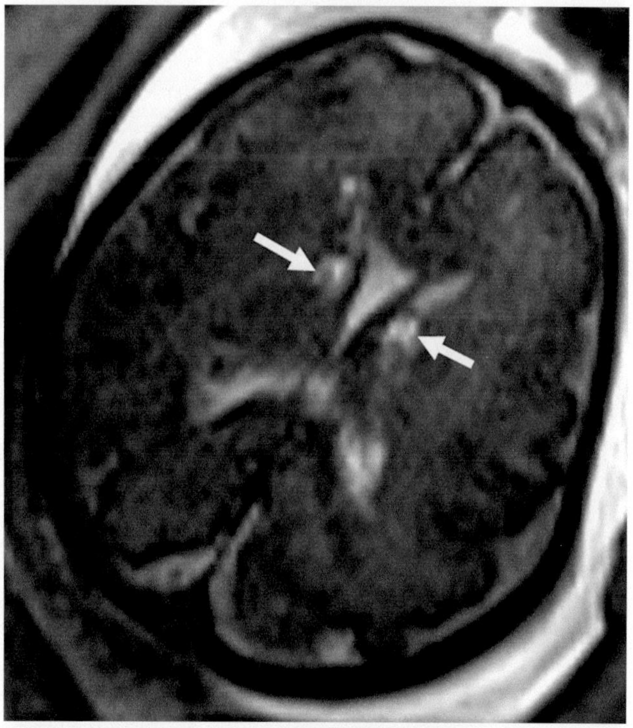

Fig. 10.4 Axial T2W image of a fetus shows bilateral periventricular cysts (arrow)

10.2 Vascular Abnormalities

These include Vein of Galen malformation and Dural venous sinus malformation.

10.2.1 Vein of Galen Malformation

Is an arteriovenous fistula, and can lead to high-output cardiac failure.

Imaging Features

- Fistulous arteries connect to the median prosencephalic vein of Markowski, which usually regresses by the 11th gestational week. If this connection persists it results in dilatation of the vein of Galen. Cerebral vascular steal can lead to brain ischemia and mass effect can result in hydrocephalus.
- MRI is useful to depict the brain parenchymal changes besides the malformation [8, 9].

10.2.2 Dural Sinus Malformation (DSM)

Definition

There is an abnormal development affecting dural sinuses/torcular Herophili.

The affected dural venous sinus shows focal dilatation. The superior sagittal, transverse, sigmoid sinuses, torcula heterophil can be involved. There is associated thrombus formation within the dilated sac.

Imaging Features

- Sonography—the dilated dural sac is seen as an echogenic or cystic lesion. Sometimes, flow is visualized in the non-thrombosed component.
- On sonography, DSM can be mistaken as a mass and MRI is useful to demonstrate the involvement of sinuses and thrombotic component.
- On MRI, the dilated dural sac appears hypointense on T2-weighted imaging and shows a triangular configuration (Fig. 10.5). The thrombus within the sac may be seen as hyperintense area on T1-weighted images or as an area of severe hypointensity on T2WI. There may be secondary intracranial hemorrhage, ischemia, or cortical malformations [10].
- Complications also include hydrocephalus and parenchymal atrophy.

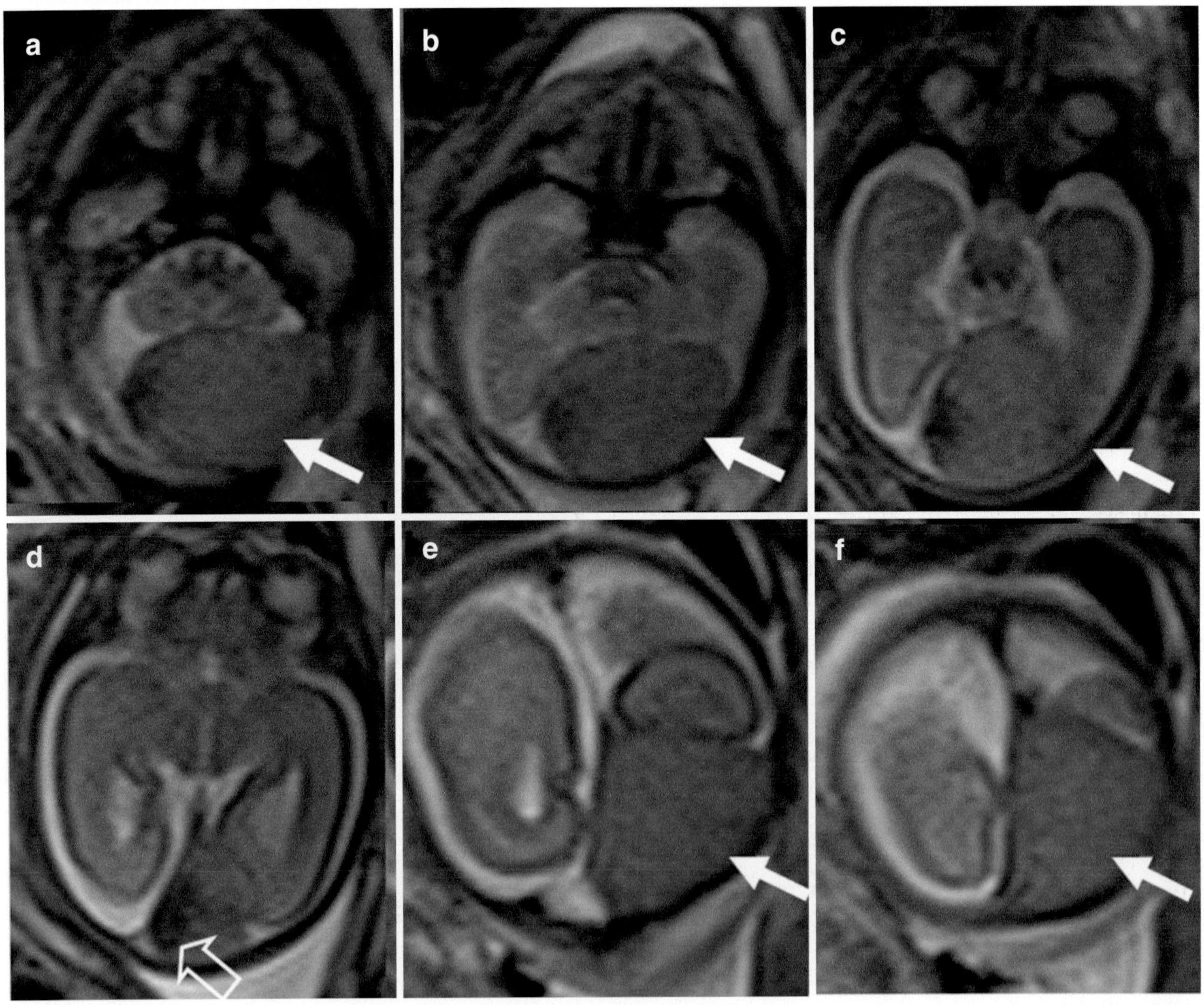

Fig. 10.5 Axial (**a–d**), coronal (**e**, **f**) T2W images of a fetus show an abnormal dilated posterior aspect of superior sagittal sinus and left transverse sinus (arrow) with a thrombus (open arrows) suggesting dural sinus malformation

Differential Diagnosis
Arachnoid cyst, hematoma, posterior fossa mass lesions.

Prognosis
- Is variable
- Good outcome, if there is no venous hypertension or ischemia and the brain is normal on MRI.
- Many of them regress spontaneously and show favorable outcome [11].
- There may be development delay postnatally in 20% of the cases.

10.3 Tumors

The common fetal brain tumors are teratoma, astrocytoma, craniopharyngioma, and primitive neuroectodermal tumor [12, 13]. Most tumors are associated with bad prognosis. Unlike children, 70% of fetal brain tumors occur in the supratentorial compartment and 30% occur in the infratentorial compartment. The most common tumor is teratoma. The etiology of tumors in fetal life is unknown. Fetal and/or maternal exposure to viruses, drugs, and radiation, may initiate tumor formation [14]. Developmental errors may also result in tumors in fetal life.

US imaging is the primary modality and demonstrates an intracranial mass with solid, cystic, or calcified components with or without hypervascularity. It is also useful to evaluate any associated fetal macrocrania [15]. MRI is useful to identify the exact site of the tumor, its extensions and the complications. MRI is also useful to differentiate tumors from hemorrhages [16]. The abnormalities associated with fetal intracranial tumors are macrocrania, intracranial hemorrhage, local skull swelling, secondary hydrocephalus, heart failure due to high-cardiac output, polyhydramnios, and hydrops [17].

10.3.1 Teratoma

- It is the commonest fetal brain tumor and the majority of them are histologically benign [18].
- It is seen as a midline irregular complex mass and can show solid, cystic, calcific components (Fig. 10.6).
- MRI is useful in assessing the remaining brain structures and in identifying the exact site of the tumor.

Differential Diagnosis
Intracranial hemorrhage—can be identified by MRI by the combination of sequences.

Prognosis—is bad. Postnatal complete resection is not possible in many cases. Termination is an option.

10.3.2 Lipoma

- Seen as an echogenic mass on ultrasound.
- It can be associated with agenesis/dysgenesis of corpus callosum.
- Seen as a curvilinear mass along the corpus callosum or as a midline lobulated mass (Fig. 10.7) in the interhemispheric region.
- T1 and T1 fat suppressed sequences are diagnostic.

Differential Diagnosis Intracranial hemorrhage.

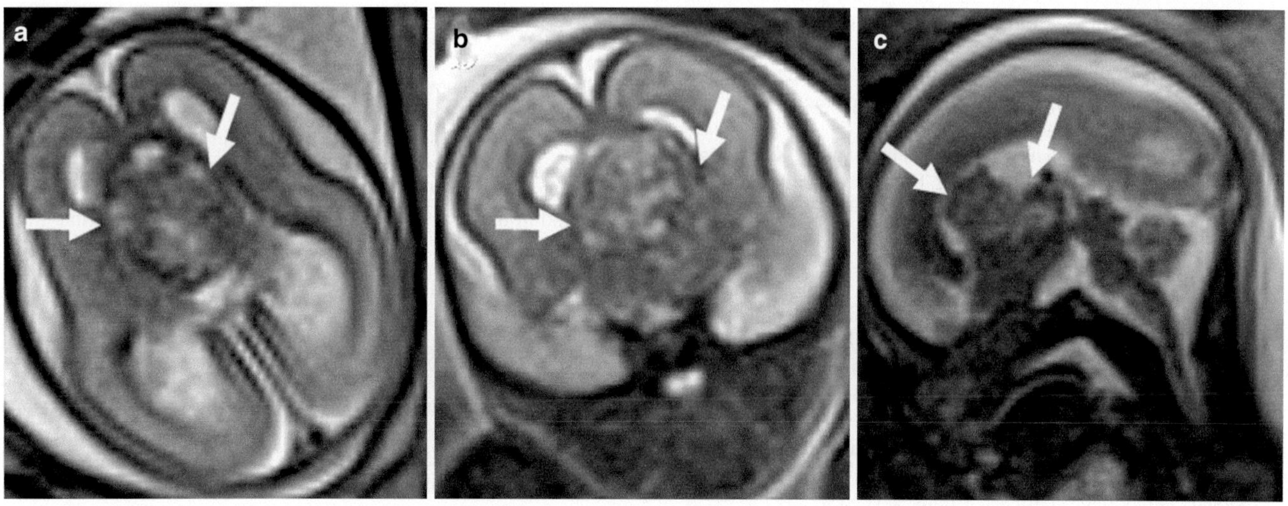

Fig. 10.6 Axial (**a**), coronal (**b**), sagittal (**c**) T2W images of a 22-week fetus show a well-defined soft tissue mass in the region of third ventricle (arrows), causing mild dilatation of bilateral lateral ventricles teratoma

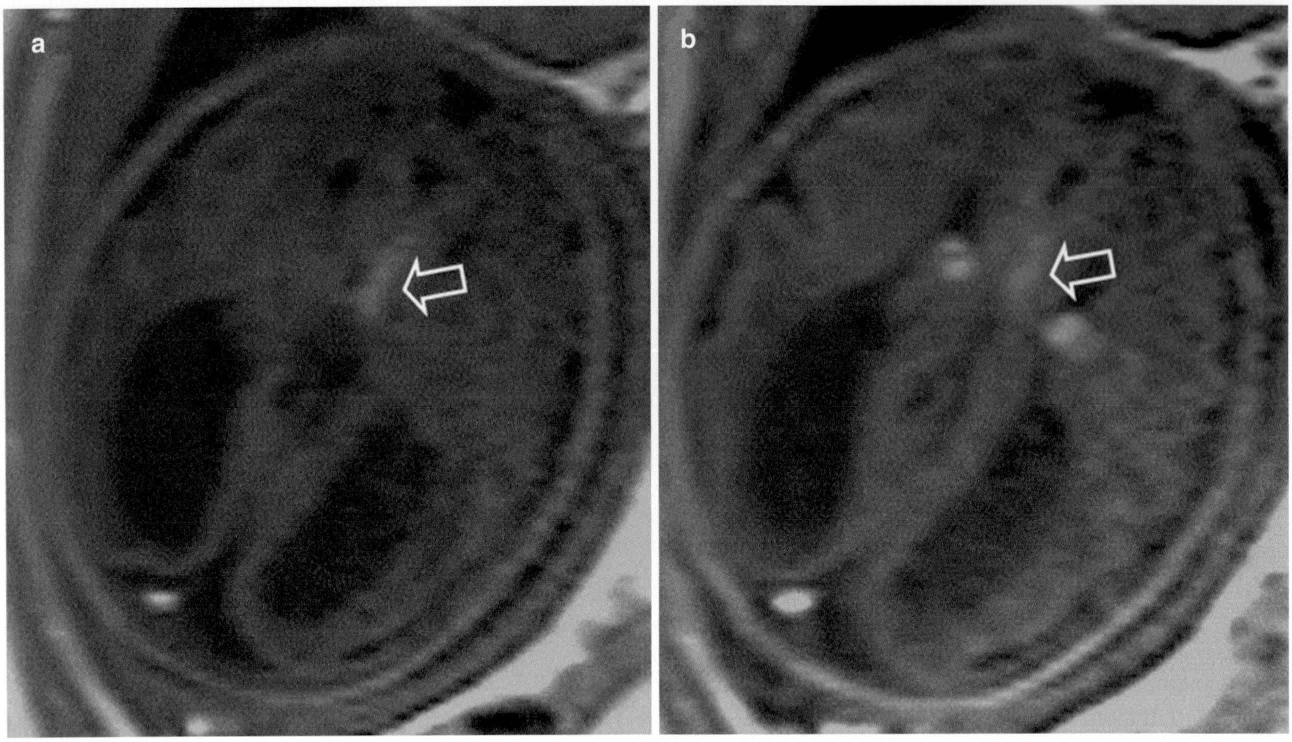

Fig. 10.7 Axial (**a**, **b**) T1W images of a 31-week fetus showing features of agenesis of corpus callosum and lipoma in the region of genu (open arrows)

References

1. Chen CP. Prenatal diagnosis of arachnoid cysts. Taiwan J Obstet Gynecol. 2007;46(3):187–98.
2. De Keersmaecker B, Ramaekers P, Claus F, Witters I, Ortibus E, Naulaers G, Van Calenbergh F, De Catte L. Outcome of 12 antenatally diagnosed fetal arachnoid cysts: case series and review of the literature. Eur J Paediatr Neurol. 2015 Mar;19(2):114–21. https://doi.org/10.1016/j.ejpn.2014.12.008.
3. Goksu E, Kazan S. Spontaneous shrinkage of a suprasellar arachnoid cyst diagnosed with prenatal sonography and fetal magnetic resonance imaging: case report and review of the literature. Turk Neurosurg. 2015;25(4):670–3.
4. Williams T, Wilkinson AG, Kandasamy J, et al. Antenatal diagnosis of intracranial haemorrhage and porencephalic cyst. Case Rep. 2015;2015:bcr2014209130.
5. Kokkinos V, Garganis K, Kontogiannis K, Zountsas B. Hemispherotomy or lobectomy? The role of presurgical neuroimaging in a young case of a large porencephalic cyst with intractable epilepsy. Pediatr Neurosurg. 2011;47(3):204–9. https://doi.org/10.1159/000330546.
6. DiPietro JA, Cristofalo EA, Voegtline KM, Crino J. Isolated prenatal choroid plexus cysts do not affect child development. Prenat Diagn. 2011;31(8):745–9. https://doi.org/10.1002/pd.2757.
7. Beke A, Barakonyi E, Belics Z, et al. Risk of chromosome abnormalities in the presence of bilateral or unilateral choroid plexus cysts. Fetal Diagn Ther. 2008;23(3):185–91.
8. Kwong Y, Cartmill M, Jaspan T, et al. Fetal MRI demonstrating vein of Galen malformations in two successive pregnancies—a previously unreported occurrence. Childs Nerv Syst. 2015;31:1033–5. https://doi.org/10.1007/s00381-015-2750-2.
9. Kalra V, Malhotra A. Fetal MR diagnosis of vein of Galen aneurysmal malformation. Pediatr Radiol. 2010;40:155. https://doi.org/10.1007/s00247-010-1813-5.
10. Merzoug V, Flunker S, Drissi C, et al. Dural sinus malformation (DSM) in fetuses. Diagnostic value of prenatal MRI and follow-up. Eur Radiol. 2008;18(4):692–9.
11. Grigoriadis S, Cohen JE, Gomori JM. Prenatal thrombosis of torcular Herophili with spontaneous resolution and normal outcome. J Neuroimaging. 2008;18(2):177–9. https://doi.org/10.1111/j.1552-6569.2007.00166.x.
12. Milani HJ, Araujo Júnior E, Cavalheiro S, et al. Fetal brain tumors: prenatal diagnosis by ultrasound and magnetic resonance imaging. World J Radiol. 2015;7(1):17–21. https://doi.org/10.4329/wjr.v7.i1.17.
13. Isaacs H. Fetal brain tumors: a review of 154 cases. Am J Perinatol. 2009;26(6):453–66.
14. Court Brown WM, Doll R, Hill RB. Incidence of leukaemia after exposure to diagnostic radiation in utero. Br Med J. 1960;2:1539–45.
15. D'Addario V, Pinto V, Meo F, Resta M. The specificity of ultrasound in the detection of fetal intracranial tumors. J Perinat Med. 1998;26:480–5.
16. Baburaj R, Rangasami R, Chandrasekharan A, Suresh I, Suresh S, Seshadri S. Utility of various ultrafast magnetic resonance sequences in the detection of fetal intracranial hemorrhage. Ann Indian Acad Neurol. 2018;21(04):275–9.
17. Pooh RK, Pooh K. Antenatal assessment of CNS anomalies, including neural tube defects. In: Fetal and neonatal neurology and neurosurgery. 4th ed. Philadelphia: Elsevier; 2009. p. 291–338.
18. Schlembach D, Bornemann A, Rupprecht T, Beinder E. Fetal intracranial tumors detected by ultrasound: a report of two cases and review of the literature. Ultrasound Obstet Gynecol. 1999;14:407–18.

11 Intracranial Hemorrhage, Destructive Pathologies, and Infection

11.1 Intracranial Hemorrhage

Definition Hemorrhage occurring within the fetal cranium. It is commonly diagnosed at 26–33 weeks.

Causes

- Alteration in fetal/maternal blood pressure.
  - Drug induced—e.g., Aspirin
  - Pre-eclampsia
  - Monochorionic twin demise
- Trauma
- Infection
- Maternal thrombocytopenia, coagulation disorders
- Placental abnormalities-insufficiency, abruption
- Fetal arteriovenous malformation

Pathology

The germinal matrix cells appear by 20 weeks. They are prone to hemorrhage due to fragile capillaries. Secondary venous infarct can also occur.

Imaging Features

Sonography: The hemorrhage appears echogenic in the hyperacute stage without color flow, isoechoic in subacute stage and later hypoechoic. There may be debris and sometimes septations within the lateral ventricles.

MR imaging: Intracranial hemorrhage can be intraparenchymal, periventricular, intraventricular, or extra-axial. Sonographic appearances of hemorrhage may sometimes be confusing and may resemble a mass. MRI is sensitive in detecting the different phases of hemorrhage from acute to chronic. MRI is useful in depicting the intraventricular/subarachnoid/intraparenchymal extensions and also the associated cyst formation, parenchymal ischemia and hydrocephalus. GRE (or EPI GRE), b0 diffusion, HASTE are important sequences to identify hemorrhage in the descending order and it is seen showing dark signal on these sequences [1]. Hemorrhage may appear hyperintense T1 and b800 sequences in subacute stage. By a combination of sequences, the age of hemorrhage can be predicted (Table 11.1) [1].

Grading of Intracranial Hemorrhage in Fetuses and Prognosis

Grade 1—isolated germinal matrix hemorrhage. Good outcome in 100% cases.

Grade 2—periventricular hemorrhage with ventricular extension. Good outcome in majority of cases (Fig. 11.1).

Grade 3—periventricular hemorrhage with ventricular extension + ventriculomegaly. Grade 4- Grade 3 hemorrhage with intraparenchymal extension (Fig. 11.2). Poor outcome in majority of cases with grade 3 and grade 4 hemorrhage.

Complications and Long-Term Effects

The complications of fetal intracranial hemorrhage are hydrocephalus intrauterine death and neonatal death. The long-term effects include developmental delay. Seizure disorder, cerebral and palsy [2, 3].

11.2 Encephalomalacia

There is focal/regional damage to the brain.

Etiology

- Ischaemia–monochorionic twin demise and ischemia in the surviving twin
- Infection–TORCH
- Placental abruption
- Arteriovenous malformation/vein of Galen malformation (vascular steal).
- Following laser treatment of twin–twin transfusion (4–7% incidence)
- Maternal trauma, hypotension

R. Rajeswaran, *MR Imaging of the Fetus*, https://doi.org/10.1007/978-981-16-9209-3_11

Table 11.1 The appearances of various stages of intracranial hemorrhage in different sequences

Stage	Duration	Hemoglobin	T1	T2	GRE
Hyperacute	<24 h	Intracellular oxyhemoglobin	Iso	Iso to hyper	Hypointense rim
Acute	1–3 days	Intracellular deoxyhemoglobin	Iso	Hypo	Hypo
Early subacute	3–7 days	Intracellular methemoglobin	Hyper	Hypo	Hypo
Late subacute	1–4 weeks	Extracellular methemoglobin	Hyper	Hyper	Central hyperintensity and peripheral hypointensity
Chronic	>4 weeks	Hemosiderin	Iso or hypo	Hypo	Hypo

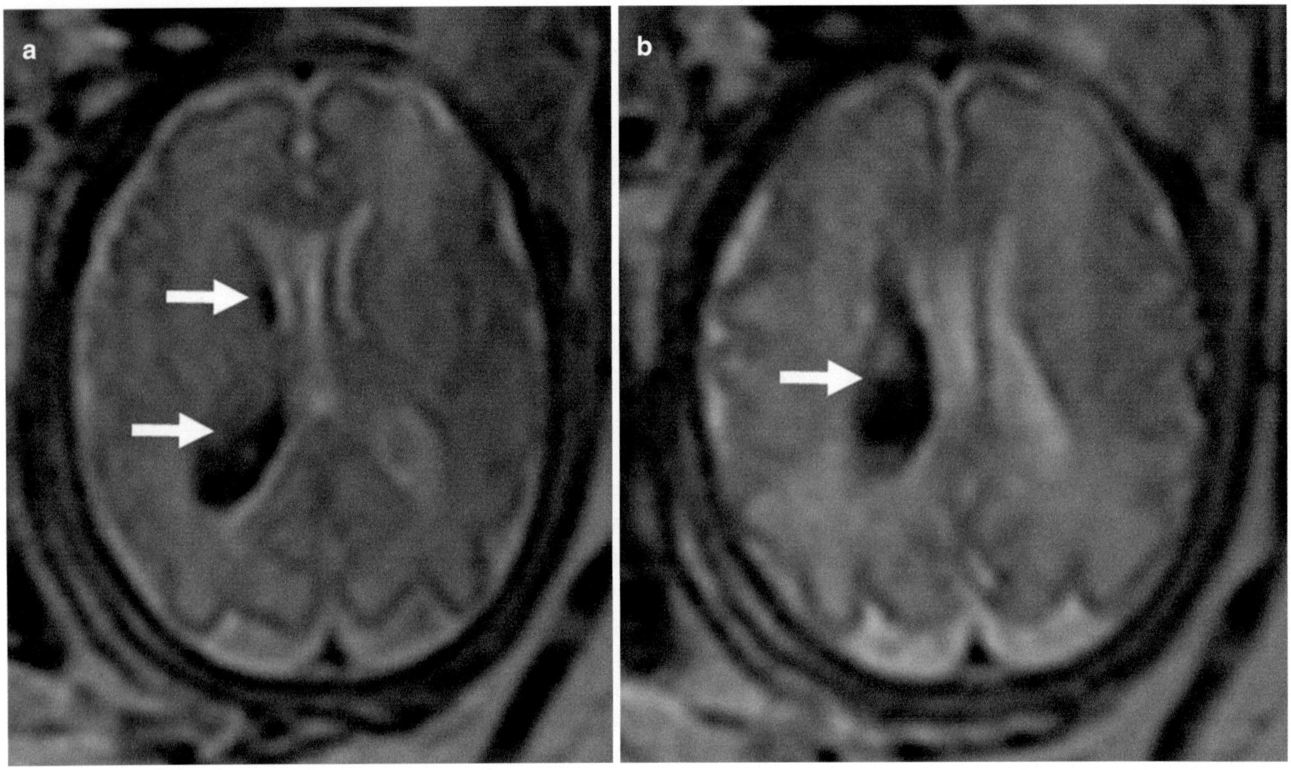

Fig. 11.1 Axial (**a**, **b**) T2W HASTE images of a 31-week fetus show a hypointense lesion in the right germinal matrix—intraventricular region (arrows)—Grade 2 Germinal matrix hemorrhage

Pathology

Following the regional/diffuse brain insult, there is astrocytic proliferation and glial septations.

Imaging Features

Sonography: In acute phase, the ultrasound may look normal. Later there may be echogenic area with irregular borders. Associated ex vacuo dilatation of the adjacent ventricle is seen.

MRI: To be done in suspected and at high-risk fetuses. There is hyperintensity in the affected brain parenchyma on T2-weighted images. There may be a hyperintensity on diffusion-weighted images in acute ischemia. Areas of hemorrhage/calcifications may be seen as hypointensities on T2-weighted images. There is associated dilatation of the adjacent ventricle.

Prognosis

- Depends on the size of the affected brain
- May be associated with developmental delay, seizures

11.3 In Utero Infections

The common in utero infections are due to TORCH (Toxoplasmosis, Other [Varicella-Zoster, syphilis], Rubella, Cytomegalovirus, Herpes), zika and parvovirus and brain abnormalities may be present. The fetus is more likely to get

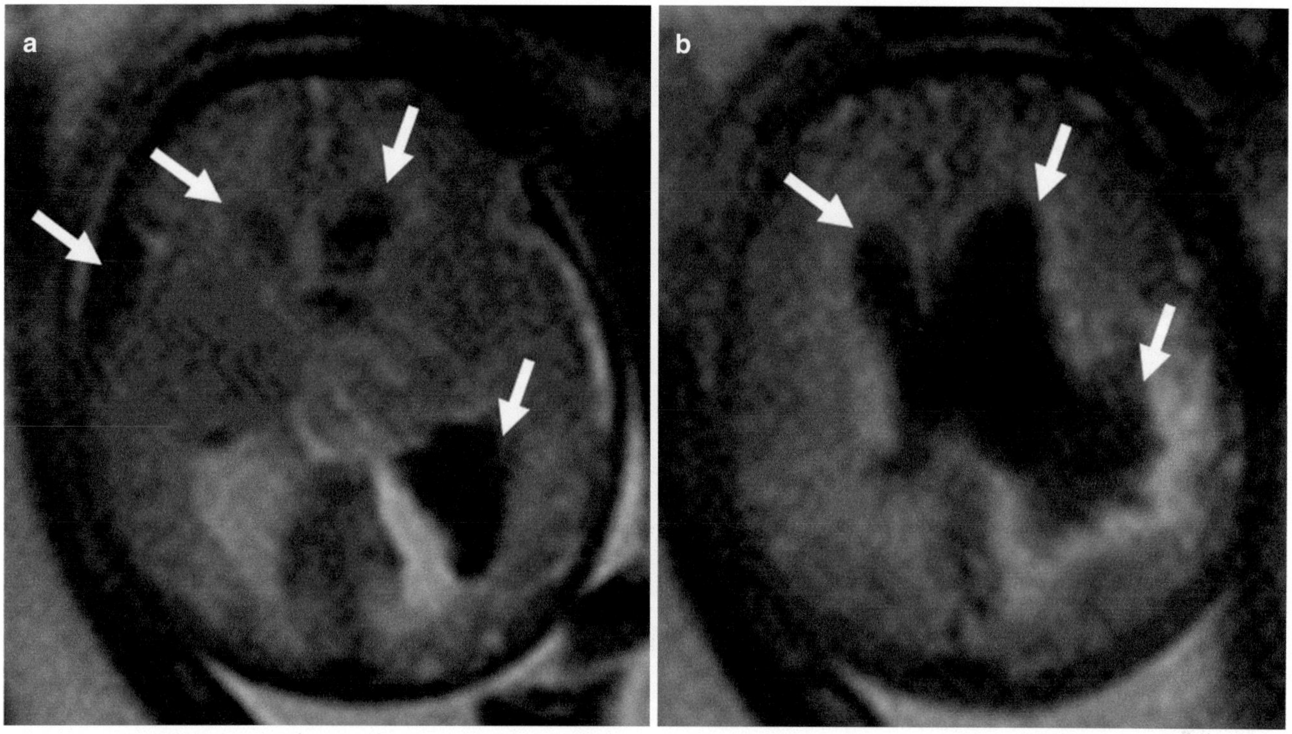

Fig. 11.2 Axial (**a**, **b**) T2W HASTE images show hemorrhage in the left germinal matrix with intraventricular/subarachnoid and intraparenchymal extension (arrows)—Grade 4 hemorrhage. There is associated mild ventriculomegaly

infected if the maternal infection happens early in gestation [4]. Once a maternal infection has been confirmed, the possibility of infection in the fetus needs to be worked up. Confirmation of fetal infection is possible by invasive testing like amniocentesis and cordocentesis. Generally, the amniotic fluid polymerase chain reaction (PCR) test will become positive after 6 weeks after the maternal infection. Fetal urination is not fully developed until 18–20 weeks' gestation, and hence amniocentesis should be delayed till 18–20 weeks' gestation, so that the virus will be present in urine (amniotic fluid) in sufficient concentrations.

Pregnant women who present with rashes, malaise, and/or other symptoms or signs suggestive of viral infection need to be investigated. The important tests utilized for diagnosing maternal infection are ELISA (enzyme-linked immunosorbent assay), paired serology tests for virus-specific immunoglobulin M (IgM) and immunoglobulin G (IgG) antibodies.

Fetal congenital infection may be suspected when some of these findings are visualized on ultrasound—microcephaly, cerebellar abnormalities, polymicrogyria, white matter signal abnormality. Multiple calcifications, parenchymal destructive lesions, cortical dysplasia, lissencephaly ventriculomegaly, hepatomegaly, splenomegaly, periventricular pseudo-cysts, and placentomegaly. Fetal MRI is extremely useful in demonstrating the brain parenchymal changes though the calcifications may not be well depicted.

Differential diagnosis: Fetal infections can be mimicked by pseudo-TORCH syndrome/Aicardi-Goutiere syndrome, a familial autosomal recessive disease that manifests with cortical malformations and calcifications.

11.3.1 Cytomegalovirus

It belongs to the human herpesvirus family and is the most common cause of congenital viral infection. It can affect multiple fetal organs.

Incidence—Approximately 0.2–2.2% of live births [5–7].

Pathology—It affects the fetus transplacentally from the mother.

Imaging Features [8–11]
Brain:

- Ventriculomegaly (Fig. 11.3a, b) can be mild to severe, the latter carrying a bad prognosis. Sometimes it can mimic aqueduct stenosis. Ventriculitis may be seen as irregularity and T1/T2 hyperintensity along the ventricular walls There may be associated intraventricular strands due to adhesions.
- Parenchymal—T2 hyperintensities in white matter and periventricular pseudocysts can occur. There may be

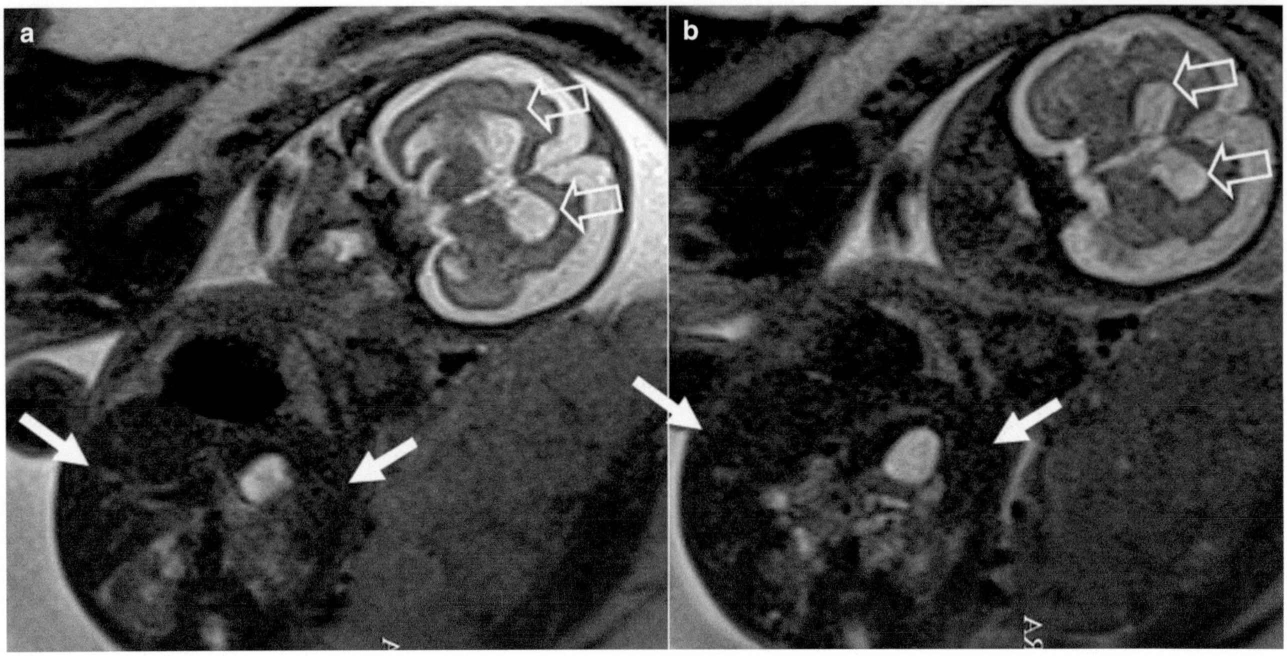

Fig. 11.3 Coronal T2W images (**a**, **b**) showing hepatosplenomegaly (arrows) in a 29-week fetus who was positive for CMV infection. Bilateral ventriculomegaly (open arrows) and cerebral atrophy are also seen in brain images

associated cortical malformations like cortical dysplasia, polymicrogyria, lissencephaly (Fig. 11.4a, b, d, e), pachygyria, and schizencephaly. Other findings include intraparenchymal calcifications (Fig. 11.4c, f), porencephaly, microcephaly, cerebellar atrophy.
- Microcephaly is associated with a poor prognosis, with the affected children having mental retardation.

Hepatosplenomegaly (Fig. 11.3a, b) may be present and low signal on T1 and T2WI may signify fibrosis.

Fetal growth retardation, Cardiomyopathy, nonimmune hydrops may be present besides poly or oligohydramnios.

The diagnosis is confirmed if the mother shows IgM antibodies or IgG antibodies (if she had been sero negative before the pregnancy). Amniocentesis can be performed to see viral secretion. However, it may take 5–7 weeks to become positive, after the infection.

Prognosis

It is important to note that the fetus need not be affected by the infection though it may have a confirmed infection. So, some of the infected fetuses may never develop structural abnormalities. Similarly, some normal-appearing infected fetuses on imaging can still manifest long-term sequelae. Seizures, neurological impairment, behavioral problems, sensorineural deafness, intellectual disability, and physical handicaps may be present postnatally. Termination is an option once the CMV infection is confirmed as it carries a bad prognosis.

11.3.2 Toxoplasmosis

This infection occurs in the mother when there is ingestion of infected meat/food due to improper cooking. The infection then spreads transplacentally and affects the fetus.

Imaging Features [12, 13]
- Brain—Ventriculomegaly may be present with intraventricular adhesions
- Intraparenchymal calcifications may be present in the basal ganglia or corticomedullary junction or periventricular locations. Sometimes obstructive hydrocephalus may be present. The other findings described are encephalomalacia, cerebral/cerebellar atrophy, microcephaly or macrocephaly due to hydrocephalus, cortical malformations, and chorioretinitis.
- Hepatic calcifications
- Fetal growth retardation

Amniocentesis can be performed and PCR test on the amniotic fluid is diagnostic.

Prognosis

For those affected fetuses, the severity of infection is related to the trimester of pregnancy when the transmission had occurred [14]. Infection during the first trimester may result in intrauterine death. Infection during the second trimester may be manifested with microcephaly, retinochoroiditis, and intellectual disability. Infection during the third trimester

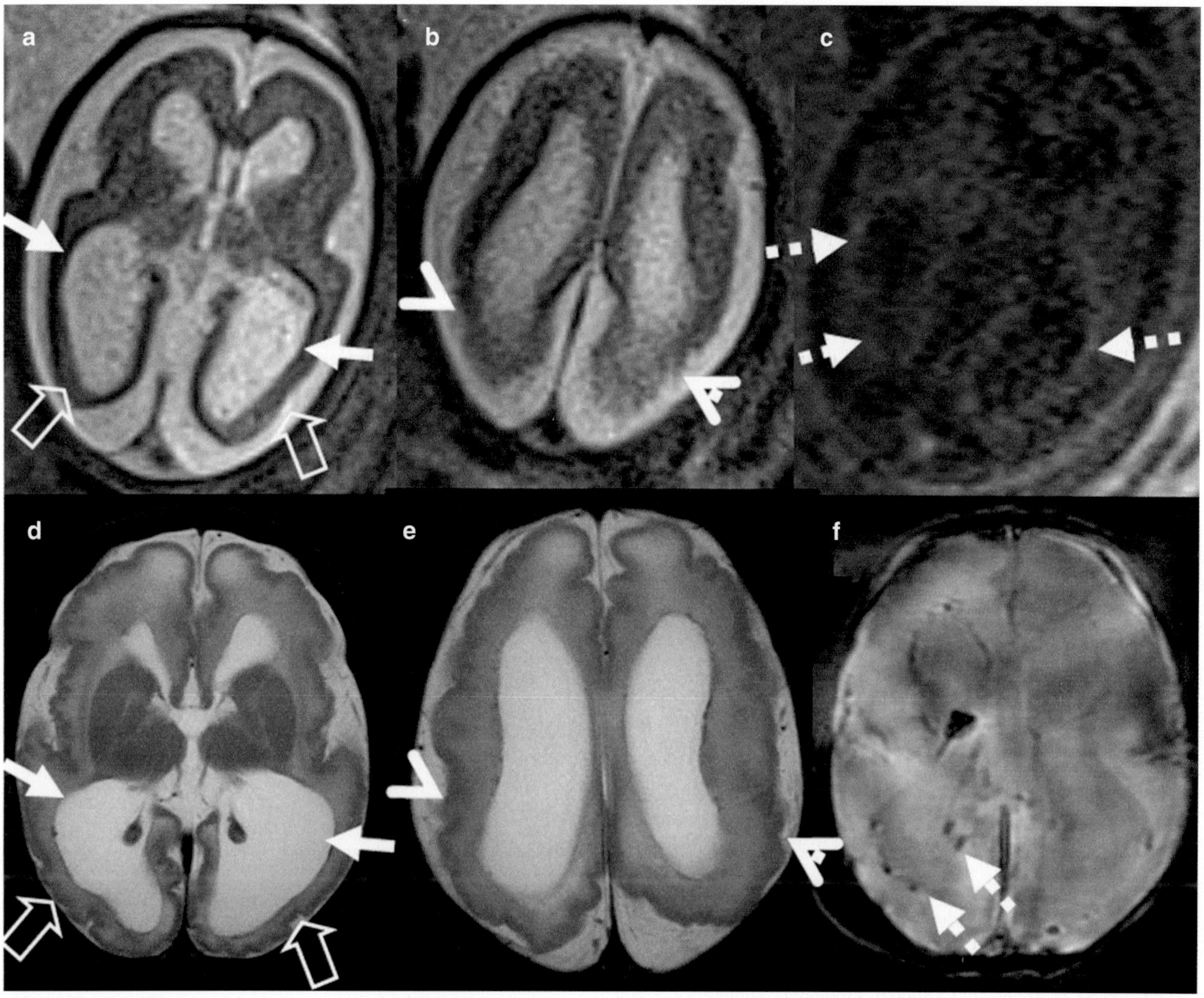

Fig. 11.4 Axial (**a**, **b**) T2W images of a 31-week CMV infected fetus shows ventriculomegaly, diffuse cerebral cortical thinning with generalized reduced sulcation and polymicrogyria (arrowheads). Axial (**c**) T1W image shows numerous small periventricular hyperintense foci (broken arrows) suggesting calcifications. Postnatal axial (**d**, **e**) T2W and GRE axial (**f**) images showing similar findings

may be manifested with lymphadenopathy, hepatosplenomegaly, ophthalmic pathologies, and brain calcifications.

Termination is an option once the infection is confirmed as it carries a bad prognosis.

11.3.3 Rubella

The imaging findings are similar to other infections and non-specific.

Imaging Features [15–17]
The important features are—Periventricular calcifications, white matter T2 hyperintensities, intraparenchymal cysts within brain, ventriculomegaly, microcephaly, congenital cataract, cardiac anomalies (especially tetralogy of Fallot and ventricular septal defect), and fetal growth restriction.

Prognosis
The affected child may have neurological/learning disabilities and sensorineural deafness.

11.3.4 Human Parvovirus B19

It is a type of in utero infection associated with fetal anemia, myocarditis, and intrauterine death. It is an inhibitor of erythropoiesis and attacks fetal erythroid progenitor cells.

Imaging Features [18, 19]
The important features are—fetal ascites, cardiomegaly, hydrops fetalis, hepatomegaly, polyhydramnios, and placentomegaly. Low resistance waveform may be seen on fetal MCA Doppler due to the presence of a fetal anemia.

Prognosis
Management consists of treating the fetal anemia, and in appropriate cases, by packed red cells transfusion into the umbilical vein. The development of hydrops fetalis carries a poor prognosis.

11.3.5 Zika Virus (ZIKV)

ZIKV belongs to the flavivirus family and is transmitted by Aedes mosquitoes or through human-to-human sexual contact. Zika virus commonly causes multiple teratogenic malformations. The developing brain is predominantly affected.

Imaging Features [20–23]
The important features are—Microcephaly, reduced cortical gyration and white-matter myelination abnormalities and cerebellar hypoplasia.

References

1. Baburaj R, Rangasami R, Chandrasekharan A, Suresh I, Suresh S, Seshadri S. Utility of various ultrafast magnetic resonance sequences in the detection of fetal intracranial hemorrhage. Ann Indian Acad Neurol. 2018;21(04):275–9.
2. Papile LA, Burstein J, Burstein R, Koffler H. Incidence and evolution of subependymal and intraventricular hemorrhage: a study of infants with birth weights less than 1,500 gm. J Pediatr. 1978;92:529–34.
3. Ghi T, Simonazzi G, Perolo A, et al. Outcome of antenatally diagnosed intracranial hemorrhage: case series and review of the literature. Ultrasound Obstet Gynecol. 2003;22:121–30.
4. Khalil A, Sotiriadis A, Chaoui R, da Silva CF, D'Antonio F, Heath PT, Jones CE, Malinger G, Odibo A, Prefumo F, Salomon LJ, Wood S, Ville Y. ISUOG practice guidelines: role of ultrasound in congenital infection. Ultrasound Obstet Gynecol. 2020;56:128–51.
5. Fowler KB, Stagno S, Pass RF. Maternal age and congenital cytomegalovirus infection: screening of two diverse newborn populations, 1980–1990. J Infect Dis. 1993;168:552–6.
6. Dollard SC, Grosse SD, Ross DS. New estimates of the prevalence of neurological and sensory sequelae and mortality associated with congenital cytomegalovirus infection. Rev Med Virol. 2007;17(355–363):5.
7. Kenneson A, Cannon MJ. Review and meta-analysis of the epidemiology of congenital cytomegalovirus (CMV) infection. Rev Med Virol. 2009;17:253–76.
8. Diogo MC, Glatter S, Binder J, Kiss H, Prayer D. The MRI spectrum of congenit al cytomegalovirus infection. Prenat Diagn. 2020;40(1):110–24. https://doi.org/10.1002/pd.5591.
9. Leruez-Ville M, Stirnemann J, Sellier Y, et al. Feasibility of predicting the outcome of fetal infection with cytomegalovirus at the time of prenatal diagnosis. Am J Obstet Gynecol. 2016;215(3): 342.e1–9.
10. Malinger G, Lev D, Zahalka N, et al. Fetal cytomegalovirus infection of the brain: the spectrum of sonographic findings. AJNR Am J Neuroradiol. 2003;24(1):28–32.
11. de Vries LS, Gunardi H, Barth PG, et al. The spectrum of cranial ultrasound and magnetic resonance imaging abnormalities in congenital cytomegalovirus infection. Neuropediatrics. 2004;35(2):113–9.
12. Antsaklis A, Daskalakis G, Papantoniou N, et al. Prenatal diagnosis of congenital toxoplasmosis. Prenat Diagn. 2002;22(12):1107–11.
13. Foulon W, Pinon JM, Stray-Pedersen B, et al. Prenatal diagnosis of congenital toxoplasmosis: a multicenter evaluation of different diagnostic parameters. Am J Obstet Gynecol. 1999;181(4): 843–7.
14. Capobiango JD, Breganó RM, Navarro IT, et al. Congenital toxoplasmosis in a reference center of Paraná, Southern Brazil. Braz J Infect Dis. 2014;18(4):364–71.
15. Sawlani V, Shankar JJ, White C. Magnetic resonance imaging findings in a case of congenital rubella encephalitis. Canadian J Infect Dis Med Microbiol. 2013;24(4):e122–3.
16. Tang JW, Aarons E, Hesketh LM, et al. Prenatal diagnosis of congenital rubella infection in the second trimester of pregnancy. Prenat Diagn. 2003;23(6):509–12.
17. Hwa HL, Shyu MK, Lee CN, et al. Prenatal diagnosis of congenital rubella infection from maternal rubella in Taiwan. Obstet Gynecol. 1994;84(3):415–9.
18. Chauvet A, Dewilde A, Thomas D, et al. Ultrasound diagnosis, management and prognosis in a consecutive series of 27 cases of fetal hydrops following maternal parvovirus B19 infection. Fetal Diagn Ther. 2011;30:41–7.
19. Dijkmans AC, de Jong EP, Dijkmans BAC, et al. Parvovirus B19 in pregnancy: prenatal diagnosis and management of fetal complications. Curr Opin Obstet Gynecol. 2012;24:95–101.
20. Brasil P, Pereira JP, Moreira ME, et al. Zika virus infection in pregnant women in Rio de Janeiro. N Engl J Med. 2016;375:2321–34.
21. Chibueze EC, Tirado V, da Silva Lopes K, et al. Zika virus infection in pregnancy: a systematic review of disease course and complications. Reprod Health. 2017;14:28.
22. Hazin AN, Poretti A, Di Cavalcanti Souza Cruz D, Tenorio M, et al. Computed tomographic findings in microcephaly associated with zika virus. N Engl J Med. 2016;374:2193–5.
23. Soares de Oliveira-Szejnfeld P, Levine D, de Oliveira Melo AS, et al. Congenital brain abnormalities and zika virus: what the radiologist can expect to see prenatally and postnatally. Radiology. 2016;281:203–18.

12 Fetal Face and Neck Anomalies

The fetal face is well demonstrated on three-dimensional ultrasound. However, in conditions like isolated cleft palate, craniosynostosis and complex craniofacial deformities occurring in holoprosencephaly MRI are complementary to sonography. MRI evaluation of the fetal face and neck includes the following sequences (a) Half-Fourier acquisition single-shot turbo spin echo (HASTE), which provides excellent visualization of the normal anatomy and the pathologies; (b) Fast Spoiled gradient echo (FSPGR) T1-weighted imaging to visualize thyroid gland, major cervical vessels, and intralesional blood products; (c) Echo planar imaging Gradient for the detection of calcification, blood products, and bony details; (d) Dynamic Steady-state sequence for assessment of swallowing.

Coronal images are useful for visualizing the nose and lips (Fig. 12.1a–c). The palate is best visualized on coronal and sagittal T2W images (Fig. 12.2) when amniotic fluid fills the fetal mouth and outlines the tongue and palate [1]. The pharynx and airway are filled with fluid and appear hyperintense on T2WI. MRI is useful in demonstrating the obstructing lesions and narrowed airway precisely, especially when ex utero intrapartum treatment (EXIT) procedures are contemplated [2]. The information on airway narrowing is useful in planning the method of delivery.

12.1 Cleft Lip and Palate

This term refers to a spectrum of clefting—usually involving the upper lip, the palate, or both with an incidence of one in 700 live births. The primary palate is formed by structures anterior to the incisive foramen—lip and alveolar ridge. The palatal structures posterior to the incisive foramen constitute the secondary palate. A cleft involving the primary palate, with or without the involvement of the secondary palate, is termed as cleft lip and palate.

Types Unilateral or bilateral or midline types.

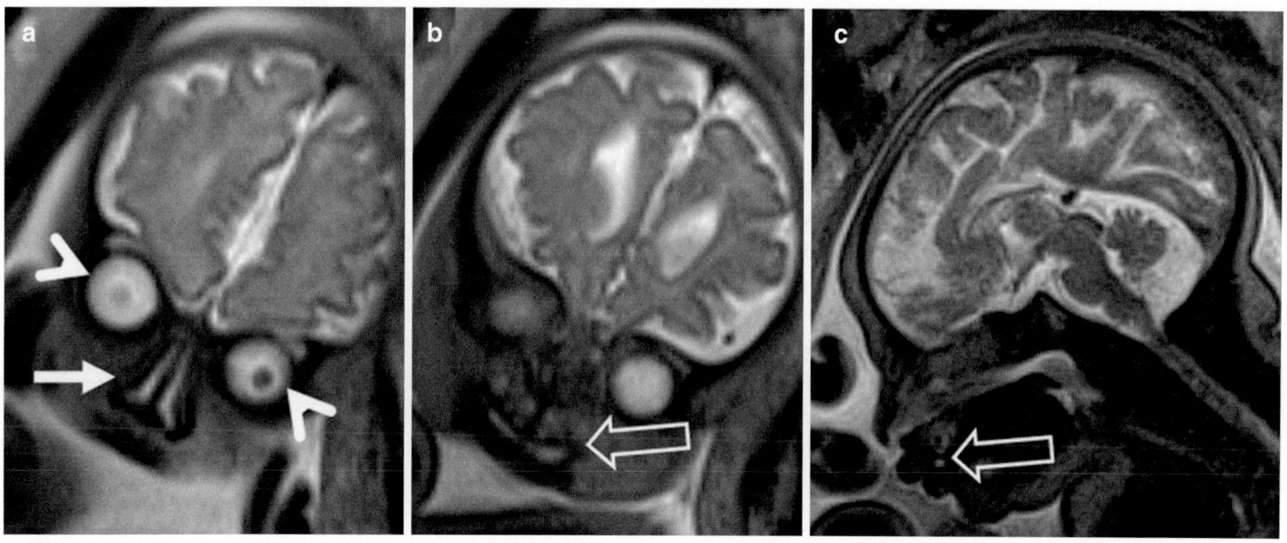

Fig. 12.1 Coronal (**a**, **b**) and sagittal (**c**) T2W images of a 34-week fetus showing normal nose (arrow), upper/lower lips (open arrows), and orbital globes (arrowhead)

R. Rajeswaran, *MR Imaging of the Fetus*, https://doi.org/10.1007/978-981-16-9209-3_12

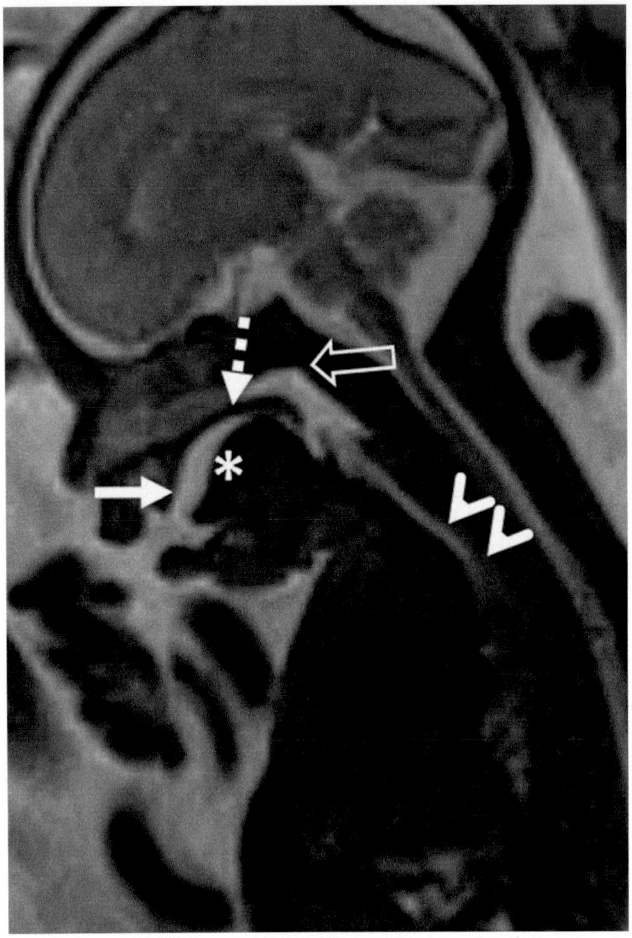

Fig. 12.2 Sagittal T2W image of the head and neck of a 22-week fetus showing normal oral cavity (arrow), nasopharynx (open arrows), oropharynx and cricopharynx. The trachea is visualized as a linear hyperintensity (arrowhead). The tongue (asterisk), palate (broken arrow), epiglottis are also visualized

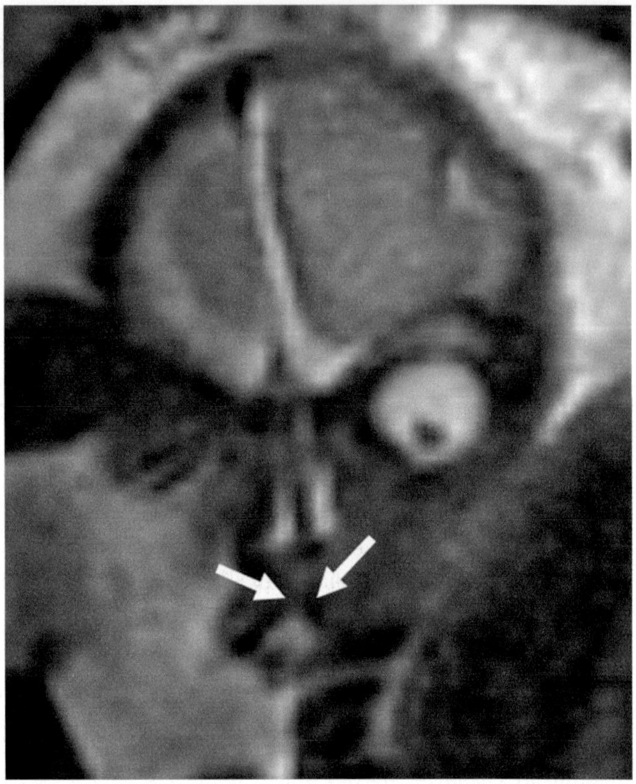

Fig. 12.3 Coronal image of a fetus showing median cleft lip (arrow)

Imaging Features [1]

- Cleft lip is seen better on 3-D ultrasound. MRI is also useful to identify the cleft lip and palate. Fluid within the nasal cavity is a clue to identify them. The tongue migrates cranially into the cleft palate.
- In unilateral cleft lip and palate, the axial and coronal images (Fig. 12.3) show the cleft directly beside the deviation of the anterocaudal portion nasal septum to the non-cleft side. In addition, the axial images show deficient or abnormal tooth buds in the medial alveolar ridge.
- In bilateral cleft lip and palate, the defect can be directly visualized on MRI (Fig. 12.4). Axial and midline sagittal images show protrusion of the premaxillary segment. In such cases, the tooth buds corresponding to the lateral incisors are deficient.
- MR is useful in identifying cleft in the soft palate, that may be difficult to demonstrate on US.
- They may be associated with hypognathism.

Prognosis It is sometimes associated with other anomalies like clubfoot, polydactyly, and congenital heart disease [3]. The prognosis is good if it is an isolated anomaly and the cleft is small. When there is a large defect, delivery in a tertiary care hospital is necessary as there may be respiratory and feeding difficulties [4].

12.2 Fetal Goiter

Definition There is enlargement of the fetal thyroid gland due to hypo- or hyperthyroidism. Normograms of sonographic thyroid circumference measurements are available.

Imaging Features [5, 6]

- The thyroid gland is diffusely enlarged in the anterior midline neck and may compress on the trachea, pharynx-esophagus (Fig. 12.5a–c).
- Sometimes, there is obstruction to swallowing leading to polyhydramnios.
- The neck may be hyperextended because of thyromegaly.
- Thyroid appears hyperintense on T1-weighted images (Fig. 12.5d) and intermediate signal on T2-weighted images.

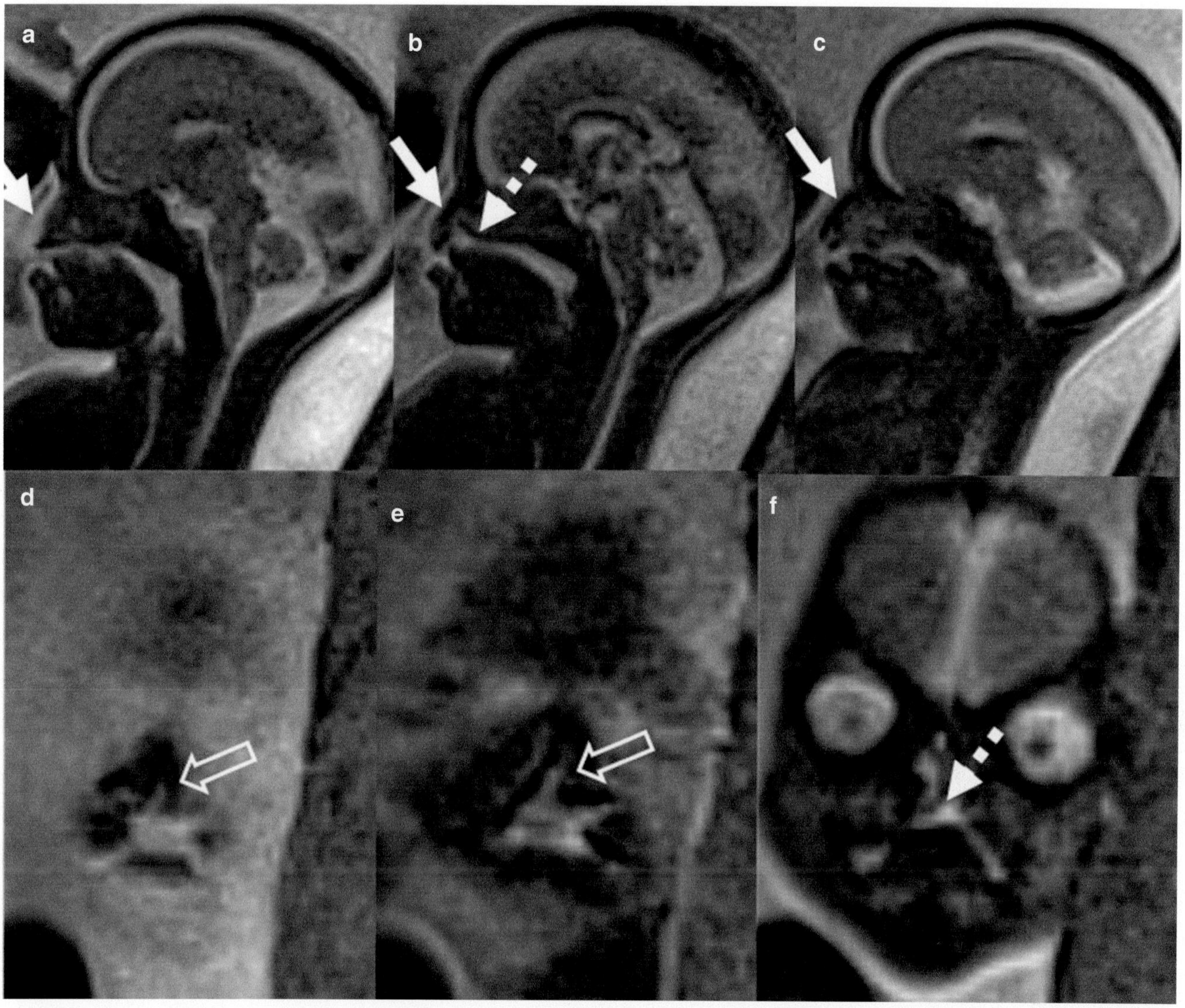

Fig. 12.4 Sagittal (**a–c**), coronal (**d–f**) images showing mid facial hypoplasia (arrows), cleft lip (open arrows) and cleft palate (broken arrow)

- MR is useful in planning in EXIT procedure in selected cases and treat appropriately.
- Fetal thyroid dysfunction can lead to cardiomegaly, high-output cardiac failure, and hydrops fetalis

Differential Diagnosis Cervical teratoma.

Prognosis
It is important to do a proper workup of maternal thyroid status and if abnormal, appropriate treatment of maternal thyroid disorder can lead to a reduction of fetal goiter. Fetal thyroid status can be assessed by umbilical cord blood sampling. If fetal hypothyroidism is present, intra-amniotic infusion of levothyroxine can be used to decrease goiter size [7]. Cesarean delivery in a tertiary care center with airway team availability/option for EXIT procedure is preferred because of the risk of airway compromise.

12.3 Cystic Hygroma

Synonym Nuchal lymphangioma.

Definition and Pathology It is a multiloculated cystic lesion due to veno-lymphatic malformation. There is a failure of the veno-lymphatic communication (between primordial lymphatic jugular sac and jugular vein). It can be associated with Turner syndrome/chromosomal abnormality/other anomalies/hydrops fetalis due to fluid overload.

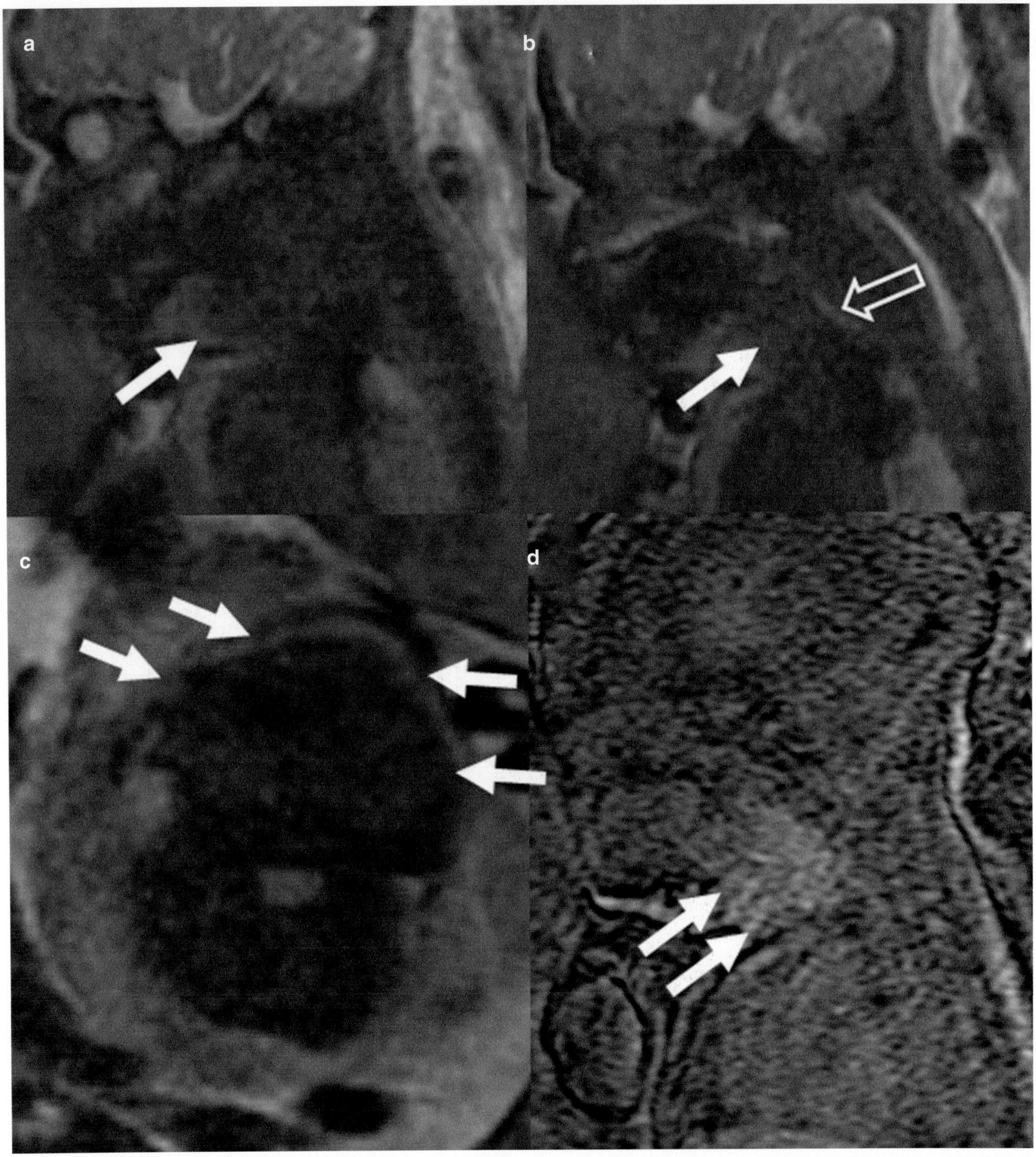

Fig. 12.5 Sagittal T2 (**a**, **b**) and axial T2W (**c**) images of a 35-week fetus shows a diffusely enlarged thyroid (appearing hypointense) with minimal intrathoracic extension—goiter. T1W sagittal image (**d**) shows hyperintensity of the lesion confirming thyroid glands. Larynx–trachea are significantly narrowed at this level (open arrows)

Imaging Features [8, 9]

- The lesion is seen in the posterior or lateral aspect of the neck and appears as a cystic lesion with multiple septations (Fig. 12.6a–d).
- The lesion appears hyperintense on T2-weighted imaging and shows an infiltrative pattern into different soft tissue planes (Fig. 12.6a–d) and mediastinum.

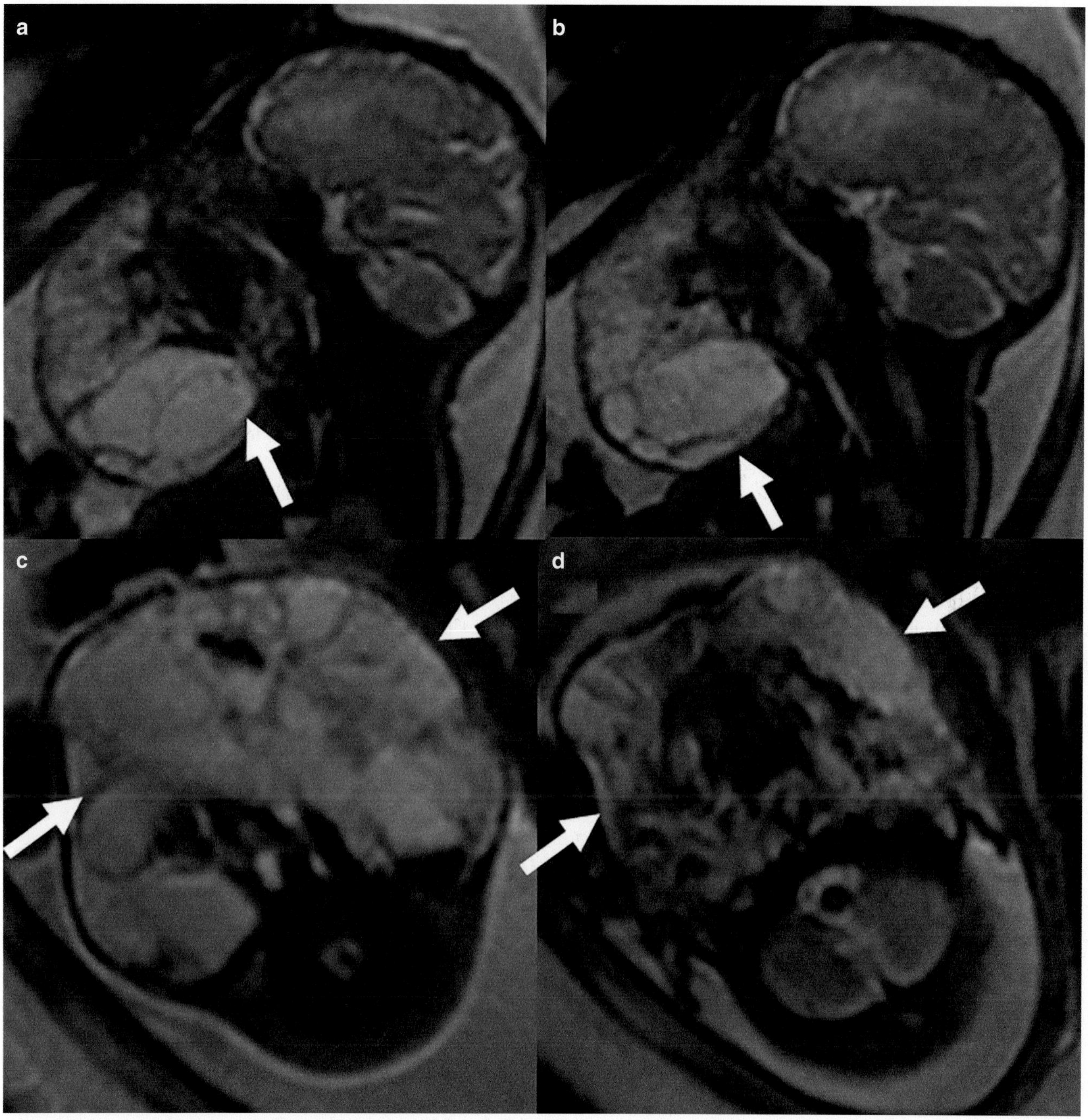

Fig. 12.6 Sagittal (**a**, **b**) and axial (**c**, **d**) T2W images of a 35-week fetus showing a large multiseptated cystic mass in the neck and inferior face in the anterior and lateral aspect—Lymphangioma (arrow)

- Four types are described based on MR appearance: Type I lesions are cystic lesions with multiple thin or thick internal septations; type II lesions are cystic lesions with less than three septations; type III lesions are purely cystic; type IV lesions have mixed cystic and solid components.

Differential Diagnosis

Meningo myelocele/Meningo encephalocele—Defect seen in the spine/cranium with herniation of the contents, better demonstrated by MRI.

Cervical teratoma—Lymphatic malformation shows an infiltrative pattern into multiple fascial planes, while teratoma tends to distort or displace surrounding tissue.

Prognosis

There is about 37% mortality when it is isolated.

There is about 75% mortality if associated with other anomalies.

In fetuses with large lesions, delivery in a tertiary care center with airway team availability/option for EXIT procedure is preferred because of the risk of airway compromise.

Prenatal sclerotherapy/aspiration of cystic components is another option. They are treated postnatally by sclerotherapy or by a combination of sclerotherapy and surgery [10–13].

12.4 Cervical Teratoma

Teratomas are classified as mature and immature types and most of them are benign and mature.

Imaging Features [8]

- It is common in the anterolateral neck, but can also be seen in the lower face, and upper mediastinum. The mass shows solid, cystic, and calcific components or may appear as a heterogenous mass.
- The fetal head may be hyperextended or turned to one side.
- Polyhydramnios is present when the pharynx/esophagus is compressed.
- Hydrops may be present when the teratoma is large.
- MRI is useful in defining the extent of mass and in demonstrating the compression of airway.
- Intratumoral necrosis and hemorrhage are associated with malignant transformation.

Differential Diagnosis

Cystic hygroma—multiseptated cystic mass present on the lateral aspect and does not show large solid component.

Goiter—homogenous mass in the thyroid location and maintaining the thyroid contour.

Prognosis

Because of the risk of airway compression, it is necessary to conduct the delivery in a tertiary care Hospital. EXIT procedure or EXIT to resection procedure may be needed if large and compressing the airway.

Termination is an option if it is diagnosed early. Postnatal resection of the lesion is curative [14].

12.5 Abnormal Orbits

The globes are visualized as rounded cysts in the upper fetal face. The lens are visualized as biconvex signal voids within them. Deviation from the normal measurements signifies some anomaly.

Interocular distance (IOD)—it is the distance between the inner margins of the orbits.

Binocular diameter (BOD)—the distance between the outer margins of the two orbits.

Ocular diameter—the diameter of single bony orbit.

Normal interocular distance = ocular diameter, i.e., an orbit should be able to be placed between two orbits.

Hypotelorism—the orbits are seen close to each other.

- The interocular diameter is less than the 5th percentile.
- May be associated with holoprosencephaly, metopic suture synostosis

Hypertelorism—the orbits are seen well apart from each other.

- The interocular diameter is greater than the 95th percentile.
- May be associated with corpus callosum dysgenesis.

Anophthalmia/microphthalmia

- The globe is absent or small and it can be unilateral or bilateral (Figs. 12.7 and 12.8).
- Can be secondary to chromosomal abnormalities, infection, and vascular insult

Dacryocystocele

- There is dilatation of the lacrimal sac/ductal system.
- Most of them resolve spontaneously.
- Seen as cystic area in the medial aspect of the orbit

12.6 Micrognathia–Retrognathia

In micrognathia, the mandible is small (Fig. 12.9) and in retrognathia there is a posterior displacement of the mandible. Mandibular abnormalities may be associated with syndromes. Sometimes, it is familial and hence it is important to check the physical appearance of the parents. In severe micrognathia, the tongue may obstruct the small oral cavity and cause polyhydramnios.

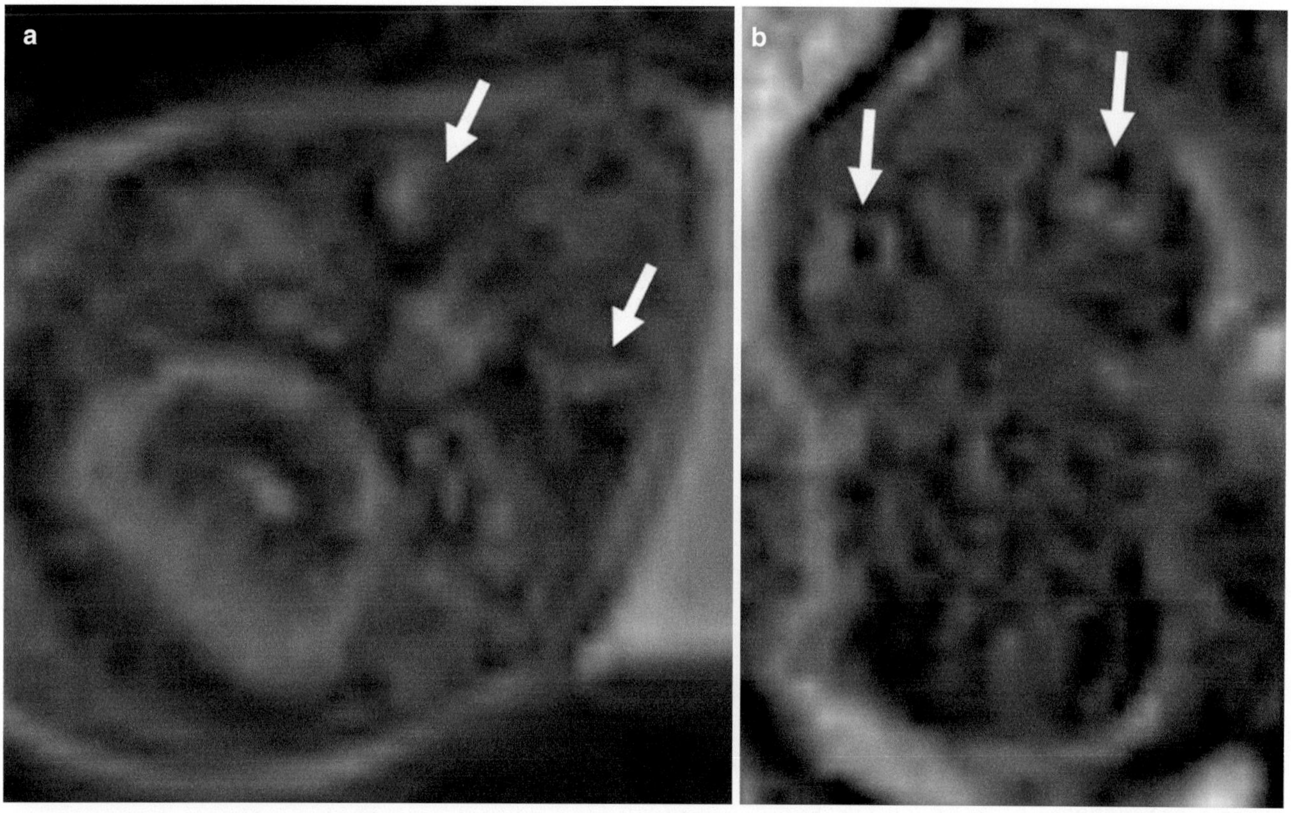

Fig. 12.7 Axial (**a**) and coronal (**b**) T2W images in an 18-week fetus, showing small orbital globes (arrows)—severe micro-ophthalmia

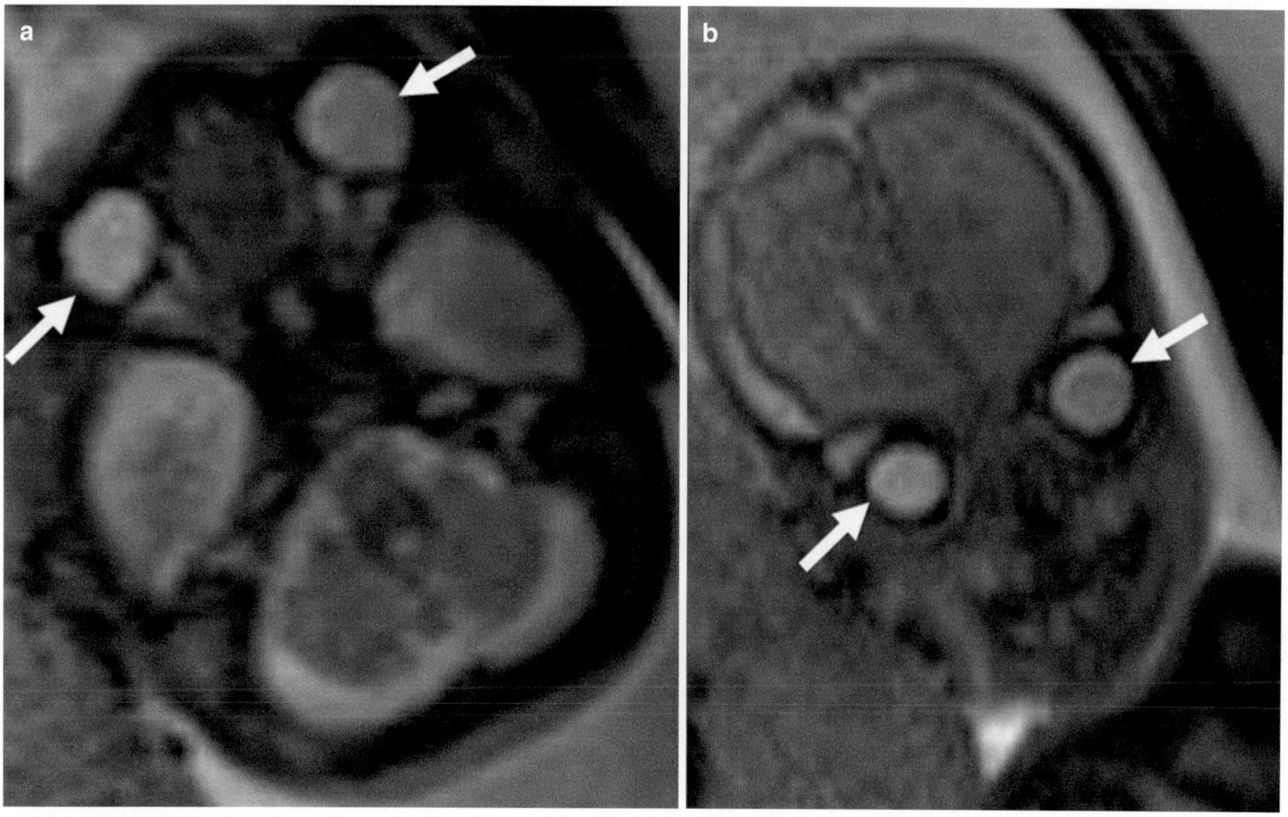

Fig. 12.8 Axial (**a**) and coronal (**b**) T2W images of a fetus, showing small orbital globes (arrows) microphthalmia and absent lens bilaterally

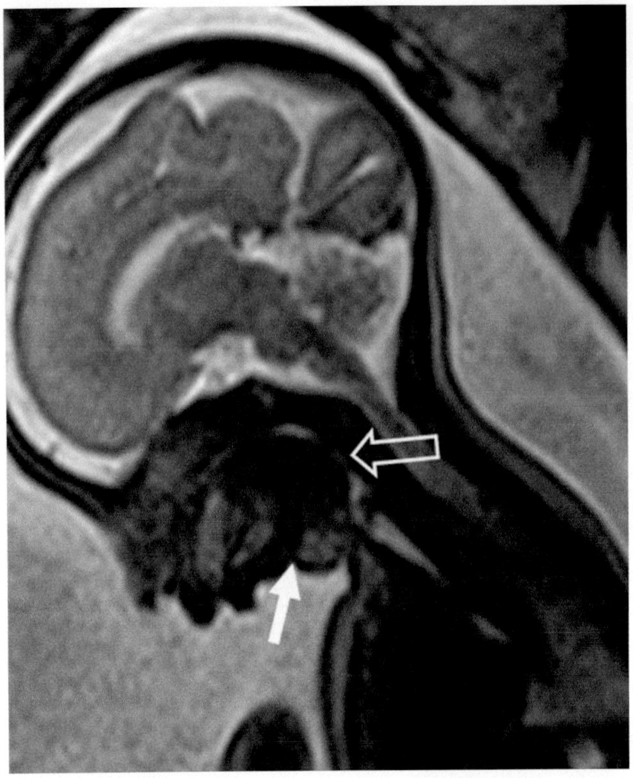

Fig. 12.9 Sagittal T2W images of a 34-week fetus showing severe retrognathism (arrow). The airway is severely narrowed (open arrows). The fetus was delivered by EXIT procedure and tracheostomy was performed subsequently

Sonographic measurements useful to assess the mandible objectively are (1) Jaw index, (2) mandibular area, (3) Mandibular width/maxillary width ratio, (4) Inferior facial angle, (5) Mandibular angle. They can be applied for MR imaging also.

Prognosis

Because of the risk of airway compression, it is necessary to conduct the delivery in a tertiary care Hospital. Neonatal mortality is very high (>80%) when there are associated abnormalities.

References

1. Stroustrup Smith A, Estroff JA, Barnewolt CE, Mulliken JB, Levine D. Prenatal diagnosis of cleft lip and cleft palate using MRI. AJR Am J Roentgenol. 2004;183(1):229–35.
2. Saleem SN. Fetal MRI: an approach to practice: a review. J Adv Res. 2014;5:507–23.
3. Hanikeri M, Savundra J, Gillett D, Walters M, McBain W. Antenatal transabdominal ultrasound detection of cleft lip and palate in Western Australia from 1996 to 2003. Cleft Palate Craniofac J. 2006;43:61–6.
4. Cohen MM. Etiology and pathogenesis of orofacial clefting. Oral Maxillofac Surg Clin North Am. 2000;12:379–97.
5. Fujii S, Nagaishi J, Mukuda N, et al. Evaluation of fetal thyroid with 3D gradient Echo T1-weighted MR imaging. Magn Reson Med Sci. 2017;16(3):203–8.
6. Harreld JH, Kilani RK, Lascola CD, Bartz SK. MR imaging of fetal goiter. AJNR Am Neuroradiol. 2011;32(8):E160.
7. Abuhamad AZ, Fisher DA, Warsoff SL, et al. Antenatal diagnosis and treatment of fetal goitrous hypothyroidism: case report and review of the literature. Ultrasound Obstet Gynecol. 1995;6(5):368–71.
8. Feygin T, Khalek N, Moldenhauer JS. Fetal brain, head, and neck tumors: prenatal imaging and management. Prenat Diagn. 2020;40:1203–19.
9. Peranteau WH, Iyoob SD, Boelig MM, et al. Prenatal growth characteristics of lymphatic malformations. J Pediatr Surg. 2017;52(1):65–8.
10. Laje P, Peranteau WH, Hedrick HL, et al. Ex utero intrapartum treatment (EXIT) in the management of cervical lymphatic malformation. J Pediatr Surg. 2015;50(2):311–4.
11. Pascoli I, Gritti A, Cutrone C, et al. EXIT (ex utero Intrapartum treatment) technique—management of a giant fetal lymphangioma. J Matern Fetal Neonatal Med. 2010;23(2):190–2.
12. Cahill AM, Nijs E, Ballah D, et al. Percutaneous sclerotherapy in neonatal and infant head and neck lymphatic malformations: a single center experience. J Pediatr Surg. 2011;46(11):2083–95.
13. Mikovic Z, Simic R, Egic A, et al. Intrauterine treatment of large fetal neck lymphangioma with OK-432. Fetal Diagn Ther. 2009;26(2):102–6.
14. Peiro JL, Sbragia L, Scorletti F, et al. Management of fetal teratomas. Pediatr Surg Int. 2016;32(7):635–47.

13 Fetal Thoracic Anomalies

The laryngotracheal tube develops from the primitive pharynx as a ventral diverticulum. It develops further to form the larynx and trachea at its cranial end and the lung buds in the distal aspect. During the 26th day of gestation onward, the lung buds continue to enlarge, divide and mature. The stages of lung development are (1) Embryonic stage (3–6 weeks), (2) Pseudoglandular stage (6–16 weeks), (3) Canalicular stage (16–28 weeks), (4) Saccular stage (28–36 weeks), and (5) Alveolar stage (36 weeks to childhood).

The trachea, carina, bronchi, and distal airways appear hyperintense on T2WI, as they are filled with fluid (Fig. 13.1). The normal fetal lungs appear homogeneous and moderately hyperintense on T2-weighted images (Fig. 13.2). With increasing gestation from 24 weeks, there is an increase in fetal lung volume and the T2 hyperintensity [1]. On coronal and sagittal images, MRI depicts the thoracic, abdominal structures, and diaphragm excellently due to its high contrast resolution [2]. The thymus is a homogeneous anterior mediastinal structure, shows intermediate signal intensity, and does not produce any mass effect on the surrounding structures. The diaphragms are seen as curvilinear hypointense bands between the lungs and the abdomen.

The commonly encountered non-cardiac thoracic anomalies are summarized in Box 13.1 [3, 4].

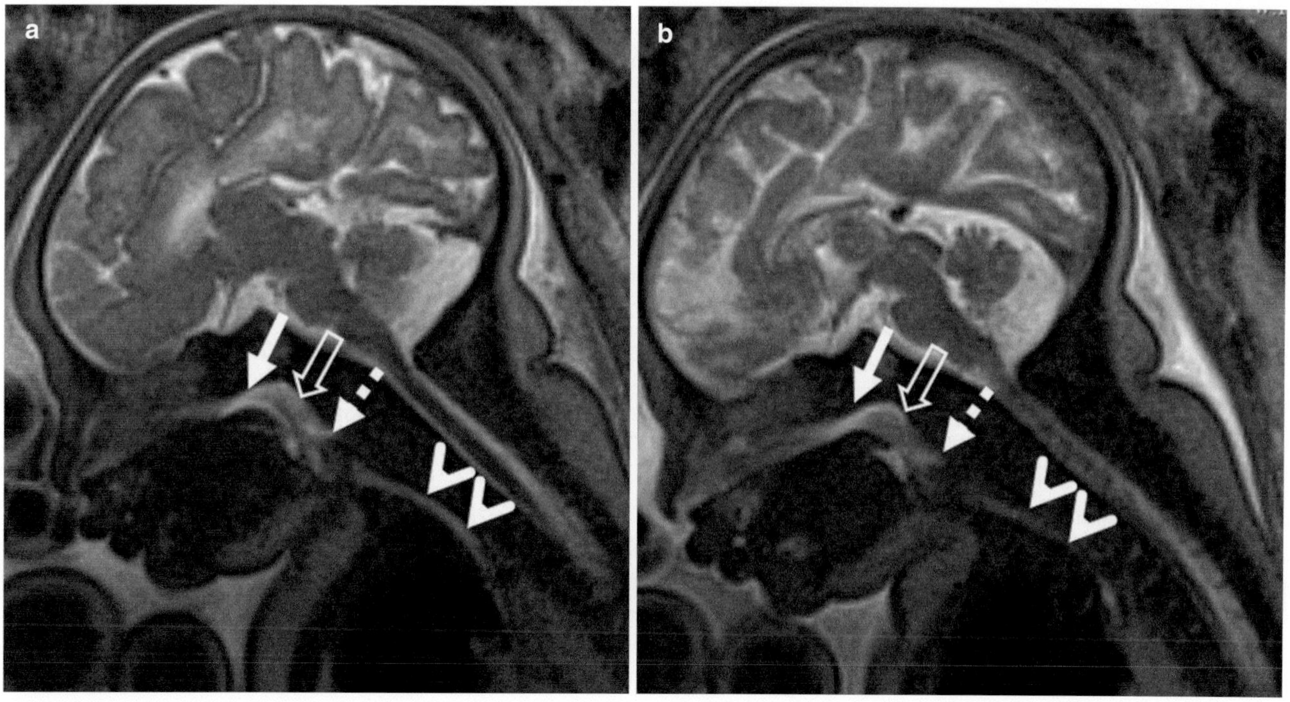

Fig. 13.1 Sagittal (**a**, **b**) T2W images of a fetus showing normal airway—nasopharynx (arrow), oropharynx (open arrows), laryngopharynx (broken arrow), and trachea (arrowhead)

R. Rajeswaran, *MR Imaging of the Fetus*, https://doi.org/10.1007/978-981-16-9209-3_13

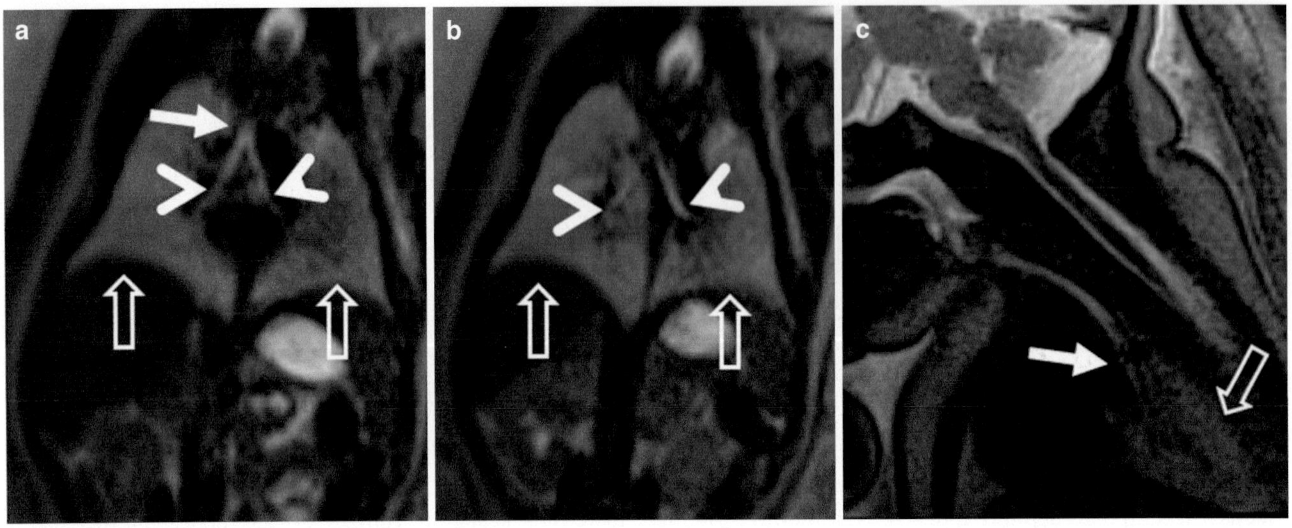

Fig. 13.2 Coronal (**a**, **b**) and sagittal (**c**) T2W images of fetal thorax showing normal tracheal bifurcation (arrow), bronchi (arrowhead), and lungs (open arrows)

Box 13.1 The Commonly Encountered Non-cardiac Thoracic Anomalies

Bronchopulmonary anomalies
Pulmonary underdevelopment (Lung agenesis-hypoplasia complex) Congenital pulmonary airway malformations (CPAM) Bronchopulmonary sequestration Congenital Lobar Overinflation Bronchogenic cyst Bronchial atresia
Vascular anomalies
Absence of the main pulmonary artery Anomalous origin of the left pulmonary artery Anomalous pulmonary venous drainage Pulmonary arteriovenous malformations.
Combined lung and vascular anomalies
Bronchopulmonary sequestration and Scimitar syndrome. Vascular abnormalities may sometimes be associated with bronchopulmonary abnormalities
Diaphragmatic anomalies
Congenital diaphragmatic hernia (with and without sac) Congenital diaphragmatic eventration
Mediastinal anomalies and masses
Esophageal duplication Thymic cyst Teratoma Neuroenteric cyst Tracheoesophageal fistula

13.1 Bronchopulmonary Anomalies

These anomalies arise due to abnormal development of the laryngotracheal tube—lung bud.

13.1.1 Pulmonary Underdevelopment

This spectrum includes Pulmonary agenesis, Pulmonary aplasia, Pulmonary hypoplasia.

Pulmonary agenesis—The lung, ipsilateral bronchus, and pulmonary artery are absent with associated ipsilateral mediastinal shift. In aplasia, rudimentary bronchus is seen on the affected side, though the other findings are similar to agenesis.

Pulmonary hypoplasia can be primary or secondary to causes like chest masses, congenital diaphragmatic hernia, eventration (Fig. 13.3), oligohydramnios, renal anomalies, and skeletal dysplasias.

Imaging Features

- The lung volume is reduced and MR is useful in the volumetric assessment of lung.
- Pulmonary vessels are reduced in size and number.
- Thoracic circumference less than the 5th percentile for the gestational age [5]. The thoracic circumference is measured in the axial plane at the level of the four-chamber view of the heart.
- Associated anomalies/oligohydramnios may be present.

13.1.2 Congenital Pulmonary Airway Malformations (CPAM)

Definition

These lesions result from the failure of a proper bronchoalveolar development with a hamartomatous development of terminal respiratory units into a glandular pattern (adenomatoid). The incidence is approximately 1 in 2500 births.

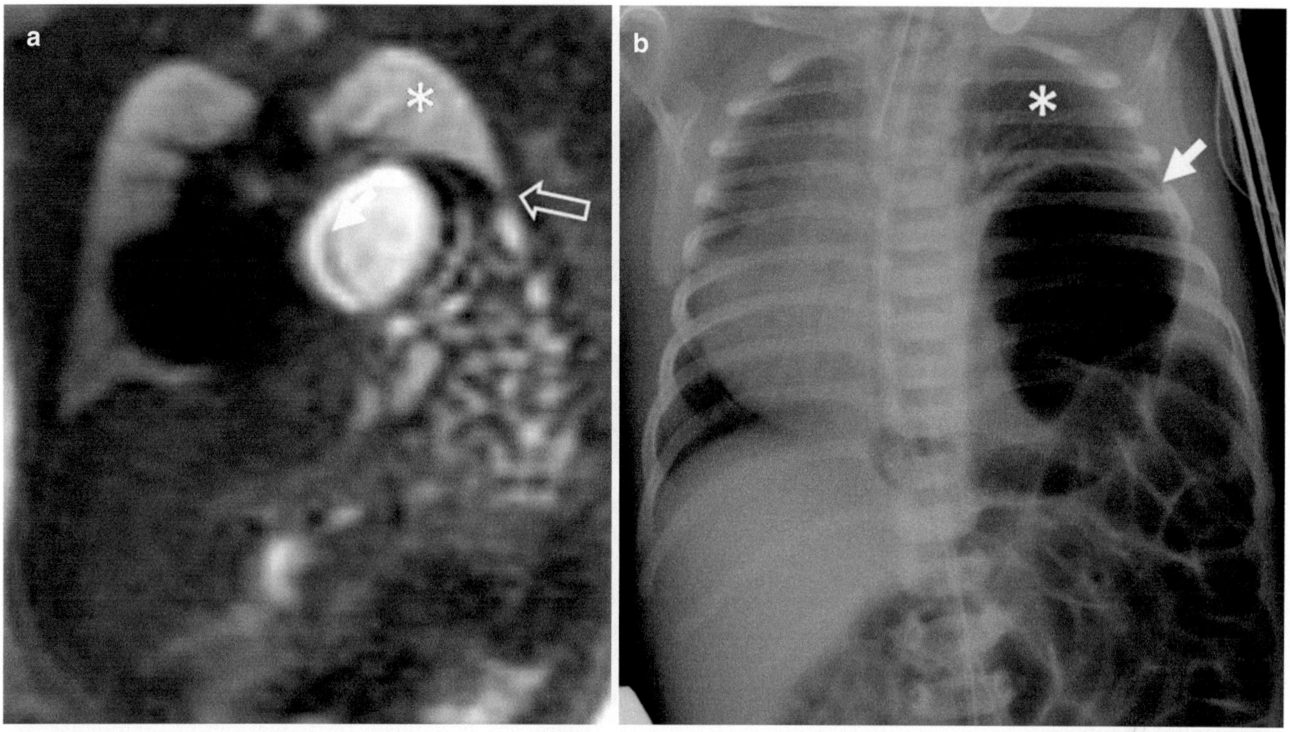

Fig. 13.3 Coronal T2 (**a**) image, showing eventration of left hemidiaphragm. The left hemidiaphragm is seen as a thin dark band (open arrow). The left lung is hypoplastic (asterisk). Postnatal chest radiograph (**b**) confirms the diagnosis of eventration (arrow) and hypoplastic left lung (asterisk)

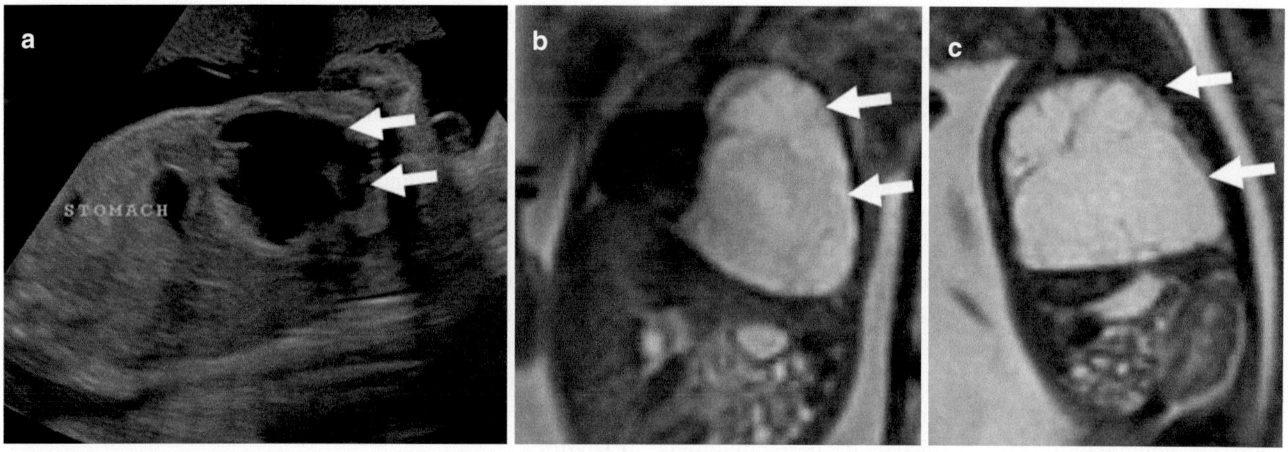

Fig. 13.4 Longitudinal sonographic image (**a**) shows multiseptated cystic lesion in the left lung (arrow). Coronal, sagittal T2W images (**b**, **c**) show a large multiseptated cystic lesion (arrow) in the left lung with mass effect suggesting Congenital pulmonary airway malformation

Imaging Features

- The imaging features depend on whether the lesions are macrocystic or microcystic.
- Macrocystic (Type 1)—1 or more cysts ≥2 cm, Cystic lesions are seen separately.
- Macrocystic (Type 2)—1 or more cysts <2 cm and >5 mm, Cystic lesions seen separately (Fig. 13.4a–c).
- Microcystic (Type 3)—1 or more cysts <5 mm Homogeneously moderately hyperintense mass on T2WI (Differential diagnosis: bronchopulmonary sequestration, that shows a feeding artery from the aorta).
- Type 4—Larger unlined cysts that are indistinguishable from Type 1 cysts
- Type 0—Very rare and lethal. Shows acinar dysgenesis or dysplasia
- *Hybrid lesions* (CPAM and bronchopulmonary sequestration)—An abnormal systemic arterial blood supply may

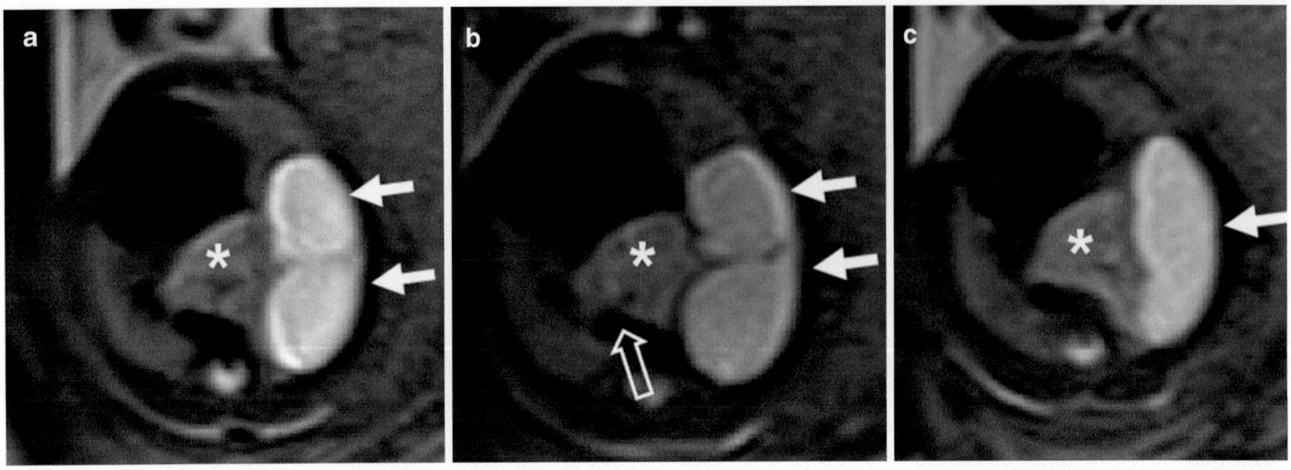

Fig. 13.5 Axial T2W images (**a–c**) show a mildly hyperintense lesion in the lower lobe of left lung (arrow) being supplied by the branch from aorta (open arrows), suggesting sequestration. Septated cystic lesion (arrow) is seen lateral to the above-mentioned lesion suggesting CPAM

be seen in macrocystic CPAMs [6]. The hybrid pathologies are better depicted on MRI due to differences in contrast (Fig. 13.5a–c).

Differential Diagnosis
Macrocystic CPAM may sometimes resemble a left-sided CDH. However, peristalsis will be present in the herniated loops of CDH with associated diaphragmatic deficiency.

The important differential diagnosis of Microcystic CPAM is BPS and CDH. BPS shows a systemic blood supply and may not show cysts.

Prognosis CPAM can grow rapidly at 20–26 weeks and then show a plateau. A rapidly-growing CPAM may cause mediastinal shift and lead to the development of hydrops and polyhydramnios. Large lesions, bilateral lung involvement, and hydrops are indicators of a poor prognosis [7, 8]. Large lesions are often complicated by pulmonary hypoplasia and cardiovascular complications and are better delivered in a tertiary hospital.

CPAM-thorax ratio of more than 0.56 or a CPAM volume ratio (i.e., volume of the mass divided by the head circumference) greater than 1.6 are predictors of the development of hydrops and poor outcome [9, 10]. Postnatally CPAMs may be asymptomatic or present with respiratory difficulty/infection. CPAMs that are symptomatic postnatally may need resection. Termination of pregnancy is an option in large masses when detected early.

13.1.3 Bronchopulmonary Sequestration (BPS)

Definition
A part of the lung does not communicate with the tracheobronchial tree and shows a systemic arterial blood supply—thoracic or abdominal aorta. Embryologically it is thought to develop from a supernumerary lung bud caudal to the normal lung bud.

Imaging Features [11]

- There are two types of sequestration—intralobar and extralobar. The extralobar type has its own pleural covering and systemic venous drainage. The intralobar type shares a common pleura with the normal lung and drains into the pulmonary venous system.
- On US, it is seen as a hyperechoic lung mass commonly in the paravertebral location (Fig. 13.6a). On MRI, it is seen as a homogeneously hyperintense lesion with a feeding vessel from the aorta (Fig. 13.6b, c).
- MRI helps in diagnosing hybrid lesions (BPS + CPAM) or when it is associated with CDH.

Differential Diagnosis
To differentiate sub diaphragmatic BPS (Fig. 13.7a, b) from neuroblastoma, the latter does not show systemic feeding artery and is heterogenous.

Prognosis
BPS can be an isolated finding or may be associated with esophageal atresia, bronchogenic cyst, pulmonary hypoplasia, CDH, cardiac anomalies, and neurenteric cyst. Isolated BPS can show regression in 80% of cases (Fig. 13.6d) [12]. Postnatally, the child can develop secondary infection or hemorrhage within the sequestrated lung and hence are electively resected.

13.1.4 Congenital Lobar Overinflation (CLO)

Definition
Congenital lobar emphysema refers to progressive lobar overexpansion, usually with compression of the remaining (ipsilateral) lung. It is thought to be secondary to an intrinsic

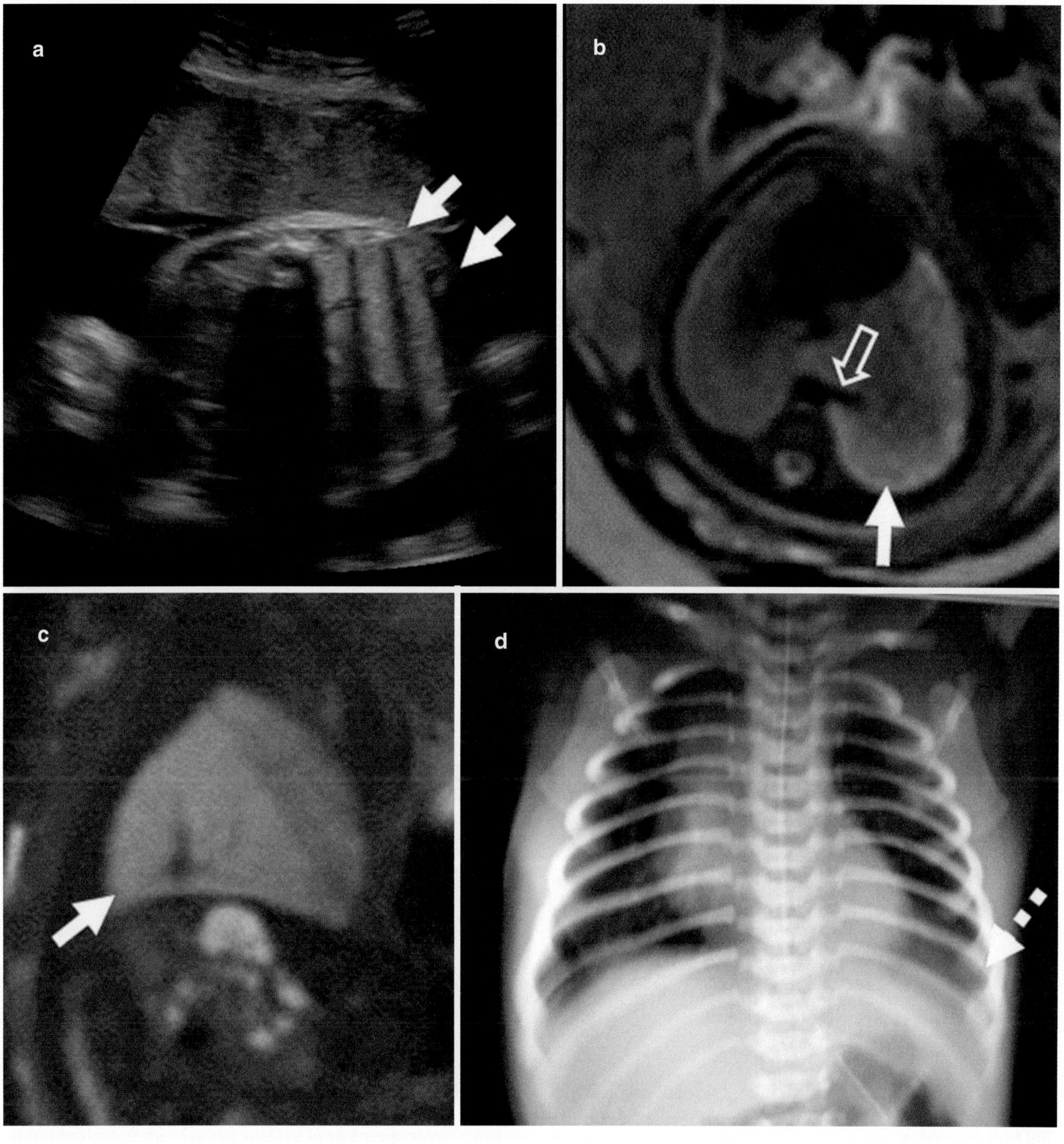

Fig. 13.6 Transverse sonographic image (**a**) showing hyperechoic lower lobe of left lung (arrow). Axial (**b**), sagittal (**c**) T2W images show hyperintense lower lobe of left lung (arrow) being supplied by the branch from aorta (open arrows), suggesting intralobar sequestration. Postnatal chest radiograph (**d**) shows significant resolution of the lesion with a small opacity in the left lung base (broken arrow)

weak or absent bronchial cartilage or due to extraneous compression of the airway. This results in a collapsed airway, acting as a one-way valve, resulting in lobar overexpansion.

Imaging Features

On US, it is seen as a homogeneous hyperechoic lung lesion commonly in the upper lobar location. On MRI, it is seen as a homogeneously hyperintense lesion (Fig. 13.8a–c). There may be compression on the adjacent lung.

Prognosis

Most neonates with CLO present with respiratory distress and the affected lobe may need to be surgically resected. For

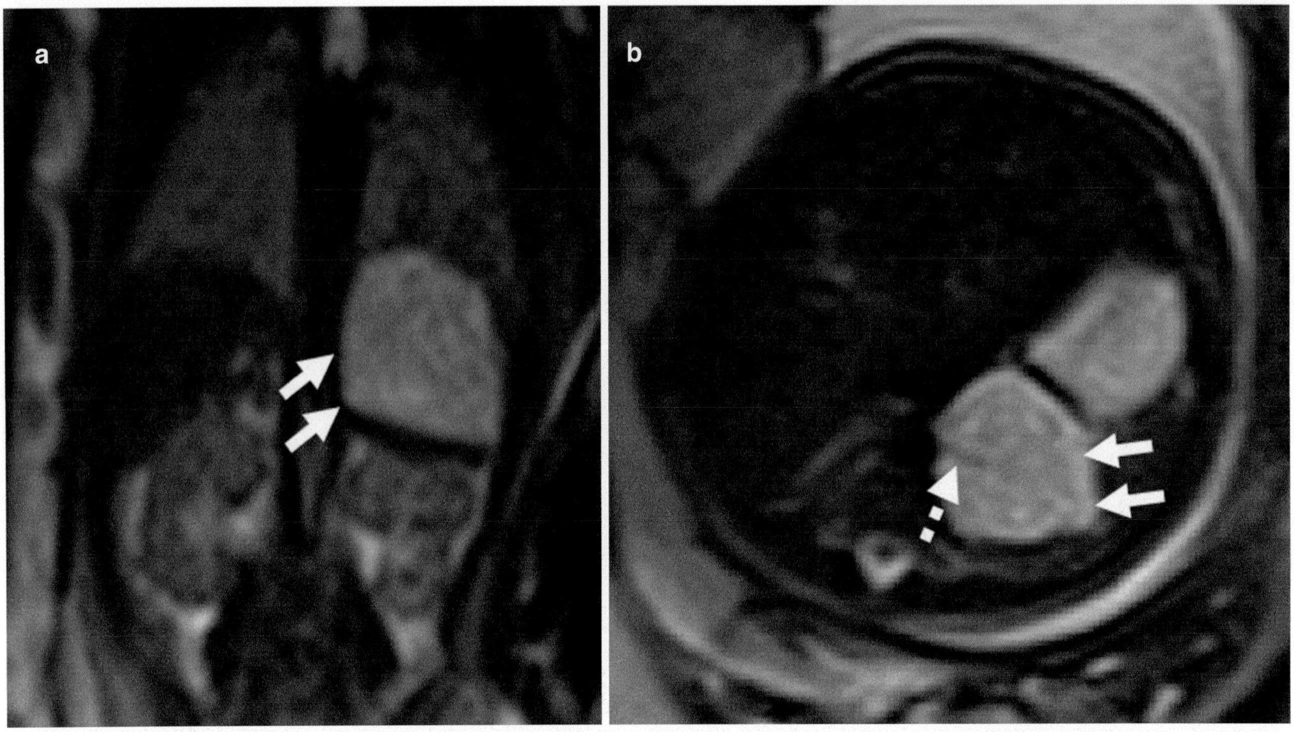

Fig. 13.7 Coronal (**a**) and Axial (**b**) T2W images show hyperintense lesion (arrow) cranial to the superior pole of left kidney and being supplied by the branch from aorta (broken arrow), suggesting extra lobar intra-abdominal sequestration

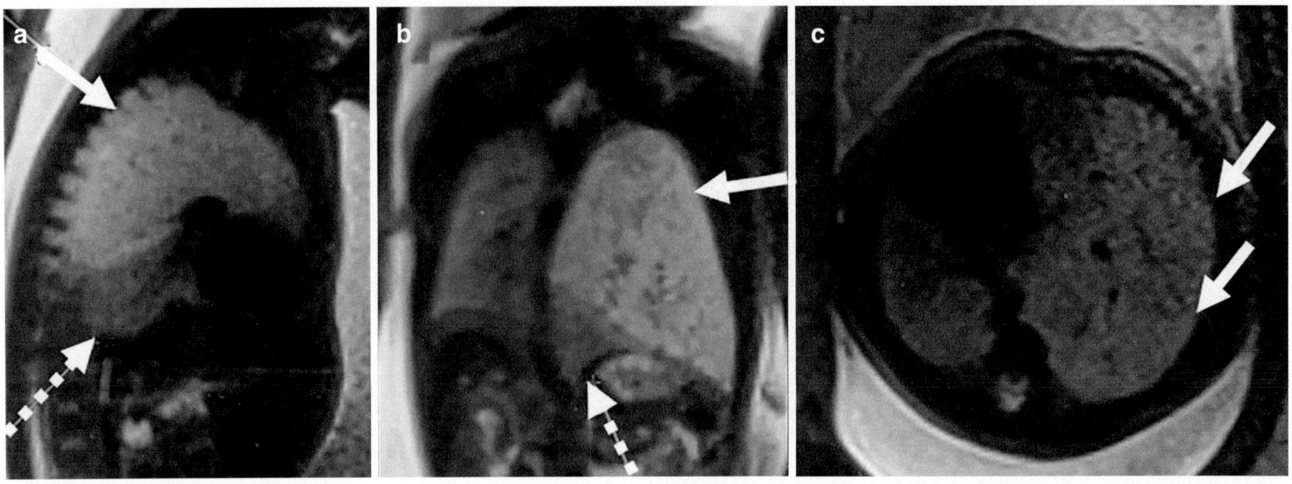

Fig. 13.8 Sagittal (**a**), coronal T2W (**b**) and axial (**c**) T2W images showing hyperintense upper lobe of left lung (arrow) with mass effect causing compression of the left lower lobe (broken arrows) and mediastinal shift to the right side—Congenital fluid overload

infants presenting with mild respiratory distress, conservative management can be tried [13].

13.1.5 Bronchogenic Cyst

Definition
It develops from the primitive foregut and may contain columnar ciliary epithelium.

Imaging Features
They can be located anywhere along the tracheoesophageal tract—Mediastinal (pericarinal being common) or intra-lung parenchymal.

Seen as unilocular thin-walled cyst (Fig. 13.9a–c) and can exert mass effect on the bronchus or esophagus if large.

Differential diagnosis: Esophageal duplication cyst, CPAM, pericardial cyst, and lymphangioma.

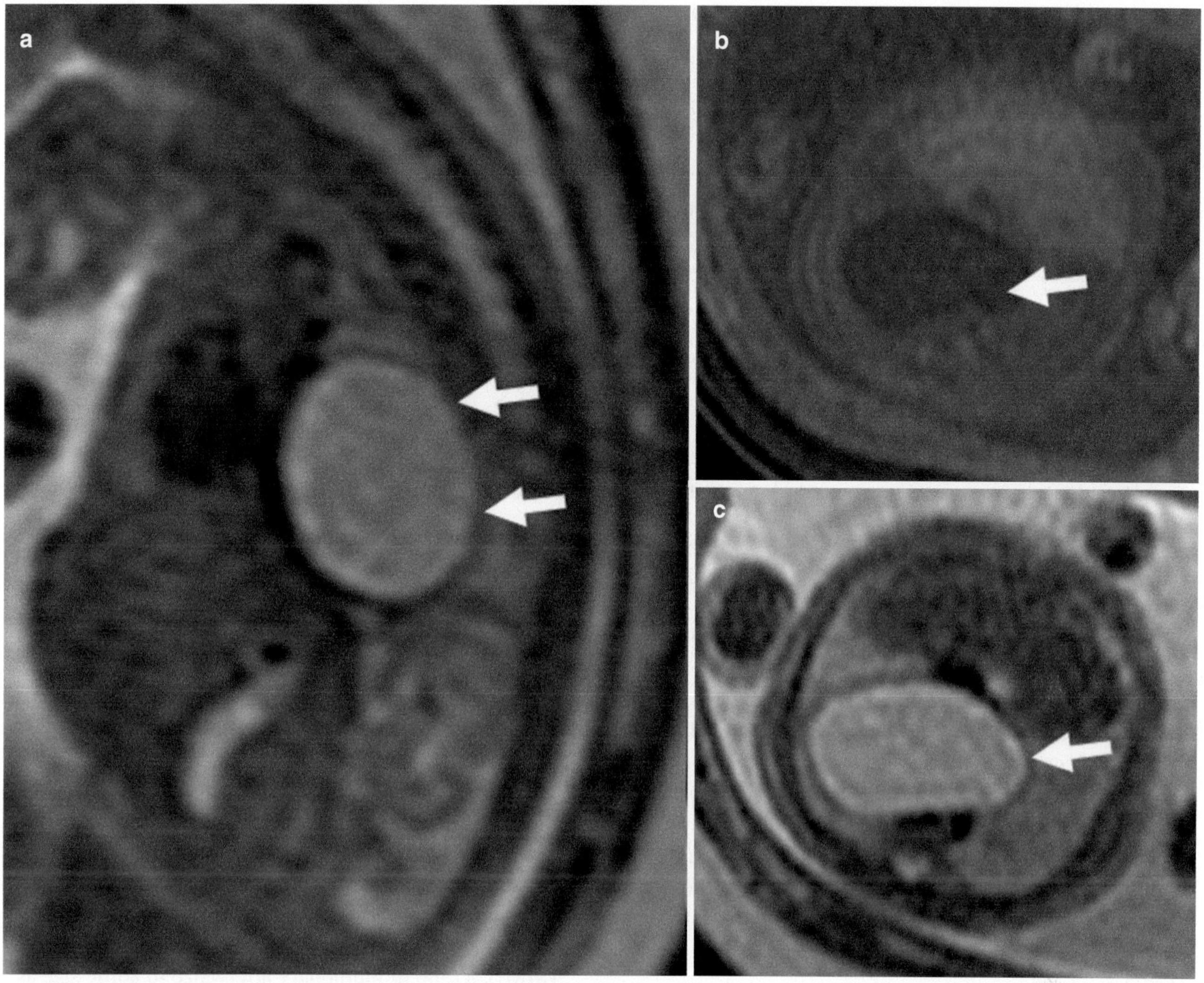

Fig. 13.9 Sagittal T2 (**a**), axial T1W (**b**) and axial (**c**) T2W images showing a cystic lesion in the subcarinal region (arrow). The lesion appears hypointense on T1 and hyperintense on T2W images—Bronchogenic cyst

Prognosis
Commonly they are asymptomatic. However, in some fetuses with large cysts, due to compression on the trachea/bronchus intubation may be needed at birth. These fetuses are better delivered in a tertiary center.

13.1.6 Bronchial Atresia

Definition
There is focal obliteration of a lobar, segmental, or subsegmental bronchus (4). The distal bronchi are dilated and filled with mucus. Due to collateral air drift, there is mild hyperinflation of the adjacent lung.

Imaging Features
On US, the fluid-filled lung distal to the atresia is seen as an echogenic lesion and may resemble other congenital lung masses. On MR imaging, it is seen as a homogeneously hyperintense lesion on T2-weighted images [14].

Prognosis
The lesion is commonly seen as an incidental finding postnatally. In case of recurrent infection, surgery may be necessary.

13.2 Diaphragmatic Anomalies

Diaphragmatic hernia and eventration are the two commonest diaphragmatic anomalies.

13.2.1 Congenital Diaphragmatic Hernia (CDH)

The diaphragm develops from four components—the septum transversum, the paraxial mesoderm of the body wall, the pleuroperitoneal membrane, and the esophageal mesenchyme. CDH occurs due to failure in the development of the diaphragmatic leaflets. CDH can occur due to defect in the posterolateral of diaphragm (Bochdalek), anterior aspect of diaphragm (Morgagni), or in the central part.

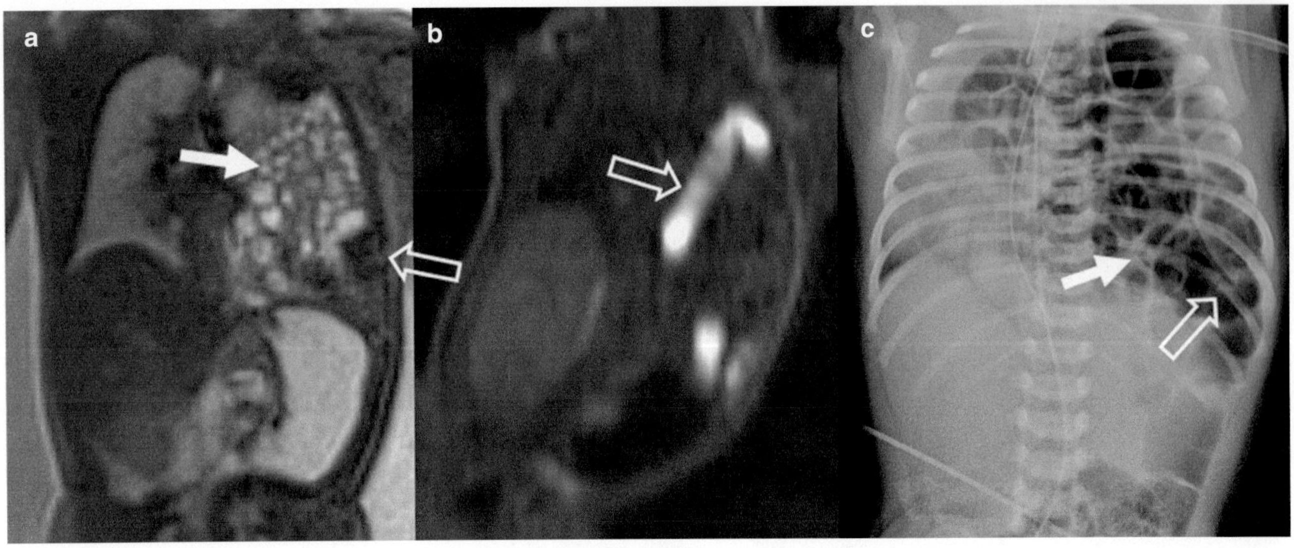

Fig. 13.10 Coronal T2 (**a**), Coronal T1W (**b**) Images of a 30-week fetus, showing congenital diaphragmatic hernia on the left side, with small bowel (arrow), large bowel (open arrows) as content. The large bowel appears hyperintense on T1W images. The observed/expected LHR was 61.4%. Postnatal chest radiograph (**c**) confirms the diagnosis. Small (arrow) and large bowel (open arrows) loops are visualized in the left thoracic cavity

CDH commonly occurs on the left side in the posterior aspect. These hernias often contain small bowel, stomach, and spleen as contents (Fig. 13.10a, b). The presence of liver as an intrathoracic content in fetuses with left-sided CDH worsens the prognosis. These hernias cause cardio-mediastinal shift to the contralateral side and lead to pulmonary hypoplasia besides pulmonary hypertension. MRI offers additional findings after sonography like:

- The visualization of the diaphragmatic defect
- The contents of the CDH can be identified individually and may not be possible on USG.
- The visualization of liver if it is an intrathoracic content (seen hyperintense on T1WI)
- Reduction in the signal intensity of lung on T2WI/ Reduction in the lung volumes are characteristic MR findings in pulmonary hypoplasia.
- Fetal lung volume is calculated by adding all the tracings of lung area and multiplying by slice thickness. At 32–34 weeks a lung volume of >40 cc is associated with 90% survival and a lung volume of <20 cc is associated with 35% survival [15].
- *Lung area to head circumference ratio (LHR)* is used to assess lung size and can be calculated by MRI. It is the ratio of the area of contralateral lung (opposite side of diaphragmatic defect) and the head circumference.
- *Observed to expected LHR ratio (o/e LHR)* is useful to assess pulmonary hypoplasia and thus predict mortality and morbidity. It is obtained by expressing the observed LHR as a percentage of the expected mean LHR for the gestational age [16–18]. Fetuses with values above 45% are likely to survive (Fig. 13.10c) as the pulmonary hypoplasia is mild.
- Presence of a hernial sac, seen as a rounded appearance in the superior most part of the hernia, carries a better prognosis [19].
- MRI is useful to obtain the modified McGoon index (MMI), a ratio of pulmonary artery size to aortic size as a prognostic indicator of survivability—infants with an MMI $\leq$1.3 have an increased (85%) mortality [20]. However, some studies have refuted this [21].

13.2.2 Congenital Diaphragmatic Eventration (CDE)

Congenital anomaly due to incomplete muscularization of the membranous diaphragm resulting in superior displacement of the hemidiaphragm.

Imaging Features

- The diaphragm is visualized but is very thin.
- Complete eventration is more common on left side (Fig. 13.11a, b).
- Partial eventration is common on the right side.
- There is partial or complete superior displacement of the hemidiaphragm.

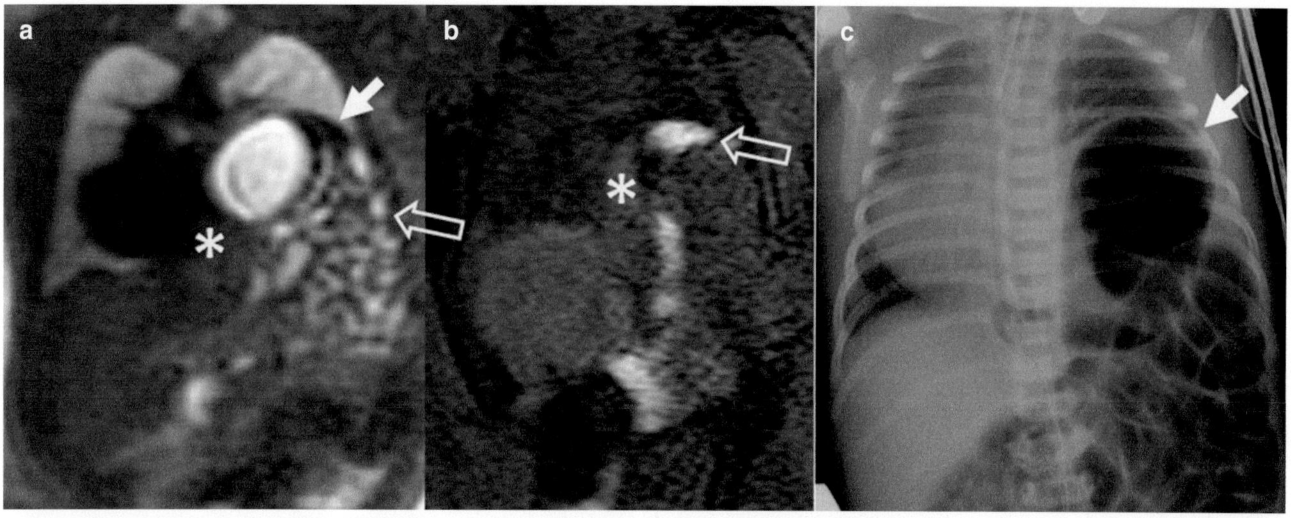

Fig. 13.11 Coronal T2 (**a**), Coronal T1W (**b**) Images, showing eventration of left hemidiaphragm. The left hemidiaphragm is seen as a thin dark band (arrow). The stomach, left lobe of liver (asterisk), small bowel, large bowel (open arrows) are seen at the level of thorax. The left lobe of liver, large bowel appear hyperintense on T1W images. Postnatal chest X-ray (**c**) confirms the diagnosis of eventration (arrow)

Prognosis

- Neonates can present with respiratory distress. Sometimes they are asymptomatic postnatally but may need surgery later on in life (Fig. 13.11c). CDE has a better prognosis and MRI helps to differentiate CDH from CDE [19, 22].

13.3 Mediastinal Cysts and Masses

They are very rare and comprise of bronchogenic cyst, esophageal duplication cyst, Neurenteric cyst, teratoma, pericardial and thymic cysts. MR is useful to characterize the mass based on the appearances on various sequences. Larger cysts may be complicated by hydrops, polyhydramnios, and respiratory distress.

Esophageal duplication cyst—It is seen as a posterior mediastinal tubular or rounded cyst and can extend below diaphragm [23]. It is seen along the course of esophagus (Fig. 13.12a–d) and may communicate with the esophagus. The cyst is lined by gastric mucosa and may show a slightly thicker wall.

Pericardial cyst—It originates from the pericardium, appears as a thin-walled, unilocular cyst in the right or left cardiophrenic angle. The cyst wall may sometimes communicate with the pericardial space.

Neurenteric cyst—may be bilobed, communicates with the spinal canal, and may be associated with adjacent spinal abnormalities.

13.4 Pleural Effusion

Causes Congenital chylothorax. Chromosomal defects. Associated with a thoracic anomaly like CDH, CDE (Fig. 13.13) or with a systemic anomaly or hydrops.

Imaging Features

On US, it is seen as an anechoic lesion surrounding the lung or in the dependent part of the thorax. On MRI it is seen as a fluid intensity lesion surrounding the lung or in the dependent part of the thorax (Fig. 13.14a, b).

Prognosis In case the pleural effusion is isolated, the prognosis is good (~90%). Prognosis becomes bad when it is associated with chromosomal defects and hydrops. Thoraco-amniotic shunting and pleurodesis (injection of sclerosants in the pleural space) are options to treat severe pleural effusion.

13.5 Fetal Cardiovascular System

MRI protocol for studying the fetal heart and the various cardiac planes have been described [24]:

- On HASTE T2WI, the heart and great vessels are seen as flow void structures (Fig. 13.15) [24].

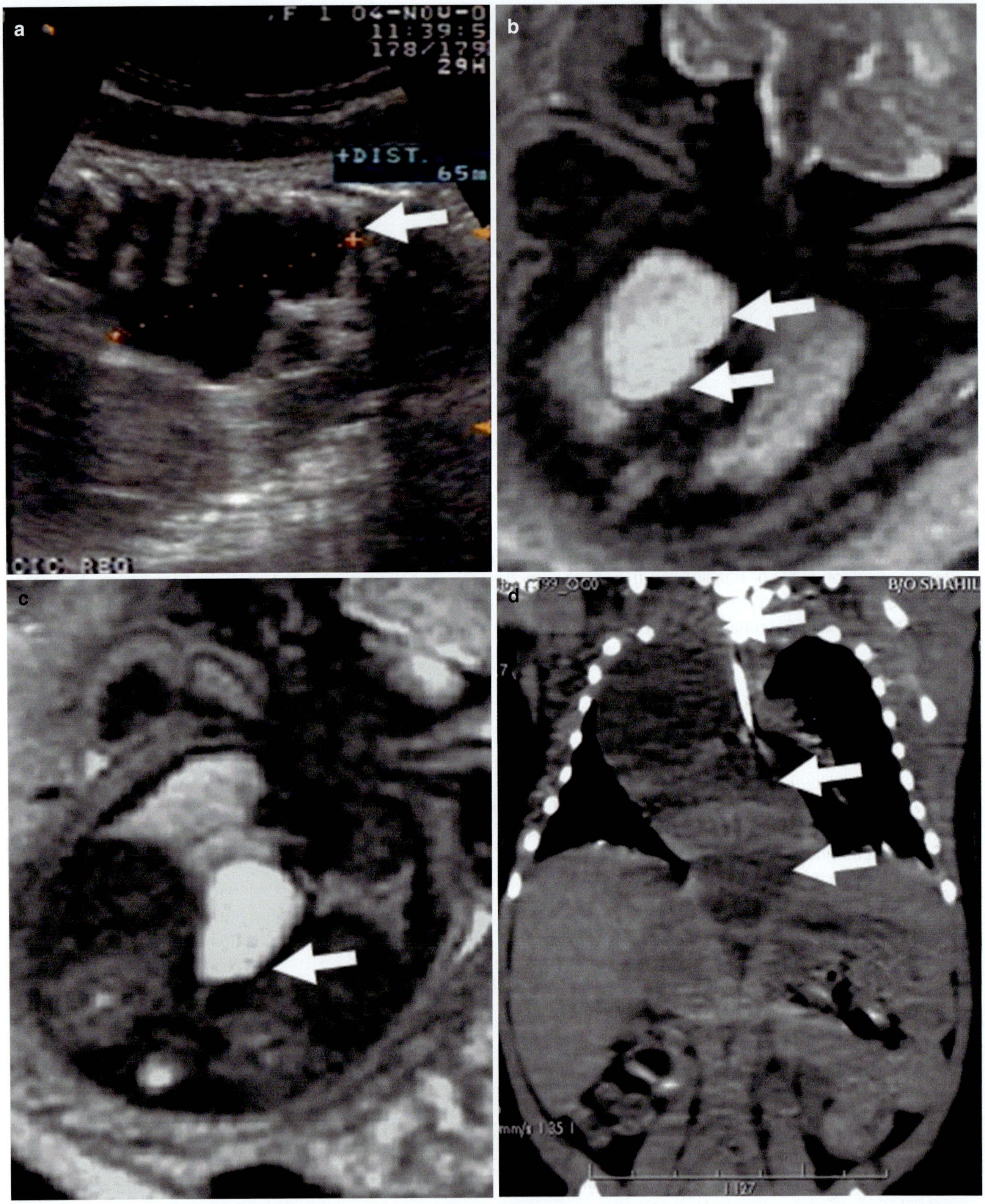

Fig. 13.12 Longitudinal sonographic image (**a**) shows an elongated mediastinal cystic lesion (arrow). Coronal T2W images (**b**, **c**) shows an elongated posterior mediastinal cystic lesion (arrows) along the course of the esophagus suggestive of esophageal duplication cyst. Postnatal coronal CT reformat (**d**) shows similar finding (arrow) and was confirmed on surgery

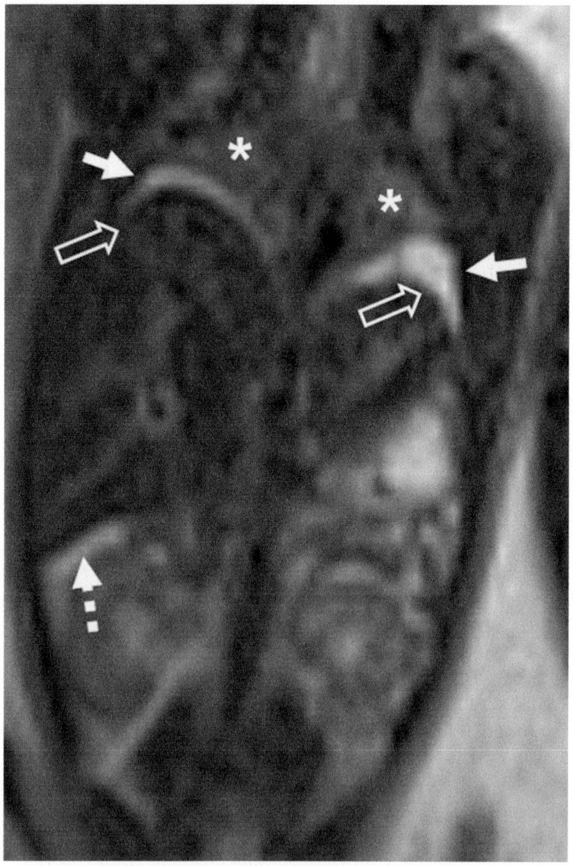

Fig. 13.13 Coronal T2W image of a 24-week fetus showing bilateral pleural effusion with associated bilateral eventration (open arrows), hypoplastic lungs (asterisk), and ascites (broken arrow)

- On steady-state free precession sequences like true-FISP the heart and vessels are seen as hyperintense structures (Fig. 13.16).
- Positional cardiac anomalies, malformations associated with cardiomegaly, sizes of the different cardiac chambers, and cardiac tumors can be studied by Fetal MRI.

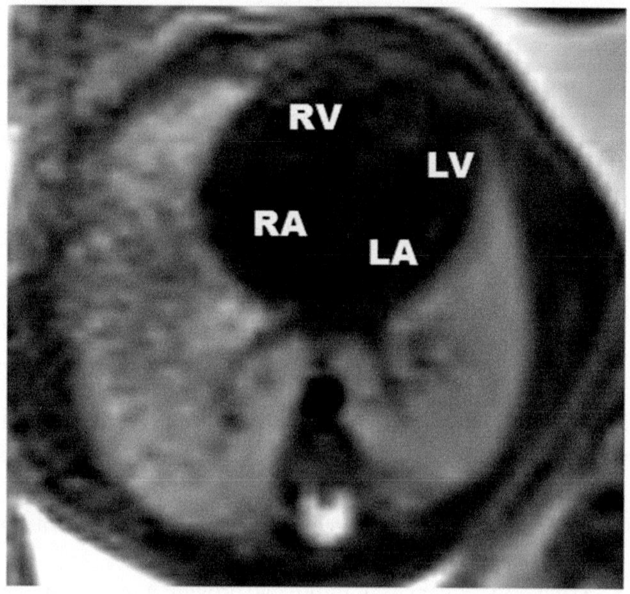

Fig. 13.15 Axial image showing four chamber view in a normal fetus. The cardiac chambers are seen as flow void on HASTE sequence

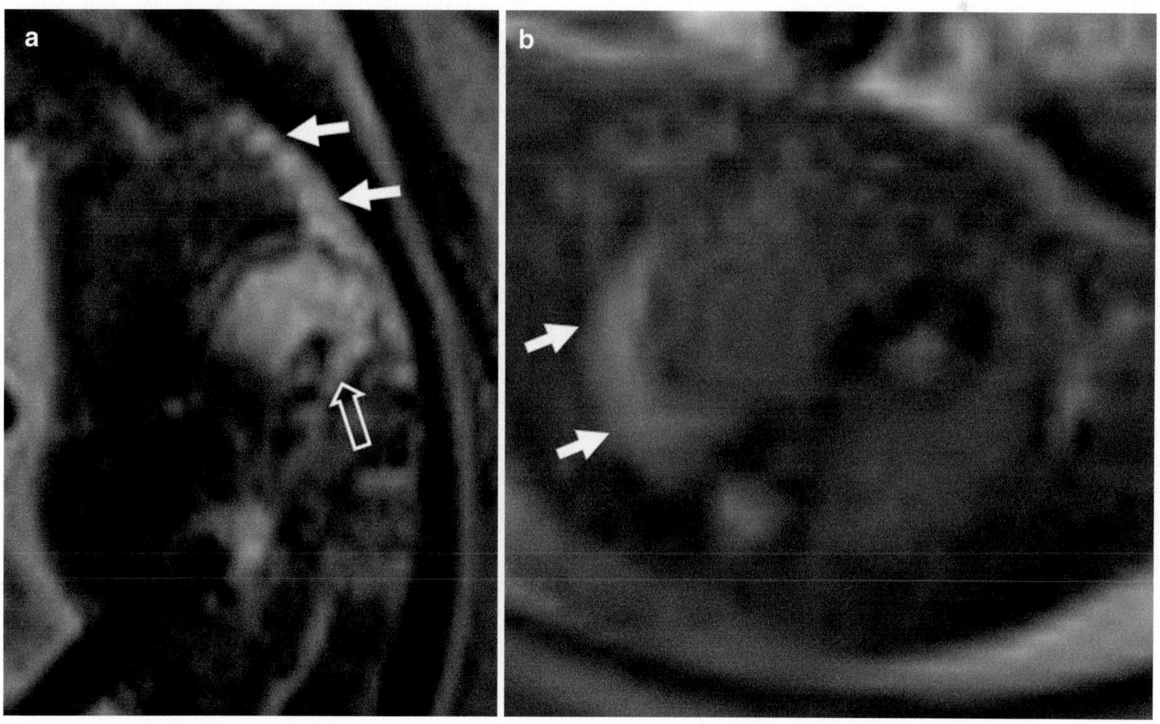

Fig. 13.14 Sagittal and axial T2W images (**a**, **b**) of a 22-week fetus showing left-sided pleural effusion (arrow) with associated congenital diaphragmatic hernia (open arrows)

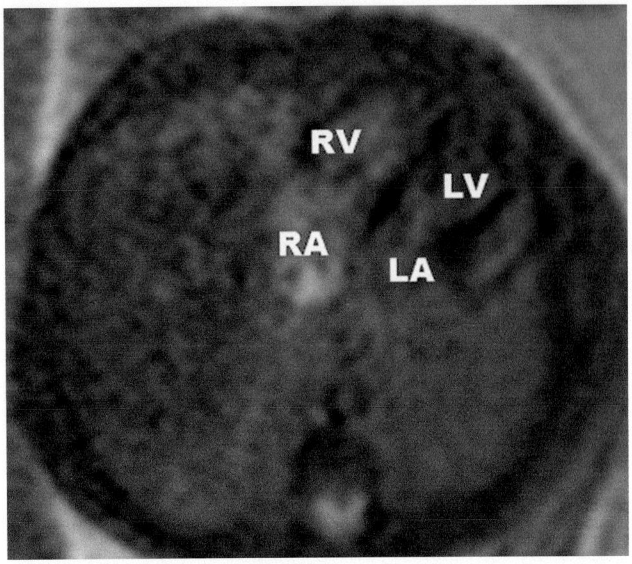

Fig. 13.16 Axial image showing four chamber view in a normal fetus. The cardiac chambers are seen hyperintense on SSFP sequence

- Malformations of the atrioventricular canal defects and great vessels can be demonstrated in larger fetuses by fetal MRI [25].
- Location, diameter of great vessels are better shown on MRI than on USG.
- Triggered sequences in future can provide fine anatomical and functional details.

References

1. Kasprian G, Balassy C, Brugger P, D. Prayer MRI of normal and pathological fetal lung development. Eur J Radiol. 2006;57:261–70.
2. Saleem SN. Fetal MRI: an approach to practice: a review. J Adv Res. 2014;5:507–23.
3. Biyyam DR, Chapman T, Ferguson MR, Deutsch G, Dighe MK. Congenital lung abnormalities: embryologic features, prenatal diagnosis, and postnatal radiologic-pathologic correlation. RadioGraphics. 2010;30(6):1721–38.
4. Berrocal T, Madrid C, Novo S, Gutiérrez J, Arjonilla A, Gómez-León N. Congenital anomalies of the tracheobronchial tree, lung, and mediastinum: embryology, radiology, and pathology. RadioGraphics. 2004;24(1):e17.
5. Chitkara U, Rosenberg J, Chervenak FA, et al. Prenatal sonographic assessment of the fetal thorax: normal values. Am J Obstet Gynecol. 1987;156(5):1069–74.
6. Langston C. New concepts in the pathology of congenital lung malformations. Semin Pediatr Surg. 2003;12(1):17–37.
7. Adzick NS, Harrison MR, Glick PL, et al. Fetal cystic adenomatoid malformation: prenatal diagnosis and natural history. J Pediatr Surg. 1985;20(5):483–8.
8. Adzick NS, Harrison MR, Crombleholme TM, Flake AW, Howell LJ. Fetal lung lesions: management and outcome. Am J Obstet Gynecol. 1998;179(4):884–9.
9. Vu L, Tsao KJ, Lee H, et al. Characteristics of congenital cystic adenomatoid malformations associated with nonimmune hydrops and outcome. J Pediatr Surg. 2007;42(8):1351–6.
10. Chen WS, Yeh GP, Tsai HD, et-al. Prenatal diagnosis of congenital cystic adenomatoid malformations: evolution and outcome. Taiwan J Obstet Gynecol. 2009;48(3):278–81.
11. Dhingsa R, Coakley FV, Albanese CT, Filly RA, Goldstein R. Prenatal sonography and MR imaging of pulmonary sequestration. AJR Am J Roentgenol. 2003;180(2):433–7.
12. García-Peña P, Lucaya J, Hendry GM, McAndrew PT, Duran C. Spontaneous involution of pulmonary sequestration in children: a report of two cases and review of the literature. Pediatr Radiol. 1998;28(4):266–70.
13. Eber E. Antenatal diagnosis of congenital thoracic malformations: early surgery, late surgery, or no surgery? Semin Respir Crit Care Med. 2007;28(3):355–66.
14. Daltro P, Werner H, Gasparetto TD, et al. Congenital chest malformations: a multimodality approach with emphasis on fetal MR imaging. RadioGraphics. 2010;30(2):385–95.
15. Lee TC, Lim FY, Keswani SG, et al. Late gestation fetal magnetic resonance imaging-derived total lung volume predicts postnatal survival and need for extracorporeal membrane oxygenation support in isolated congenital diaphragmatic hernia. J Pediatr Surg. 2011;46(6):1165–71. https://doi.org/10.1016/j.jpedsurg.2011.03.046.
16. Peralta CF, et al. Assessment of lung area in normal fetuses at 12–32 weeks. Ultrasound Obstet Gynecol. 2005 Dec;26(7):718–24.
17. Jani J, et al. Observed to expected lung area to head circumference ratio in the prediction of survival in fetuses with isolated diaphragmatic hernia. Antenatal-CDH-Registry Group. Ultrasound Obstet Gynecol. 2007;30(1):67–71.
18. Peralta CF, et al. Left and right lung volumes in fetuses with diaphragmatic hernia. Ultrasound Obstet Gynecol. 2006;27(5):551–4.
19. Heiwegen K, van Heijst AF, Daniels-Scharbatke H, van Peperstraten MC, de Blaauw I, Botden SM. Congenital diaphragmatic eventration and hernia sac compared to CDH with true defects: a retrospective cohort study. Eur J Pediatr. 2020;179(6):855–63.
20. Casaccia G, Crescenzi F, Dotta A, et al. Birth weight and McGoon Index predict mortality in newborn infants with congenital diaphragmatic hernia. J Pediatr Surg. 2006;41(1):25–8.
21. Weitzel B, Holmes G, Moran R. The modified McGoon index does not predict mortality in infants with congenital diaphragmatic hernia. 2009. https://digitalrepository.unm.edu/ume-research-papers/95brought to you by COREView metadata, citation and similar papers at core.ac.uk provided by University of New Mexico
22. Mahalingam H, Babu B, Rangasami R, et al. Fetal magnetic resonance imaging in the evaluation of congenital diaphragmatic anomalies. Egypt J Radiol Nucl Med. 2020;51:221. https://doi.org/10.1186/s43055-020-00340-w.
23. Rajeswaran R, Chandrasekharan A, Archana L, Santhosh J. Case report: antenatal MRI diagnosis of esophageal duplication cyst. Indian J Radiol Imaging. 2009;19:75–7.
24. Saleem SN. Feasibility of magnetic resonance imaging (MRI) of the fetal heart using balanced steady-state-free-precession (SSFP) sequence along fetal body and cardiac planes. AJR Am J Roentgenol. 2008;191:1208–15.
25. Saleem SN. In: Bajraktari G, editor. Fetal cardiac magnetic resonance (CMR), echocardiography—new techniques, vol. 10. InTech; 2012. p. 167–84. Isbn:978-953-307-762-8. Available from: http://www.intechopen.com/articles/show/title/fetalcardiac-magnetic-resonance-cmr.

Fetal Gastrointestinal and Abdominal Wall Anomalies

14

MR evaluation of the fetal gastrointestinal system requires both T1- and T2-weighted sequences in three orthogonal planes with respect to the fetal abdomen. T1-weighted imaging provides additional information regarding the meconium contained large bowel and size/location of the fetal liver. The fetal visceral situs is determined by looking at the orientation of stomach, descending aorta, and cardiac apex (being located on the fetal left side) and liver, inferior vena cava (being located on the fetal right side).

The esophagus (Fig. 14.1), stomach, jejunum appear hypointense on T1 and hyperintense on T2WI because of the ingested amniotic fluid (Fig. 14.2) [1, 2]. After 25 weeks, the ileum appears intermediate to hyperintense on T2WI and hyperintense on T1WI. The colon appears hyperintense on

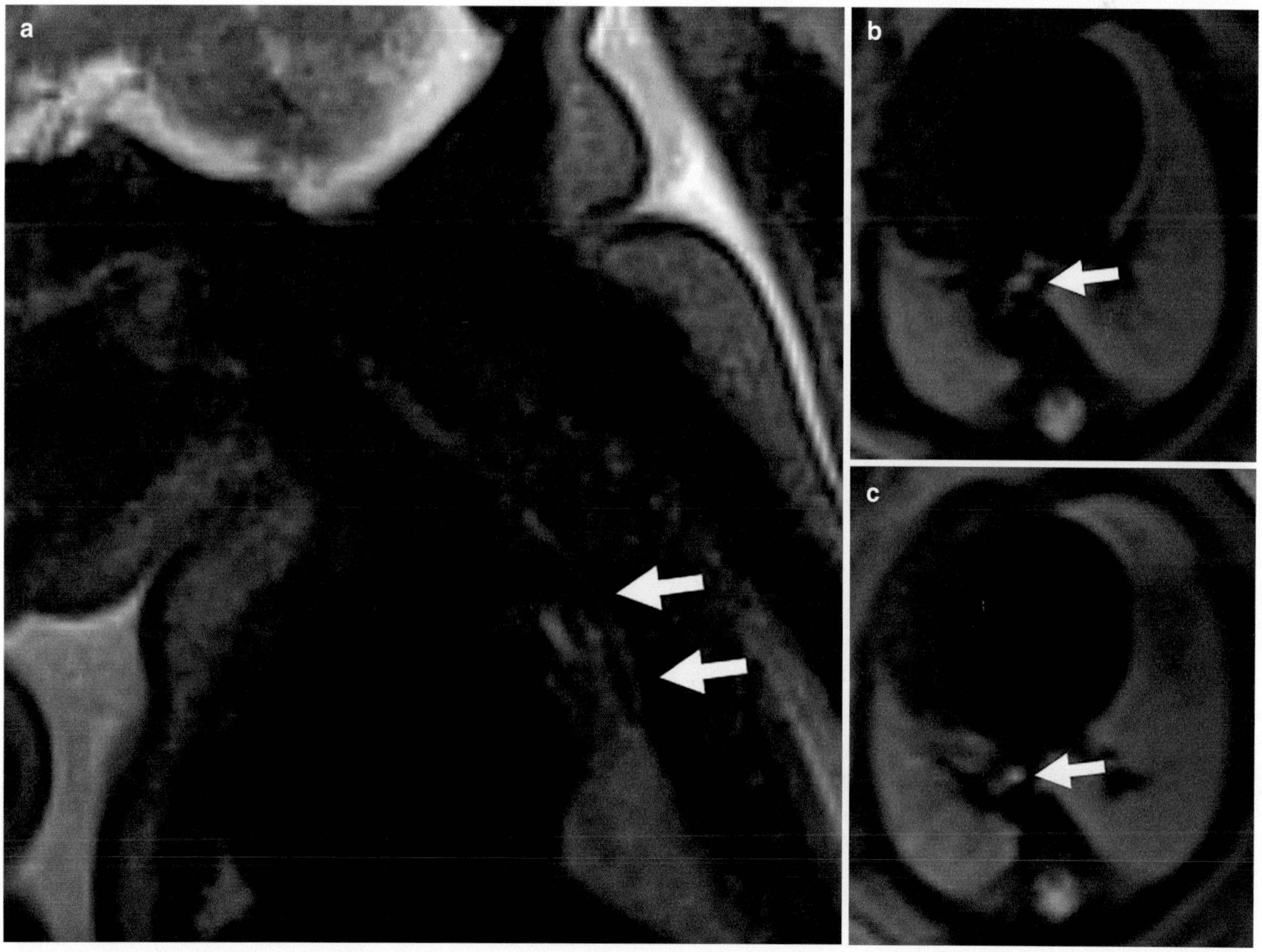

Fig. 14.1 Sagittal (**a**) and axial (**b**, **c**) T2W images of a 34-week fetus showing normal esophagus as a hyperintense tubular structure (arrows)

R. Rajeswaran, *MR Imaging of the Fetus*, https://doi.org/10.1007/978-981-16-9209-3_14

T1 (Fig. 14.3e, f) and hypointense on T2 weighted images due to the intraluminal meconium which is rich in minerals and protein (Fig. 14.2c). The small and large intestinal caliber increase with the advancing gestational age. At 20 weeks, the small bowel measures 2 mm, and the large bowel measures 3–4 mm in diameter. By 35 weeks of gestational age, small bowel measures 5–7 mm, and the large bowel measures 9–15 mm in diameter [1, 3].

The erythropoiesis in early fetal life occurs predominantly in the liver. The fetal liver is hyperintense on T1 (due to protein content and minerals like copper, and zinc) (Fig. 14.3d–f) and hypointense on T2 WI (due to iron content) (Fig. 14.3a, b).

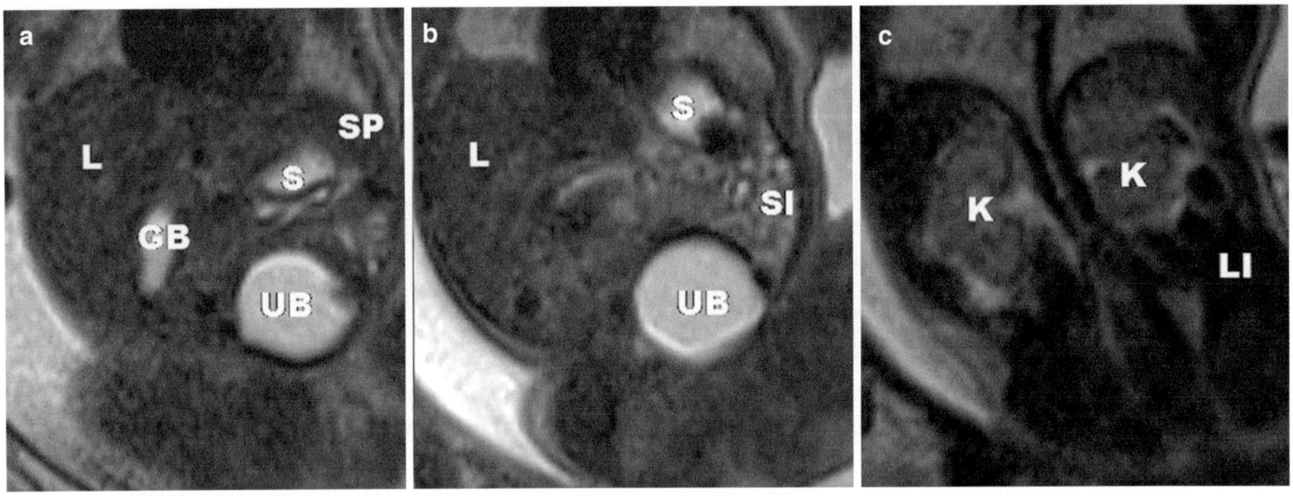

Fig. 14.2 Coronal (**a–c**) T2W images of a 30-week fetus showing normal abdominal structures. *L* liver, *GB* gall bladder, *S* stomach, *SI* small intestines, *LI* large intestines, *SP* spleen, *K* kidneys, and *UB* bladder

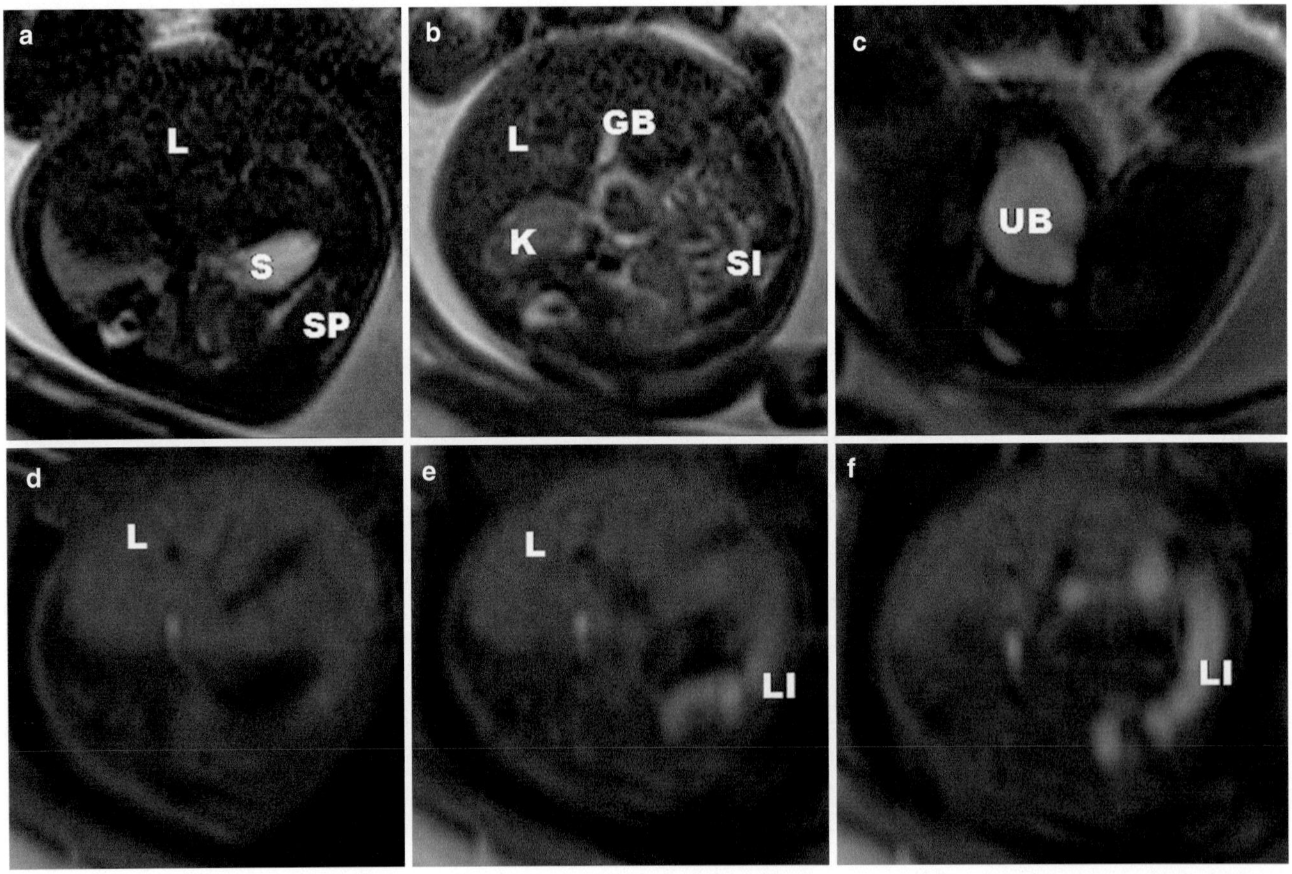

Fig. 14.3 Axial T2W (**a–c**) and T1W (**d–f**) images of a 30-week fetus showing normal abdominal structures. *L* liver, *GB* gall bladder, *S* stomach, *SI* small intestines, *SP* spleen, *K* kidneys, and *UB* bladder. Large intestine is seen hyperintense on T1WI due to meconium

The spleen is visualized by 20 weeks and shows decreasing hypointensity on T2WI with increasing gestational age (Fig. 14.3a). The gall bladder is demonstrable from 18 weeks onward. The normal intrahepatic biliary radicles are not demonstrable on MRI.

14.1 Esophageal Atresia

Definition It is a malformation of the tracheoesophageal septum leading to the absence of a segment of the esophagus. It shows an incidence of 1 in 2500 to 1 in 4000 live births. It may be associated with tracheoesophageal fistula and VACTERL anomalies.

Imaging Features

- Esophageal atresia may be suspected when there is a small stomach and Polyhydramnios (Fig. 14.4b).
- "Pouch sign"—dilated proximal pouch of esophagus may be demonstrated on USG and MRI (Fig. 14.4a, b) [4, 5]. There may be failure to demonstrate the entire course of esophagus.
- However, the entire course of esophagus and its patency may not be demonstrated on MRI even in some normal fetuses.
- Both the modalities are poor in predicting tracheoesophageal fistula.
- There may be associated, fetal growth retardation.

Prognosis

Perinatal approach consists of karyotype analysis and searches for other associated anomalies. The birth should be planned in a tertiary care center with a neonatal intensive care unit considering the high risk of prematurity (due to polyhydramnios) and morbidity due to aspiration. Perinatal approach consists of surgical reconstruction of the esopha-

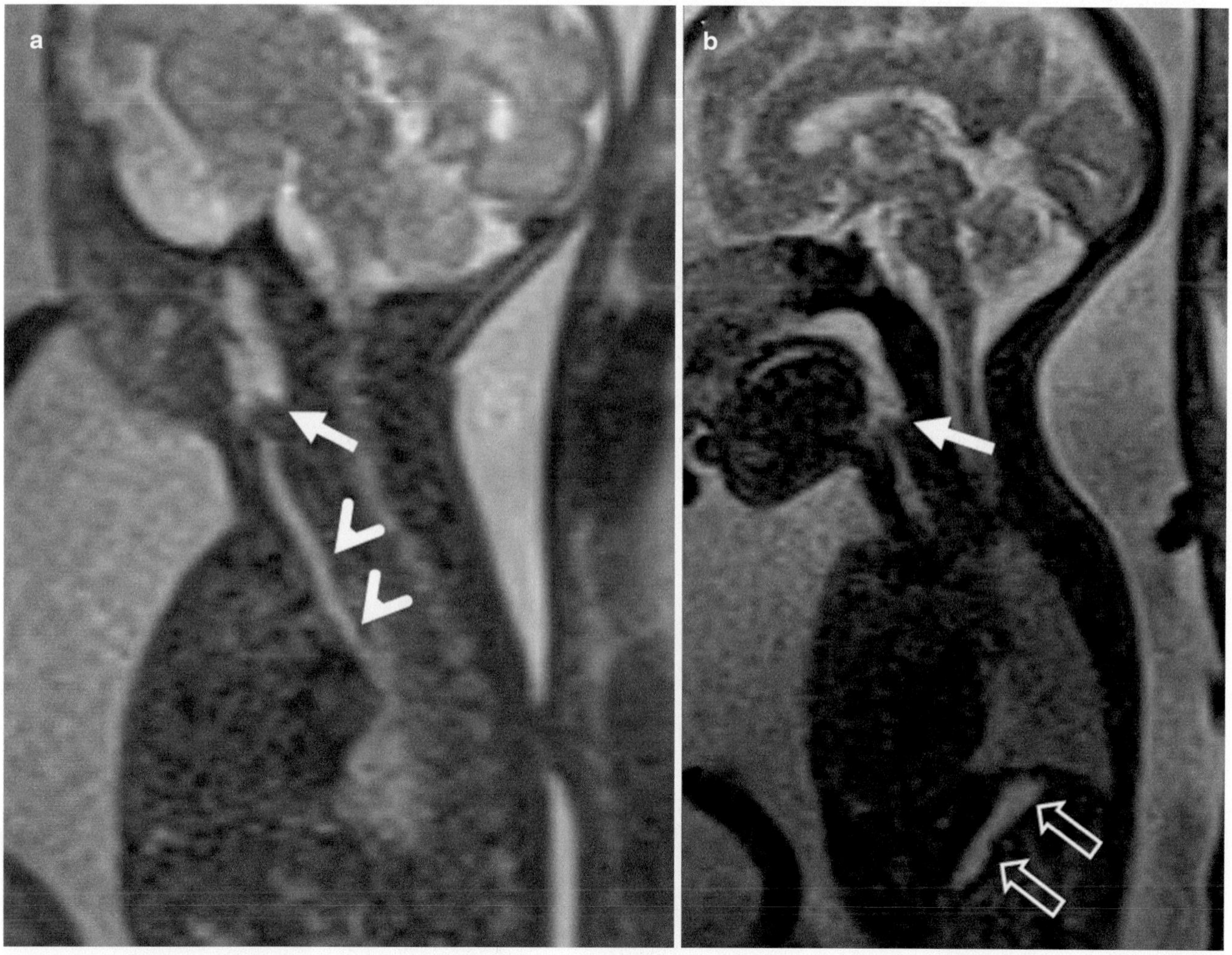

Fig. 14.4 Sagittal (**a**, **b**) T2W images of a 29-week fetus showing dilated esophageal pouch (arrow) posterior to the trachea (arrowhead) with associated small stomach (open arrows) and polyhydramnios—esophageal atresia

gus and the survival rates are 90–95% [6]. The prognosis depends on the gestational age at birth and the association with other anomalies [7].

14.2 Duodenal Atresia

Definition Deficient duodenal canalization due to web/stenosis/atresia with an incidence of 1 in 10,000 births [8]. It can be associated with chromosomal abnormalities, Down's syndrome, and VACTERL anomalies [9].

Imaging Features

- The fluid-filled stomach and proximal duodenum give a double bubble appearance (Fig. 14.5a–c).
- Polyhydramnios may be present.
- MR is useful to assess the other bowel segments. T1 W images depicting meconium in the colon can exclude additional atretic small bowel segments, as the patent small bowel distal to the atresia produces sufficient intestinal secretions, allowing normal distension of the colon with T1 hyperintensity.

Differential Diagnosis Abdominal cysts like choledochal cyst, hepatic cyst, intestinal duplication, and mesenteric cyst.

Prognosis Depends on the associated malformation with mortality ranging from 15 to 40%.

14.3 Jejunal/Ileal Atresia

Definition One or more segments of narrowing seen involving the small bowel with an incidence of 1 in 1500 to 1 in 12000 births [10, 11]. It is presumed to be due to ischemia resulting from interruption of mesenteric arterial blood supply [12].

Imaging Features

- Pre stenotic dilatated fluid-filled loops are visualized. The normal small bowel loop is less than 8 mm in diameter.
- When the obstruction is at the level of the jejunum, the dilated small bowel loops are seen hyperintense on T2WI and hypointense on T1WI (Fig. 14.6a–c). Conversely, when the obstruction is at the level of distal ileum, the dilated small bowel loops show intermediate signal intensity on T2WI and hyperintensity on T1WI.
- In jejunal atresia "triple bubble sign" is seen. Associated polyhydramnios is sometimes present.
- Swirling signal voids due to hyperperistalsis may be present within the dilated small bowel loops on T2WI.
- The colon shows decreased caliber with reduced or no meconium.

Complications Perforation in ileal atresia, meconium peritonitis, ascites, fetal growth retardation.

Differential Diagnosis

Meconium ileus—The obstruction is secondary to the impaction of meconium in the distal ileum. In some cases, associated cystic fibrosis is present. In Ileal atresia, the dilated small bowel loops demonstrate T1 hyperintensity and T2 hypointensity, whereas in meconium ileus the dilated small bowel loops show moderately increased signal intensity T1WI and intermediate signal intensity on T2WI [13].

Anal atresia: Dilated small and large bowel loops are seen.

Malrotation: There is a displacement of bowel loops with associated change of caliber in some of them.

14.4 Colonic Atresia

Definition One or more segments of the colon has narrowing/atresia.

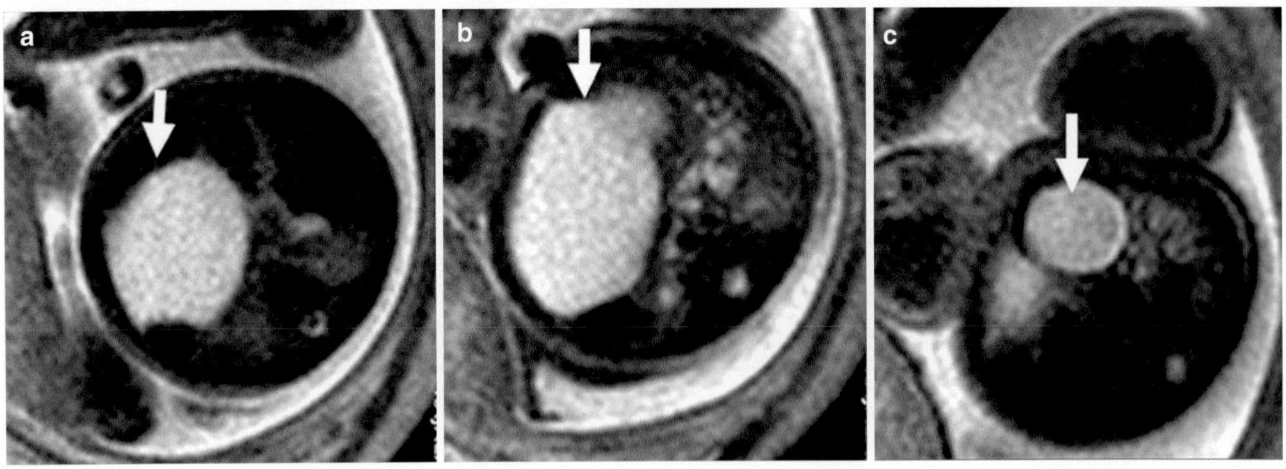

Fig. 14.5 Axial T2 W (**a**–**c**) images of a fetal abdomen showing a grossly dilated stomach (arrows) and nondilated small bowel loops suggesting duodenal atresia

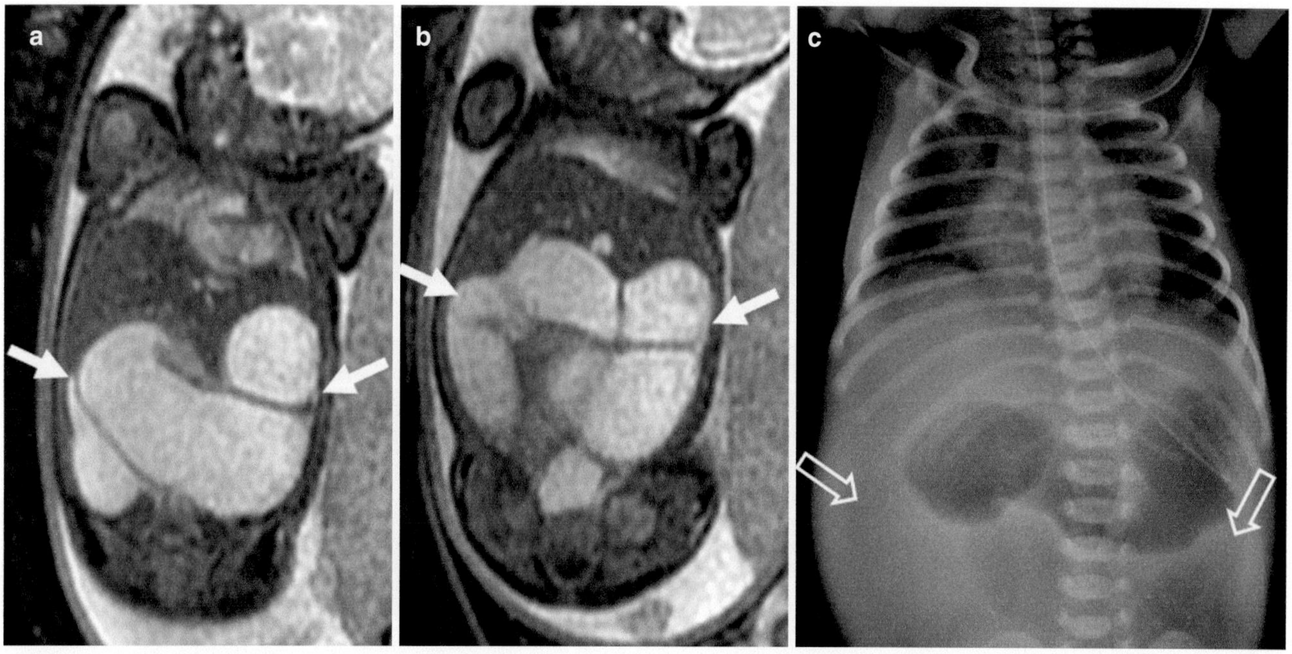

Fig. 14.6 Coronal T2 W (**a**, **b**) images of a fetal abdomen showing grossly dilated proximal jejunal loops suggesting jejunal atresia. Postnatal radiograph (**c**) shows distended proximal jejunal loops (open arrows) confirming the diagnosis

Imaging Features Dilated proximal small and large bowel loops are seen. Large bowel is identified by its T1 hyperintensity and presence of haustra. It can be associated with Hirschsprung disease. Stenotic segments do not show usual meconium signals and are less hyperintense on T1WI [14, 15].

Differential Diagnosis Anal atresia, jejunal atresia.

Prognosis Depends on the associated malformations and the length of the stenotic segment.

14.5 Anal Atresia

Definition Atresia involving the anal canal with an incidence of 1 in 2000 births. It is termed "high" if it occurs above the levator ani and low when it occurs below levator ani [16, 17]. It may be associated with VACTERL anomalies and several syndromes [18].

Imaging Features

- Prenatal detection is difficult with detection rate being 8–10% [19].
- Commonly presents in the III trimester. There is the absence of anal dimple with associated dilated fluid-filled dilated bowel loops are seen (Normal large measures 8 mm in diameter by 24 weeks and 16–18 mm by 35–38 weeks). Normal rectum is hyperintense on T1 and hypointense on T2WI and is seen opposed to the urinary bladder. Inferiorly it should be seen 10 mm below bladder neck from 20 weeks. If there is associated recto urinary fistula, rectum shows hyperintensity on T2WI due to urine.
- Pitfalls—A prominent rectum can be a normal variant and a non-dilated colon does not rule out anal atresia.

Prognosis Isolated anal atresia has a good prognosis.

14.6 Cloaca

Definition Spectrum of malformation arising due to abnormality in the partitioning of the cloaca (genital, urinary, and intestinal tracts). There is communication of the urogenital sinus with rectum [20, 21]. This condition is very rare, with an incidence of 1 in 50,000 births. It may be associated with VACTERL anomalies, duplication of uterus, vagina, bladder, urethra, and caudal dysgenesis.

Types

In the severe form—cloacal dysgenesis—there is no opening.

Presence of single opening—with coalescence of urethra, vagina, and hindgut.

Presence of two openings—urogenital sinus and hindgut.

Imaging Features

There is absence of anal dimple. Uterus and vagina are duplicated in 80% of cases. The vagina is distended (hydrocolpos) and appears as a cystic area posterior to the urinary bladder (Fig. 14.7a–c). There is a loss of T1 hyperintensity within the rectum due to its distension with urine. There

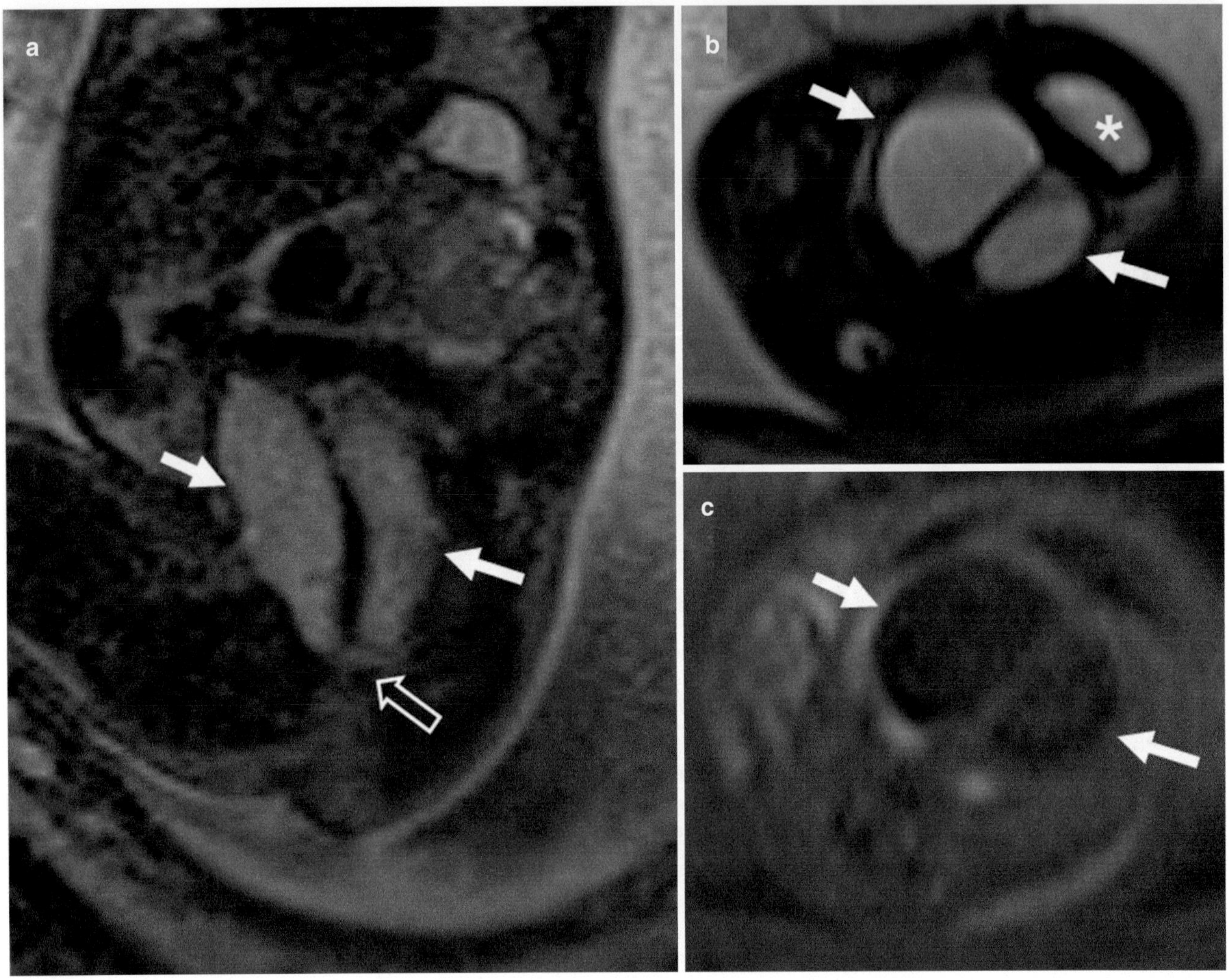

Fig. 14.7 Coronal (**a**), axial T2W (**b**) and axial T1W (**c**) fetal images show two tubular cystic areas (arrows) behind the bladder (asterisk) representing hydrometrocolpos and distended rectum. These three structures are seen to communicate in the inferior aspect (open arrows)—Persistent cloaca

may be urinary ascites due to spillage of urine through the fallopian tube.

Differential Diagnosis

Isolated hydrocolpos: The vagina is not duplicated, appears unilocular and there is preserved rectal anatomy and T1 hyperintensity.

Ovarian Cyst—Is seen in one side of the lower abdomen.

Enteric duplication cyst: The cyst wall shows layered appearance—"gut signature."

Prognosis

Prognosis is poor with cloacal dysgenesis.

Cloaca with short common channel <3 cm: The continence is better after surgery (70% cases).

Cloaca with short common channel >3 cm: The continence is not good after surgery in majority of cases.

Presence of two openings—with a normally placed anus shows a good prognosis.

14.7 Choledochal Cyst

Definition Cystic dilatation of the intra-/extrahepatic bile duct.

Imaging Features Cyst is seen in the course of bile ducts. They may show communication with biliary tree [22].

Differential diagnosis: Congenital hepatic cyst—They are unilocular and do not communicate with biliary tree.

14.8 Hepatic Tumors and Hemochromatosis

14.8.1 Congenital Hepatic Hemangioma

It is a rare benign lesion resulting from the proliferation of the vascular endothelium and is commonly associated with spontaneous involution. It has two types—(1) Rapidly Involuting congenital hemangioma (RICH) and (2) Non-involuting congenital hemangioma (NICH).

Imaging features: They are solid lesions appearing hypointense on T1 and hyperintense on T2WI. Sometimes they may show necrosis, fibrosis, or hemorrhage within.

Prognosis: Most of them show involution postnatally in the first one and half years.

Larger tumors may show arteriovenous shunts resulting in high-output cardiac failure. Other complications include hepatic dysfunction, fetal non-immune hydrops, hemolytic anemia, coagulopathy, and tumor rupture. Larger lesions are treated postnatally with corticosteroids, drugs with strong antiangiogenic effect (e.g., alpha-interferon, cyclophosphamide, vincristine, or actinomycin D), and irradiation.

14.8.2 Mesenchymal Hepatic Hamartoma

It is a rare benign tumor resulting from excessive focal overgrowth of mature normal hepatic cells and stroma.

Imaging Features It appears as a cystic lesion or as a mixed solid-cystic mass lesion. It is seen as a hyperintense lesion with a hypointense stroma on T2WI.

Prognosis There is 70% survival postnatally after surgical resection. Early presentation, rapidly growing tumor, polyhydramnios, and compression of arteries are poor prognostic indicators [23].

14.8.3 Hepatoblastoma

Definition
It is a very rare solid hepatic tumor.

Imaging Features

- On US, hepatoblastoma appears as well-defined, solid, echogenic lesions with a spoke-wheel appearance. Doppler may reveal hypervascularity within the tumor.
- On MRI it shows a variable signal intensity mass, with mild hyperintensity on DWI. Fetal MRI is useful to identify the extent of the tumor and its relationship with adjacent organs [24].

Prognosis
The prognosis is generally poor. Complications are Polyhydroamniosis, nonimmune fetal hydrops, rupture of mass, and respiratory distress due to pressure of the mass on the adjacent lung. There is 60% survival postnatally after chemotherapy and surgical resection.

14.8.4 Neonatal Hemochromatosis

It is a very rare disease that manifests as cirrhosis and intra- and extrahepatic siderosis.

Imaging Features MRI is useful to assess noninvasively in the prenatal period though sonography is normal. It is seen as a diffusely hypointense fetal liver on T2* images relative to fetal spleen and maternal liver (Fig. 14.8) [25].

14.9 Omphalocele

Definition
Midline abdominal wall defect, where there is herniation of the abdominal contents into the base of the umbilical cord. The contents are covered by a membrane and the usual contents are small/large bowel and liver. Rarely spleen and bladder are seen in the contents [26, 27].

Imaging Features MRI is useful to assess the normalcy of cord insertion site (Fig. 14.9). When omphalocele is present, MRI is useful to show the contents (Fig. 14.10a–d)—Large bowel may show hyperintensity on T1WI due to meconium. Fluid-filled small bowel loops are hyperintense, liver is hyperintense on T1 and hypointense on T2WI. Sometimes there may be associated ascites.

14.10 Heterotaxy

Synonym Situs ambiguous.

Definition
There is alteration in the usual left-right distribution of the abdominal and thoracic organs. It is in between situs solitus and situs inversus [28].

Etiology Most cases occur sporadically. It occurs due to early embryological developmental disturbance and may be associated with cardiac anomalies. Immotile cilia syndrome is seen in 25% of cases.

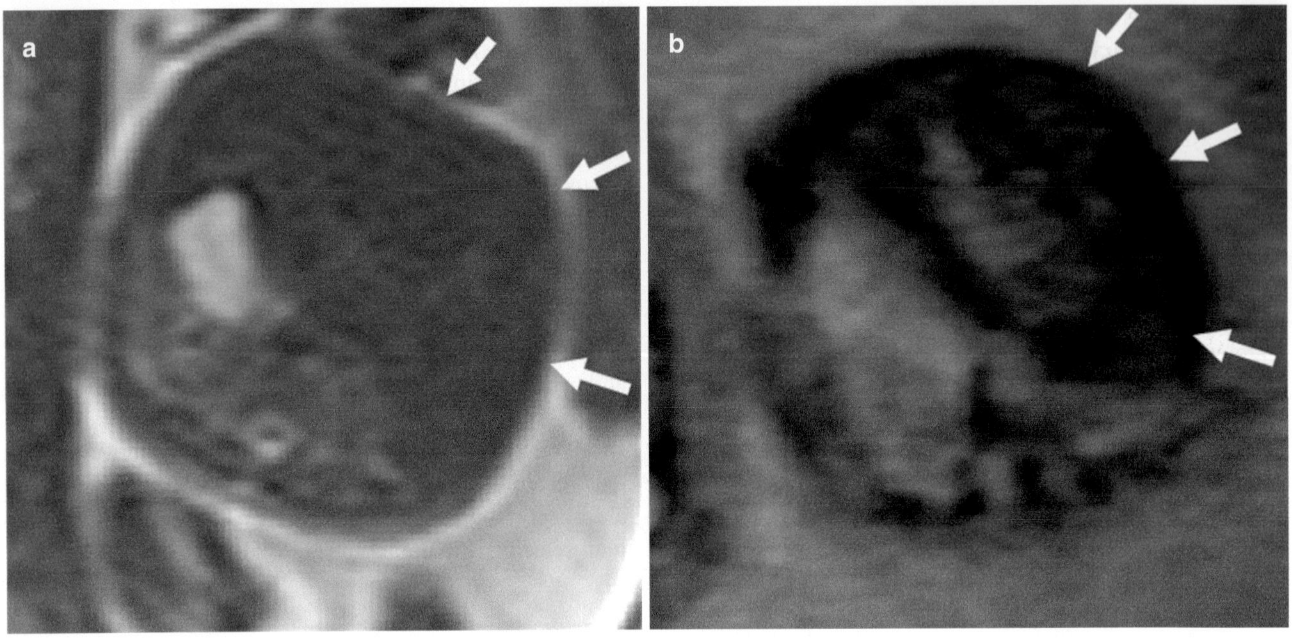

Fig. 14.8 Axial T2 (**a**) and T2* (**b**) images showing darkening of liver in a 21-week fetus with hemochromatosis on GRE images (arrows)

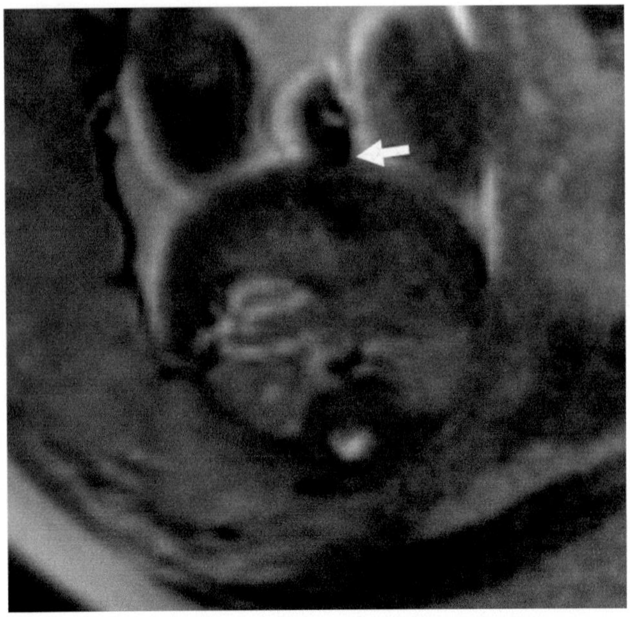

Fig. 14.9 Axial T2W image showing normal umbilical cord insertion site

Imaging Features MRI is useful to assess the position and size of liver, diaphragm, and the location of various organs. It is also useful to assess the absence or multiplicity of spleen. Complex cardiac malformations, absent spleen are often associated with a bad prognosis.

14.11 Fetal Ascites

It represents the presence of free fluid in the fetal abdomen. Many of its causes are similar to those of hydrops fetalis. Other causes include fetal urinary ascites (Fig. 14.11), intrauterine infection, bowel perforation, ovarian cyst rupture, severe pulmonary abnormality (Fig. 14.12), and idiopathic.

Imaging Features Free fluid is seen in the abdominal cavity as T2 hyperintensity with bowel loops floating within it.

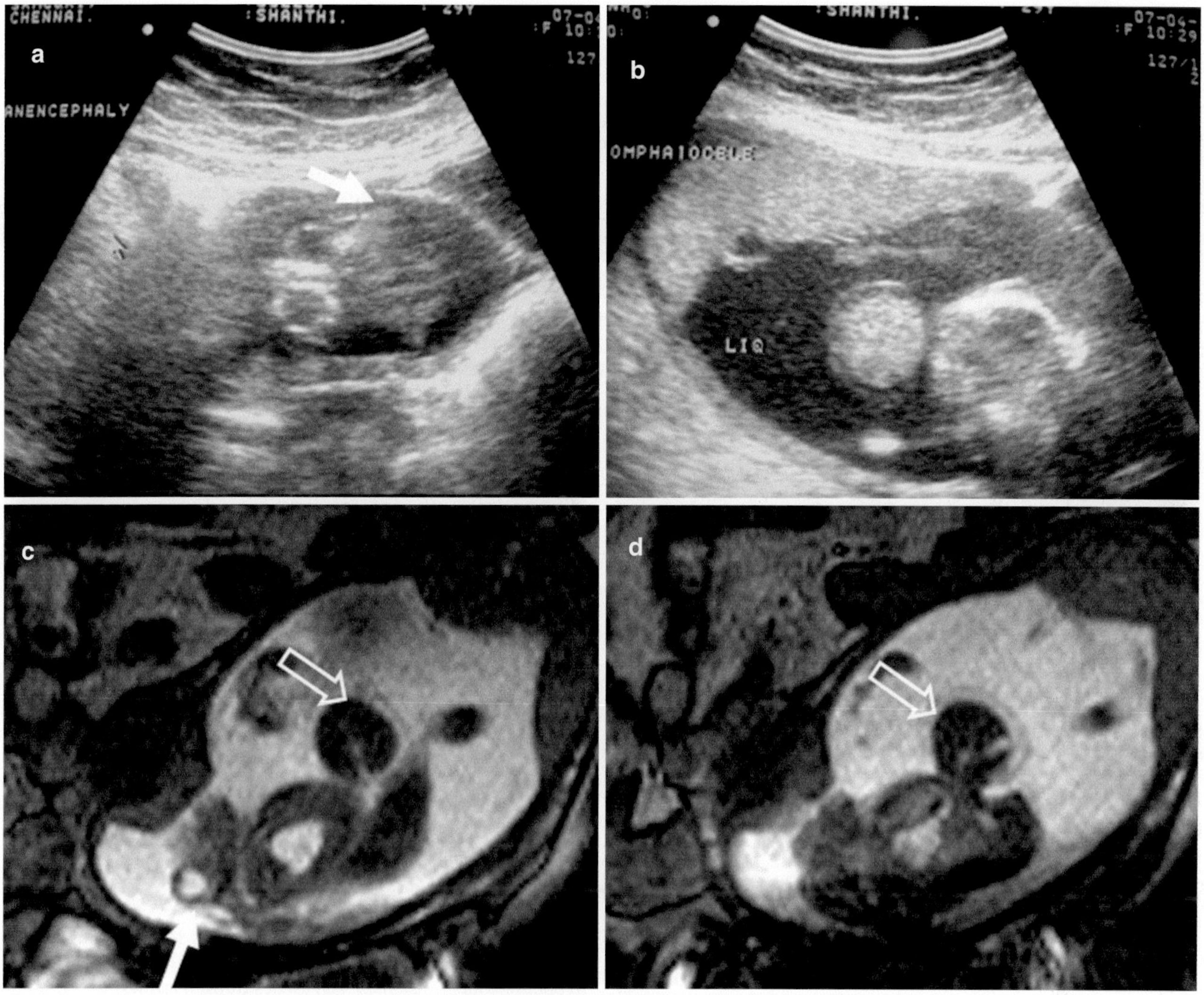

Fig. 14.10 Sonographic (**a**, **b**) and T2w MR images (**c**, **d**) showing anencephaly (arrow) and omphalocele (open arrows)

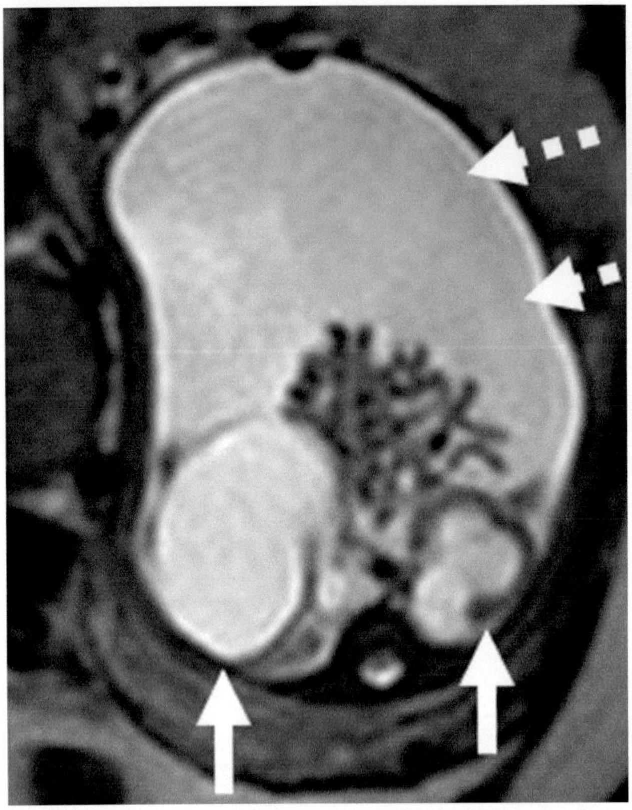

Fig. 14.11 Axial T2 W image of a fetus showing bilateral hydronephrosis (arrows), overdistended bladder (open arrows), and urinary ascites (broken arrows)

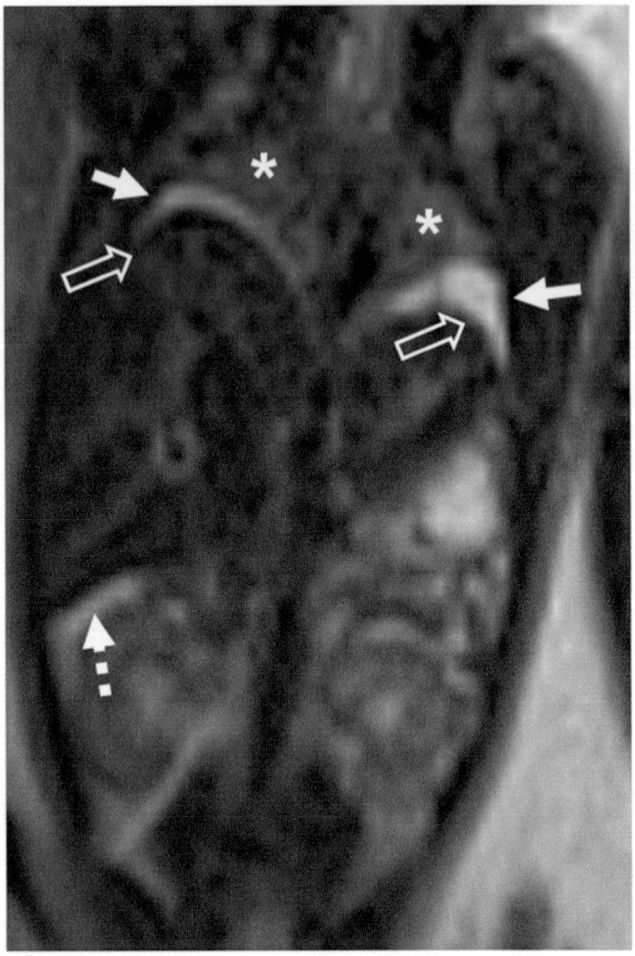

Fig. 14.12 Coronal T2W image of a 24-week fetus showing bilateral pleural effusion with associated bilateral eventration (open arrows), hypoplastic lungs (asterisk), and ascites (broken arrow)

References

1. Furey EA, Bailey AA, Twickler DM. Fetal MR imaging of gastrointestinal abnormalities. Radiographics. 2016;36(3):904–17.
2. Saleem SN. Fetal MRI: an approach to practice: a review. J Adv Res. 2014;5:507–23.
3. Brugger PC. MRI of fetal abdomen. In: Prayer D, editor. Fetal MRI. Berlin: Springer; 2011. p. 361–401.
4. Hochart V, Verpillat P, Langlois C, et al. The contribution of fetal MR imaging to the assessment of oesophageal atresia. Eur Radiol. 2015;25:306–14. https://doi.org/10.1007/s00330-014-3444-y.
5. Ethun CG, Fallon SC, Cassady CI, et al. Fetal MRI improves diagnostic accuracy in patients referred to a fetal center for suspected esophageal atresia. J Pediatr Surg. 2014;49(5):712–5.
6. Malinger G, Levine A, Rotmenschi S. The fetal esophagus: anatomical and physiological ultrasonographic characterization using a high-resolution linear transducer. Ultrasound Obstet Gynecol. 2004;24:500–5.
7. Kunisaki SM, Bruch SW, Hirschl RB, et al. The diagnosis of fetal esophageal atresia and its implications on perinatal outcome. Pediatr Surg Int. 2014;30:971–7. https://doi.org/10.1007/s00383-014-3562-2.
8. Chen QJ, Gao ZG, Tou JF, Qian YZ, Li MJ, Xiong QX, Shu Q. Congenital duodenal obstruction in neonates: a decade's experience from one center. World J Pediatr. 2014;10(3):238–44. https://doi.org/10.1007/s12519-014-0499-4.
9. Brantberg A, Blaas H-GK, Salvesen KÅ, Haugen SE, Møllerløkken G, Eik-Nes Fetal SH. Duodenal obstructions: increased risk of prenatal sudden death. Ultrasound Obstet Gynecol. 2002;20:439–46.
10. Virgone C, D'antonio F, Khalil A, Jonh R, Manzoli L, Giuliani S. Accuracy of prenatal ultrasound in detecting jejunal and ileal atresia: systematic review and meta-analysis. Ultrasound Obstet Gynecol. 2015;45(5):523–9. https://doi.org/10.1002/uog.14651.
11. Best KE, Tennant PW, Addor MC, et al. Epidemiology of small intestinal atresia in Europe: a register-based study. Arch Dis Child Fetal Neonatal Ed. 2012;97(5):F353–8.
12. Rubesova E. Fetal bowel anomalies—US and MR assessment. Pediatr Radiol. 2012;42(Suppl 1):S101–6.
13. Carcopino X, Chaumoitre K, Shojai R, Panuel M, Boubli L, D'Ercole C. Use of fetal magnetic resonance imaging in differentiating ileal atresia from meconium ileus. Ultrasound Obstet Gynecol. 2006;28(7):976–7.
14. Cox SG, Numanoglu A, Millar AJ, Rode H. Colonic atresia: spectrum of presentation and pitfalls in management. A review of 14 cases. Pediatr Surg Int. 2005;21(10):813–8. https://doi.org/10.1007/s00383-005-1488-4.

15. Adams SD, Stanton MP. Malrotation and intestinal atresias. Early Hum Dev. 2014;90(12):921–5. https://doi.org/10.1016/j.earlhumdev.2014.09.017.
16. Podberesky DJ, Towbin AJ, Eltomey MA, Levitt MA. Magnetic resonance imaging of anorectal malformations. Magn Reson Imaging Clin N Am. 2013;21(4):791–812. https://doi.org/10.1016/j.mric.2013.04.010.
17. Gindes L, Weissmann-Brenner A, Weisz B, Tzadikevitch Geffen K, Zajicek M, Achiron R. OC24.04: 3-dimensional ultrasound demonstration of fetal anal canal and sphincter. Ultrasound Obstet Gynecol. 2010;36:44. https://doi.org/10.1002/uog.7903.
18. Cuschieri A, EUROCAT Working Group. Anorectal anomalies associated with or as part of other anomalies. Am J Med Genet. 2002;110(2):122–30.
19. Stoll C, Alembik Y, Dott B, Roth MP. Evaluation of prenatal diagnosis of congenital gastro-intestinal atresias. Eur J Epidemiol. 1996;12(6):611–6.
20. Livingston JC, Elicevik M, Breech L, Crombleholme TM, Peña A, Levitt MA. Persistent cloaca. J Ultrasound Med. 2012;31:403–7. https://doi.org/10.7863/jum.2012.31.3.403.
21. Levitt MA, Peña A. Cloacal malformations: lessons learned from 490 cases. Semin Pediatr Surg. 2010;19(2):128–38. https://doi.org/10.1053/j.sempedsurg.2009.11.012.
22. Jensen KK, Sohaey R. Antenatal sonographic diagnosis of choledochal cyst: case report and imaging review. J Clin Ultrasound. 2015;43(9):581–3. https://doi.org/10.1002/jcu.22256.
23. Kodandapani S, Pai MV, Kumar V, Pai KV. Prenatal diagnosis of congenital mesenchymal hamartoma of liver: a case report. Case Rep Obstet Gynecol. 2011;2011:932583. https://doi.org/10.1155/2011/932583.
24. Ergin H, Yildirim B, Dagdeviren E, Yagci B, Ozen F, Sen N, Duzcan E. A prenatally detected case of congenital hepatoblastoma. Pathol Oncol Res. 2008;14(1):97–100. https://doi.org/10.1007/s12253-008-9001-8.
25. Martí-Bonmatí L, Baamonde A, Poyatos CR, Monteagudo E. Prenatal diagnosis of idiopathic neonatal hemochromatosis with MRI. Abdom Imaging. 1994;19(1):55–6. https://doi.org/10.1007/BF02165863.
26. Pakdaman R, Woodward PJ, Kennedy A. Complex abdominal wall defects: appearances at prenatal imaging. Radiographics. 2015;35(2):636–49. https://doi.org/10.1148/rg.352140104.
27. Torres US, Portela-Oliveira E, Braga Fdel C, Werner H Jr, Daltro PA, Souza AS. When closure fails: what the radiologist needs to know about the embryology, anatomy, and prenatal imaging of ventral body wall defects. Semin Ultrasound CT MR. 2015;36(6):522–36. https://doi.org/10.1053/j.sult.2015.01.001.
28. Applegate KE, Goske MJ, Pierce G, et al. Situs revisited: imaging of the heterotaxy syndrome. Radiographics. 1999;19(4):837–52.

15 Fetal Genito Urinary System Anomalies and Miscellaneous Conditions

15.1 Genito Urinary System Anomalies

Normal kidneys are visualized from 15weeks and appear as elliptical paravertebral organs. The parenchyma shows intermediate signal intensity and the pelvicalyceal system appears hyperintense on T2-weighted HASTE images (Fig. 15.1). The renal cortex appears mildly hypointense as compared to the medulla with the renal corticomedullary differentiation becoming more and more prominent as the gestational age advances [1, 2]. The true-FISP sequence is helpful in the better delineation of obstructive changes in the urinary tract. T1W images are useful in differentiating dilated ureters from adjacent bowel loops as meconium-filled large bowel appear hyperintense as compared to the hypointense dilated ureter [2]. Kidneys appear hyperintense on DWI due to the high cellularity (Fig. 15.2a, b). DWI are very useful in the detection of renal parenchyma and in the assessment of renal functionality. A diseased fetal kidney shows reduced brightness on DWI due to decreased cellularity. Hence, increased ADC values of renal parenchyma are indicative of impaired renal functions. MRI is also helpful in the assessment of associated VATER (vertebral, anal atresia, trachea-esophageal fistula, renal) and pulmonary anomalies. Urinary tract abnormalities can impact fetal lung maturity and thus affect the prognostic implications. MRI is complementary to US when the evaluation is hampered due to oligohydramnios, maternal obesity, and overlying bones.

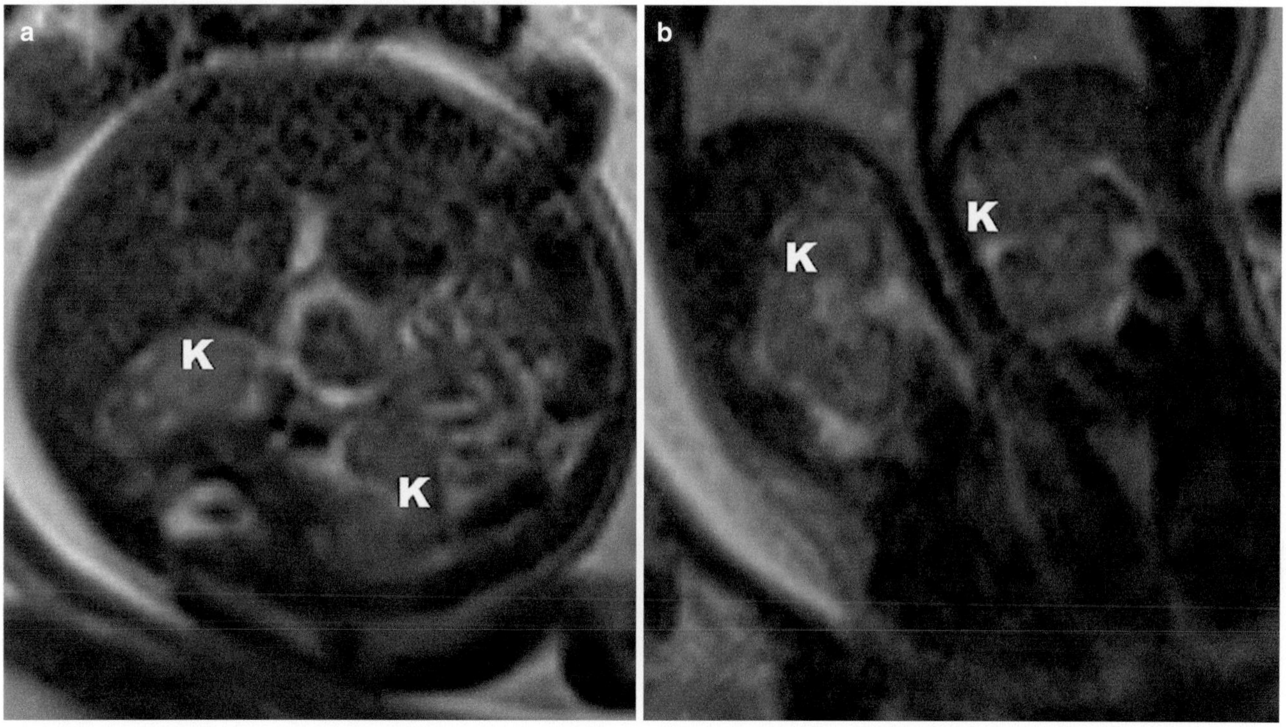

Fig. 15.1 Axial (**a**) and coronal (**b**) T2W images of a 30-week fetus showing normal kidneys. *K* kidneys

R. Rajeswaran, *MR Imaging of the Fetus*, https://doi.org/10.1007/978-981-16-9209-3_15

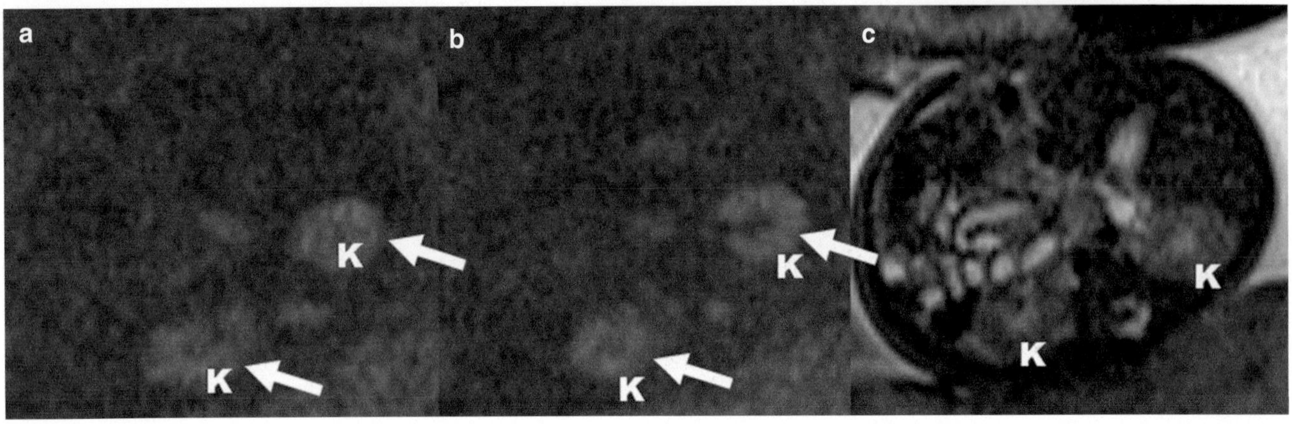

Fig. 15.2 Axial DW images (**a**, **b**) and axial T2W image (**c**) of a 29-week fetus showing normal kidneys. The kidneys appear hyperintense on DWI (arrows). *K* kidneys

15.1.1 Unilateral Renal Agenesis

Definition Absent kidney on one side.

Ultrasound and doppler are diagnostic. Presence of renal artery is useful to pinpoint the presence of kidney and *MRI* is rarely done.

Imaging Features

- Kidneys appear hyperintense on DWI and they are easily located on MRI.
- The ipsilateral renal fossa is empty with absent DWI hyperintense signal elsewhere in the abdomen favors agenesis.
- The contralateral kidney shows compensatory hypertrophy.
- MRI is also useful to differentiate bowel from kidney when there is doubt on sonography.
- MRI is useful when there is associated oligohydramnios [3, 4].

Differential Diagnosis Globular adrenal may mimic a kidney.

Colonic loop may mimic a kidney.

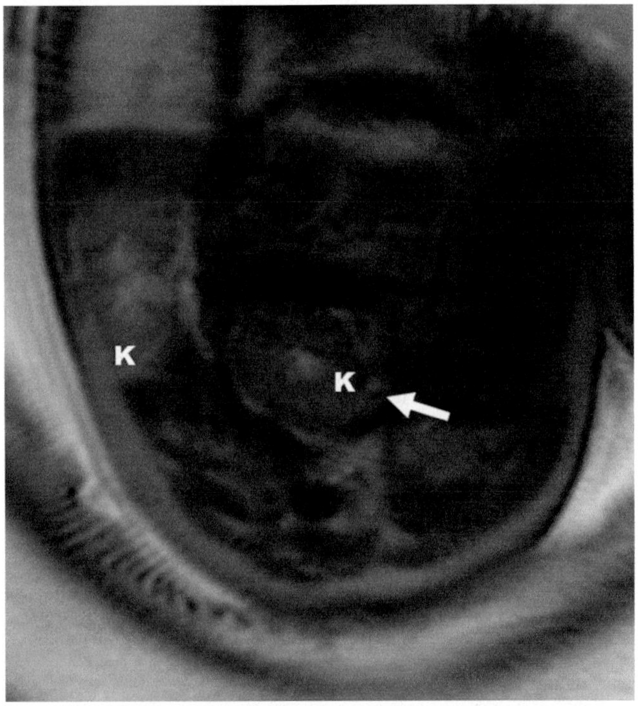

Fig. 15.3 Coronal T2W images of a 34-week fetus showing ectopic left kidney (arrows), *K* kidneys

15.1.2 Ectopic Kidney

- MRI is useful to identify ectopic kidney (Fig. 15.3). It is helpful to differentiate bowel from kidney when there is doubt on sonography [5].
- The ipsilateral renal fossa is empty with the presence of extrarenal/pelvic location of DWI bright signal favors ectopia.

15.1.3 Fusion Abnormality of Kidneys

- Sometimes fusion abnormality may appear as a mass on sonography, MRI is useful to identify the abnormality.
- Crossed fused ectopia (Fig. 15.4), horseshoe kidney (Fig. 15.5) are well seen on MRI.

15.1.4 Multicystic Dysplastic Kidney

Definition The kidney is replaced by noncommunicating cysts of varying sizes. It is due to atresia of the ureter or renal pelvis.

Imaging Features

- MRI is useful in complex/bilateral cases.

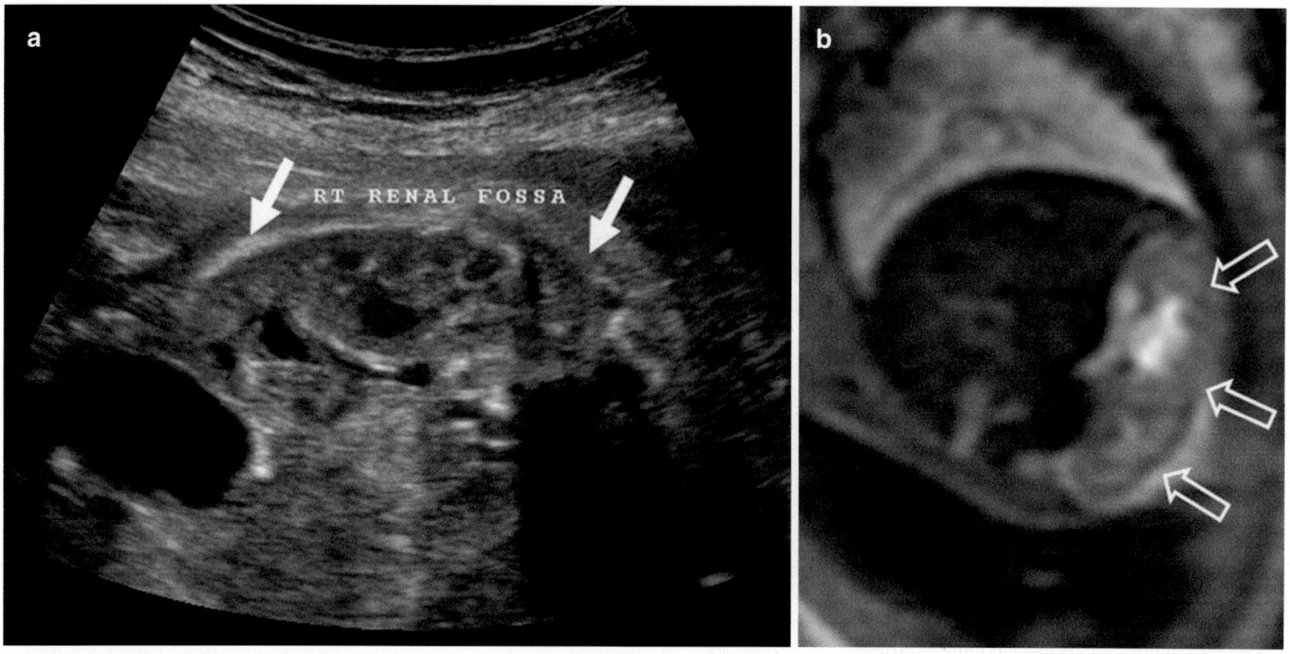

Fig. 15.4 Sonographic (**a**) image shows an enlarged kidney in the right renal fossa (arrow). Sagittal T2w MR image (**b**) shows crossed fused ectopia of the left kidney (open arrows)

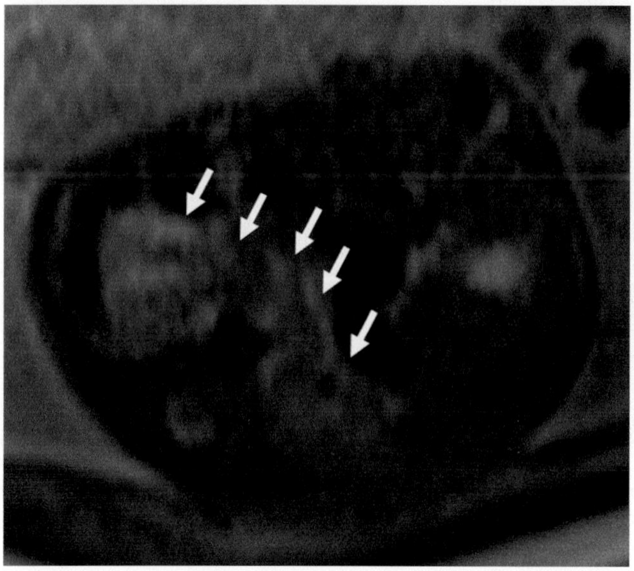

Fig. 15.5 Axial T2W image showing horseshoe kidney (arrows)

- The affected kidney shows the absence of reniform shape. Noncommunicating peripheral and central cysts seen replacing the kidney (Fig. 15.6).
- The lack of normal renal parenchyma results in hypointensity on diffusion-weighted images.
- Bilateral renal involvement may lead to anhydramnios and pulmonary hypoplasia.

Differential Diagnosis

Lymphangioma—multi-septated cyst showing infiltrative features.

Enteric/Duodenal duplication cyst—may resemble perinephric fluid collection, shows laminated bowel signature.

Urinoma—Urine collection within Gerota's fascia due to leakage of urine from severe hydronephrosis. Seen as unilocular cyst that displaces the kidney.

Hydronephrosis due to pelvi-ureteric junction obstruction—The centrally placed dilated renal pelvis shows intercommunication with the peripherally placed dilated calyces.

Mesenteric cyst, Meconium pseudocyst are the other differential diagnoses.

15.1.5 Obstructive Uropathy

The common causes of fetal urinary tract dilatation are Pelviureteric junction obstruction, posterior urethral valves (PUV), ureterocele (usually associated with a duplication anomaly), vesicoureteric reflux disease, urethral atresia, and megacystis microcolon hypoperistalsis syndrome.

Oligohydramnios and pelvic bone ossification may obscure details on sonography. MRI is useful to identify perineal structures like the rectum, vagina, and uterus besides the features like over distended bladder, dilated ureters, and dilated pelvicalyceal system on MRI. Rectum, large bowel appear hyperintense on T1WI due to meconium.

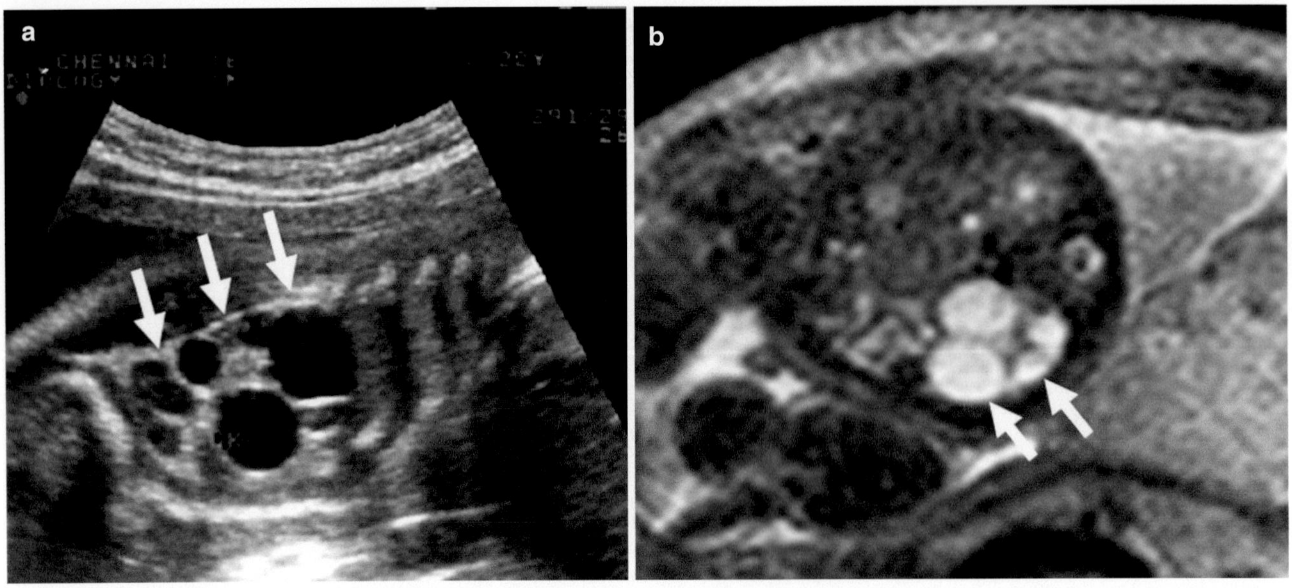

Fig. 15.6 Sonographic (**a**) and axial MR T2W (**b**) images of fetal abdomen show an enlarged kidney with multiple non-communicating cysts suggesting multicystic dysplastic kidney (arrows)

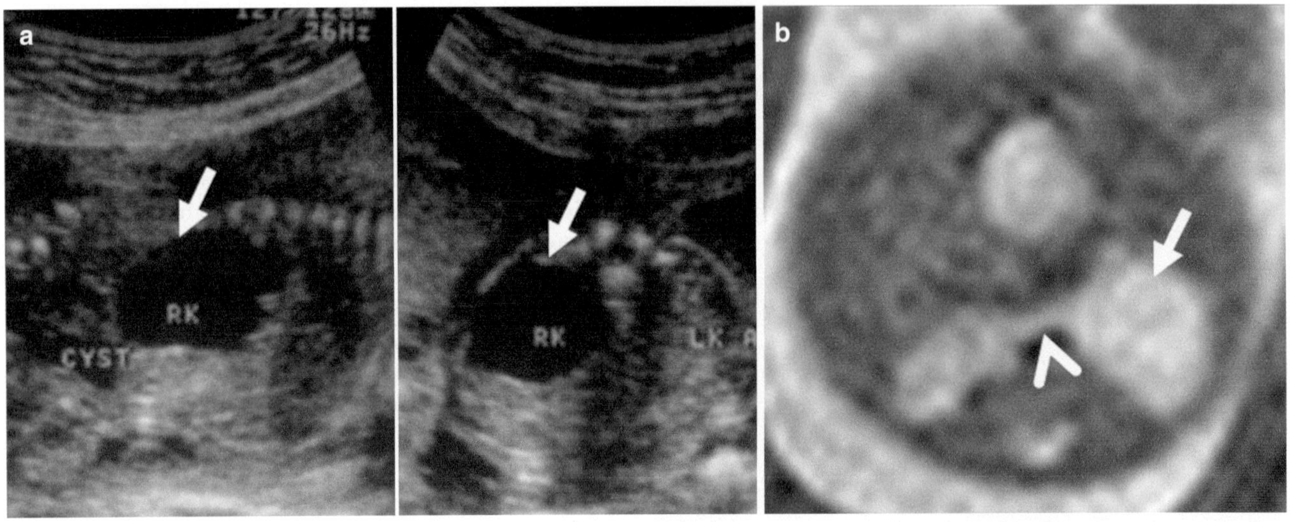

Fig. 15.7 Sonographic (**a**) and axial MR T2W (**b**) images of fetal abdomen show horseshoe kidney (arrowhead). Hydronephrosis with pelvic ureteric junction obstruction is seen in the right limb (arrows). The bridging tissue could not be appreciated on USG

Cloacal abnormalities, posterior urethral dilatation, and ectopic ureteral insertional anomalies are better diagnosed by MRI [6, 7]. MRI can also be utilized for providing additional useful information on other renal features like cortical thickness and signal intensity of renal parenchyma. MRI is also useful to demonstrate cortical thinning in severe hydronephrosis. Dysplastic changes in the kidney lead to increased parenchymal T2 hyperintensity.

Pelvi-Ureteric Junction Obstruction

- Hydronephrosis with narrowing at Pelvi-ureteric junction (Fig. 15.7).
- Presence of communicating cysts within the kidney [7].

Prognosis

Prognosis depends on the contralateral kidney; milder anomaly being associated with a good prognosis. Vesico ureteric reflux, obstruction can be present in the contralateral kidney. Nonfunctioning kidney may involute postnatally.

Posterior Urethral Valve

- Bilateral ureters and pelvicalyceal system may be dilated (Fig. 15.8a).
- Dilated posterior urethra is seen as a "Keyhole." Urinary bladder appears distended (Fig. 15.8b).
- MRI is also useful to demonstrate cortical thinning in severe hydronephrosis.

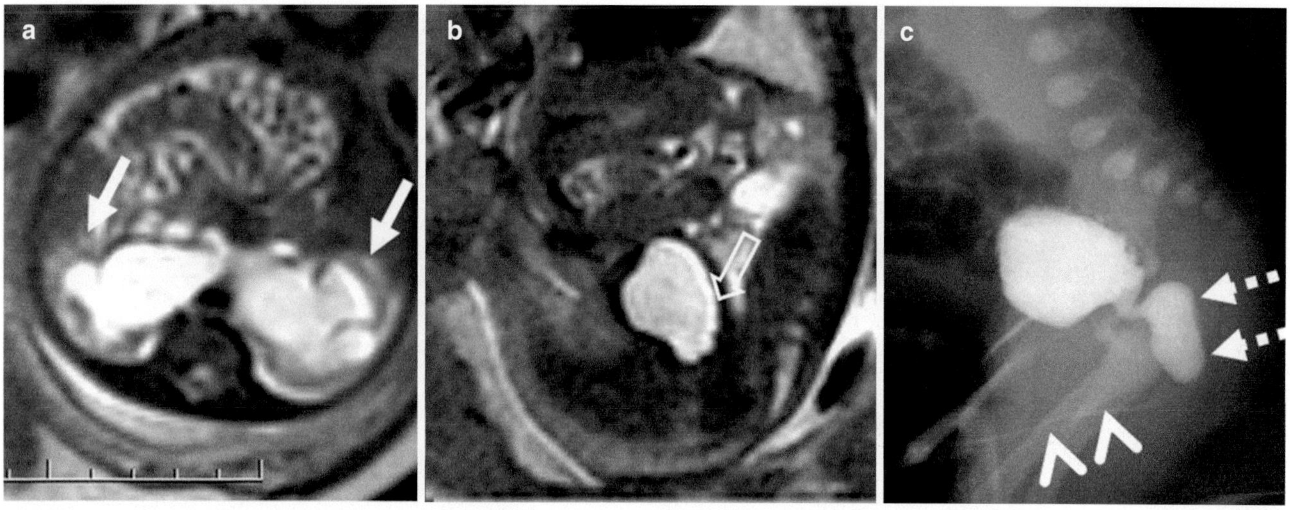

Fig. 15.8 Axial (**a**) and sagittal (**b**) T2 W images of a fetal abdomen showing bilateral hydronephrosis (arrow) and an overdistended bladder (open arrows). Postnatal MCU (**c**) shows dilated posterior urethra (broken arrows), thin stream in anterior urethra (arrowhead) confirming the diagnosis of posterior urethral valve

- There may be urinary ascites when there is a leak from the distended urinary tract (Fig. 15.9).

Differential Diagnosis

Prune belly syndrome—There is a triad of large hypotonic bladder, deficiency of the abdominal wall musculature with anterior abdominal wall distension and bilateral cryptorchidism (Fig. 15.10).

15.1.6 Mesoblastic Nephroma

Definition Hamartoma of fetal kidney. It is a benign spindle cell containing tumor arising from the renal mesenchyme.

Imaging Features [8, 9]

Sonography: Solid mass with increased vascularity. Associated hypoechoic "ring sign" seen surrounding the tumor. Hydrops may be present.

MRI—Is useful to identify the organ of origin. The "Claw sign" is often seen suggesting intrarenal origin. The lesion is mildly hyperintense on T2WI. Larger masses may displace the bowel loops.

Differential diagnosis: Crossed fused ectopia, duplex collecting system, adrenal mass.

Prognosis: Better to be monitored in tertiary care hospital. Postnatal resection with margins is curative. Local recurrence or distant metastasis is rare.

15.1.7 Adrenal Neuroblastoma

Definition Malignant tumor comprising of neuroblasts, arises from adrenal medulla or sympathetic chain.

Pathology Normal fetal adrenal has neuroblastic nodules similar to neuroblastoma. These nodules involute normally. When they do not involute and keep growing, they evolve into neuroblastoma.

Staging:

Stage 1: Confined to the adrenal gland.

Stage 2: Showing extra-adrenal extension but does not cross midline.

Stage 3: There is extension across midline.

Stage 4: Distant metastases.

Stage 4S (Special): Shows good prognosis with metastases to liver, skin, bone marrow, and not bone.

Imaging Features

Sonography: Solid echogenic mass or complex cystic mass with thick septae and doppler flow. Hydrops may be present [10–12].

MRI—Useful to identify the organ of origin and to assess locoregional spread.

Solid mass—Hypo on T1 and moderately hyperintense on T2WI.

Cystic mass—Hypo on T1 and very hyperintense on T2WI.

Differential Diagnosis

1. Extra-lobar sequestration—common on left side (90%). It appears as a homogenous hyperintense mass on T2WI with a prominent feeding vessel from the aorta. A normal adrenal gland may be seen separately.
2. Adrenal hemorrhage: Very rare, showing blooming on GRE/EPI GRE images. By the signal characteristics, it is possible to identify the stage of hemorrhage.
3. Duplex Collecting system: The hydronephrotic upper moiety may resemble a cystic suprarenal mass. The

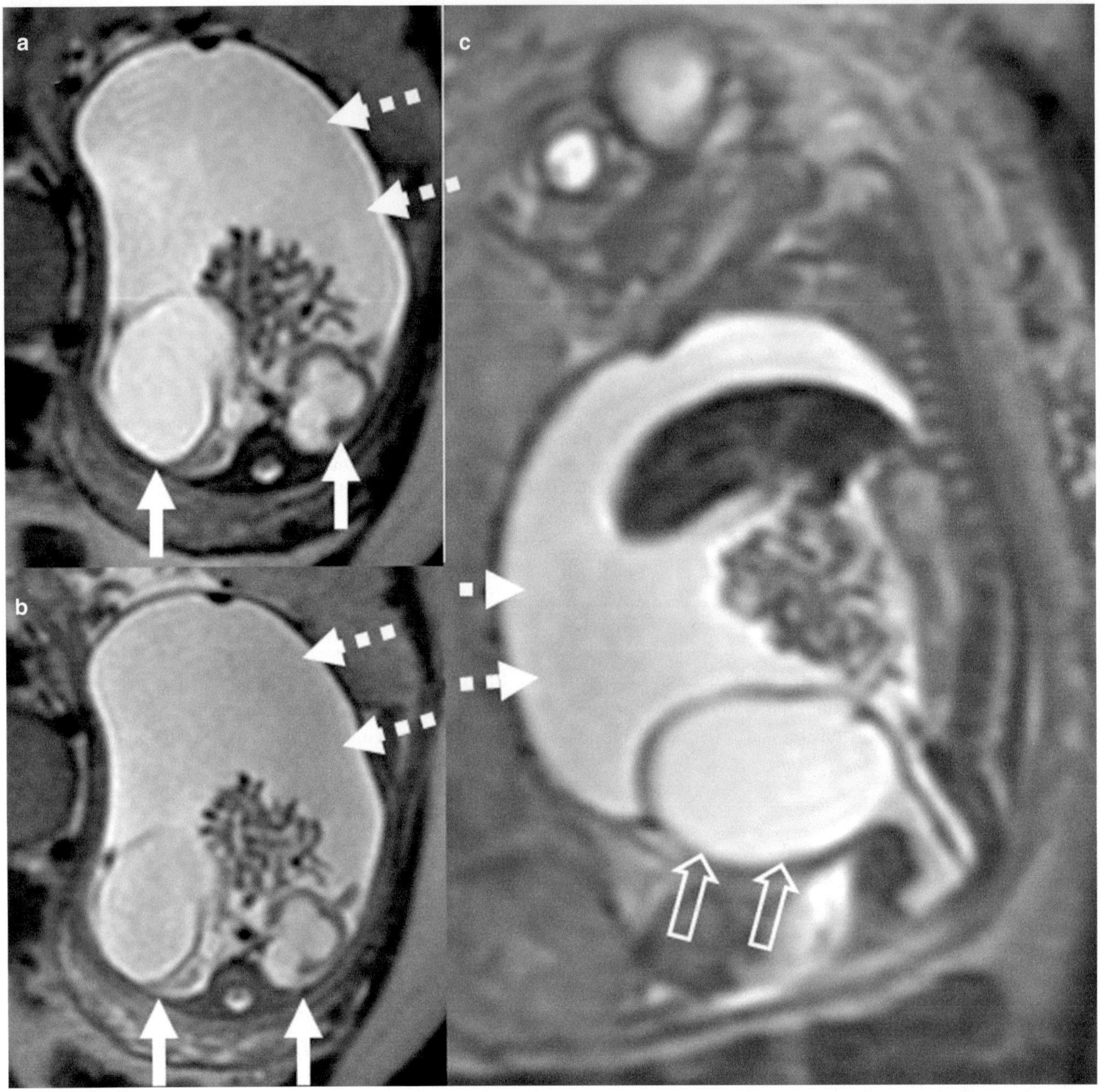

Fig. 15.9 Axial (**a**, **b**) and sagittal (**c**) T2 W images of a fetal abdomen showing bilateral hydronephrosis (arrows), overdistended bladder (open arrows), and urinary ascites (broken arrows)

hydronephrotic upper moiety may be associated with ectopic ureterocele. MRI is useful to identify a normal adrenal gland separately.

Prognosis Is variable with many of them remaining stable and some them showing resolution. Few of them can develop hydrops, extensive disease, and death.

Treatment

Postnatally stable masses less than 5cm size are followed up. Surgery is performed when masses are larger than 5 cm. Chemotherapy is the option when there is a widespread disease.

15.1.8 Ovarian Cyst

Definition Commonly a benign cyst arising from the ovary.

Imaging Abdominal/pelvic cyst with imperceptible wall, with or without daughter cyst (Fig. 15.11) and may show attachment to the ovary. When there is torsion, the cyst may

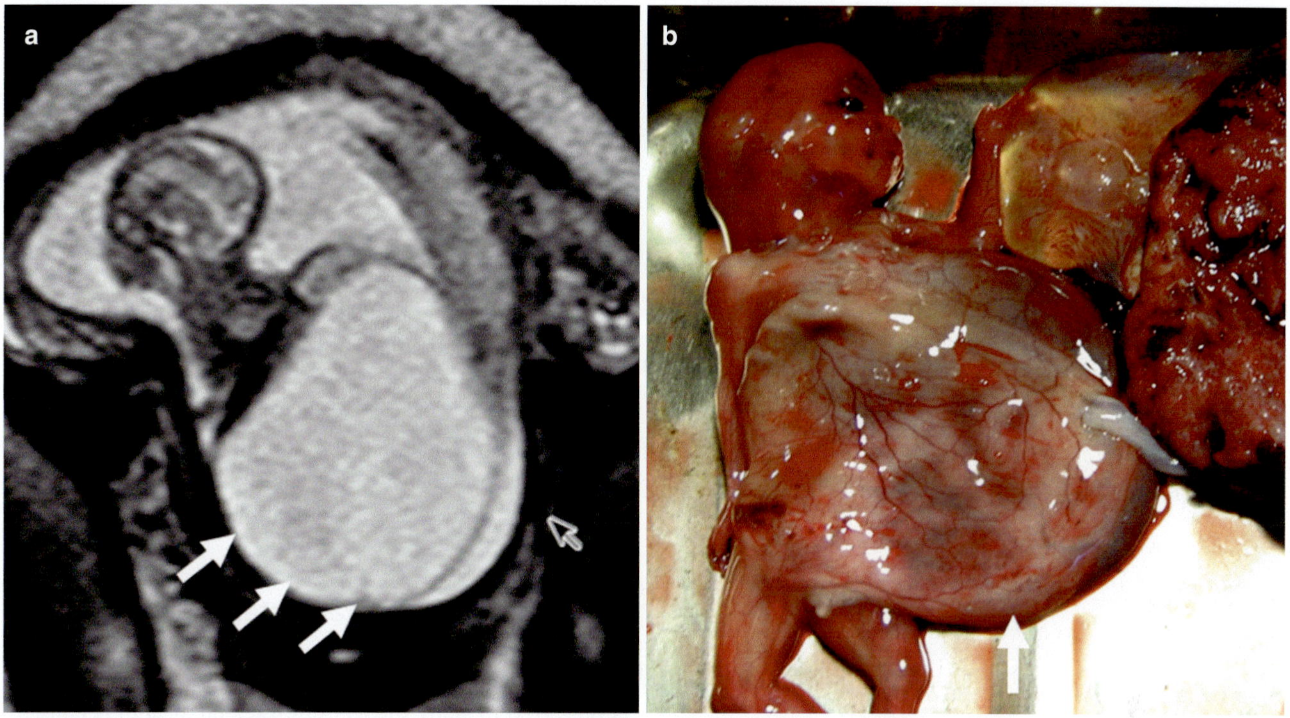

Fig. 15.10 MR (**a**) T2W image of a 17-week fetus shows a large bladder (arrow) due to Prune belly syndrome, that was confirmed postnatally (**b**)

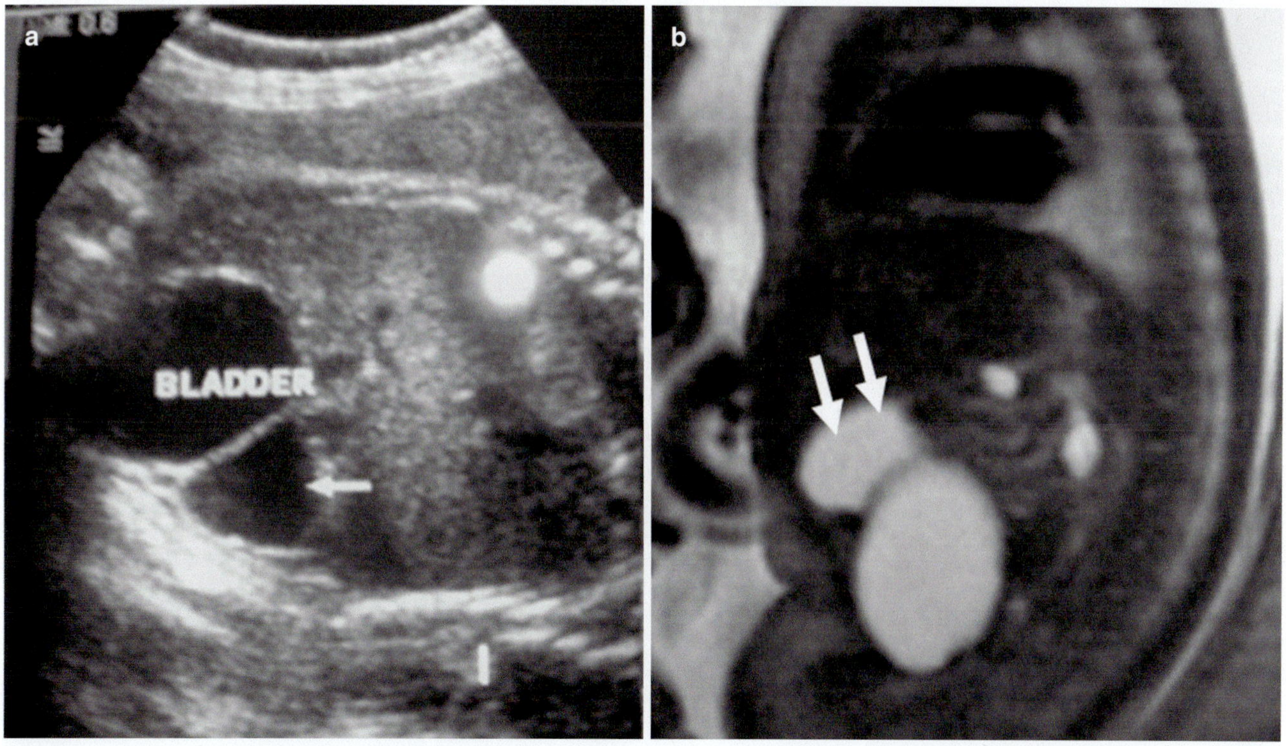

Fig. 15.11 Sonographic (**a**) and sagittal MR T2W (**b**) images of fetal abdomen show an abdominopelvic cyst on left side (arrow)—ovarian cyst. The cyst resolved on postnatal follow-up US scans

show fluid–fluid level and debris with associated free fluid in the abdomen [13, 14].

MRI is useful to identify the anatomy, complexity, and details like intracystic hemorrhage.

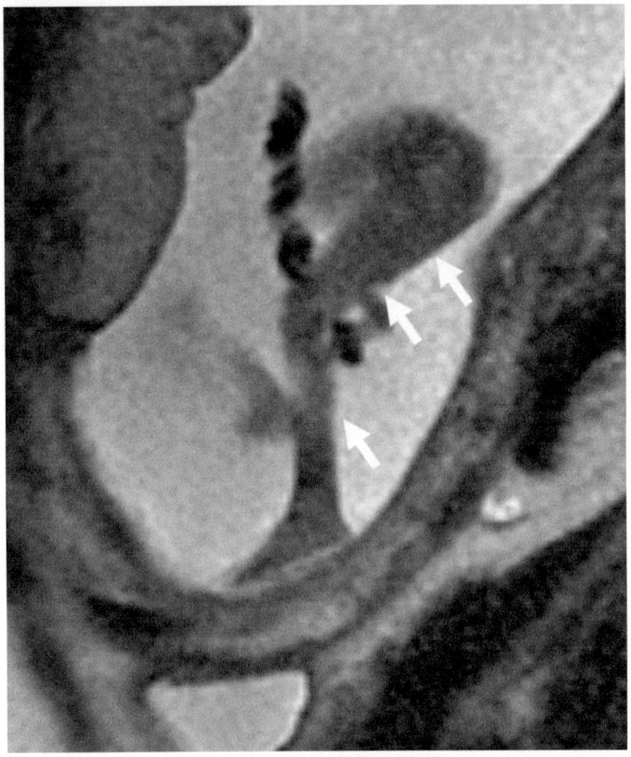

Fig. 15.12 T2W image in a 22-week fetus shows normal lower limb (arrow). The foot is seen at right angle to leg and is seen in profile

Differential Diagnosis Urachal cyst—midline cyst between bladder and cord insertion site.

Enteric duplication cyst—Presents in II trimester and shows "gut signature".

Mesenteric cyst—very rare and can resemble ovarian cyst, may be seen in midline [14].

Hydrocolpos—Midline and is seen posterior to bladder.

Prognosis Cysts less than 5 cm in size may resolve spontaneously. Cysts larger than 5 cm in size are unlikely to resolve and are prone to torsion. They can be treated by in utero- or postnatal aspiration.

Complication Torsion, Infarction/hemorrhage within the cyst can occur. They rarely cause intestinal obstruction because of the mass effect on the bowel [13, 15].

15.2 Musculoskeletal System

Ultrasonography, especially with three-dimensional imaging is preferred to study the Musculoskeletal system because of rapid limb movements. Apart from the usual HASTE sequence (Figs. 15.12 and 15.13) Echoplanar imaging (EPI), thick slab T2 sequences, and dynamic sequences can provide information about the skeleton and muscles. EPI is also useful to obtain an overview of the fetal thorax and skeleton.

Congenital Talipes Equinovarus

Normally in sagittal sections of the leg, the foot is seen at right angle and is seen in profile. In talipes equinovarus, in

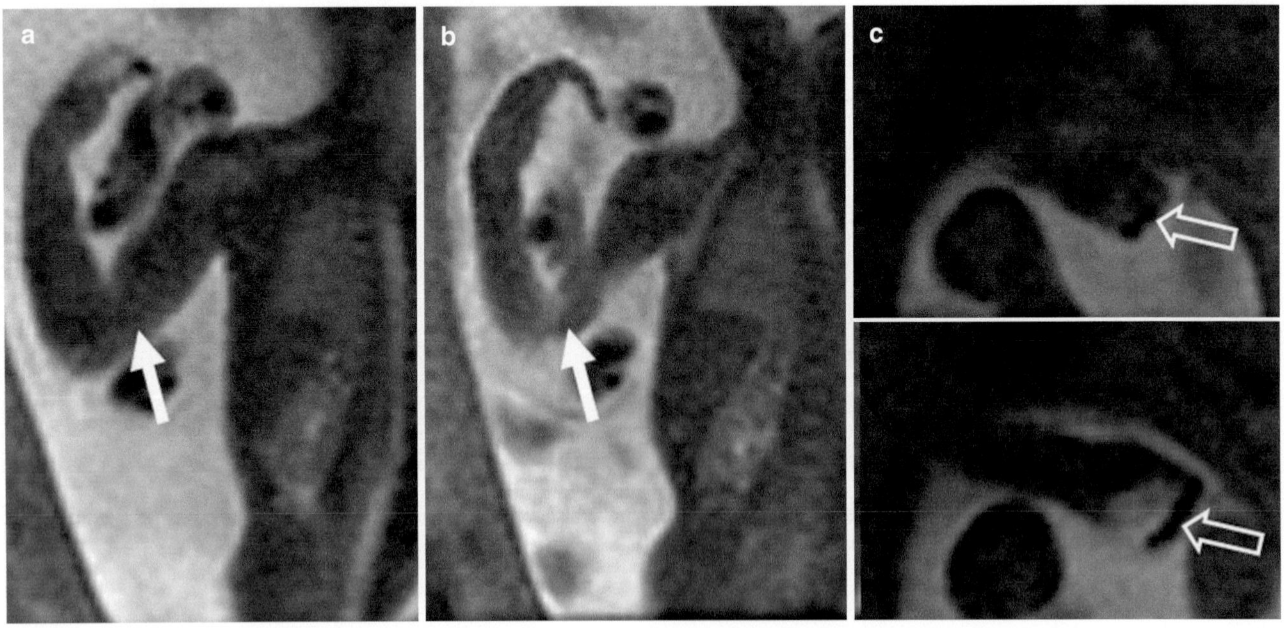

Fig. 15.13 T2W images (**a**–**c**) in a 22-week fetus show normal upper limb (arrows) and hands (open arrows)

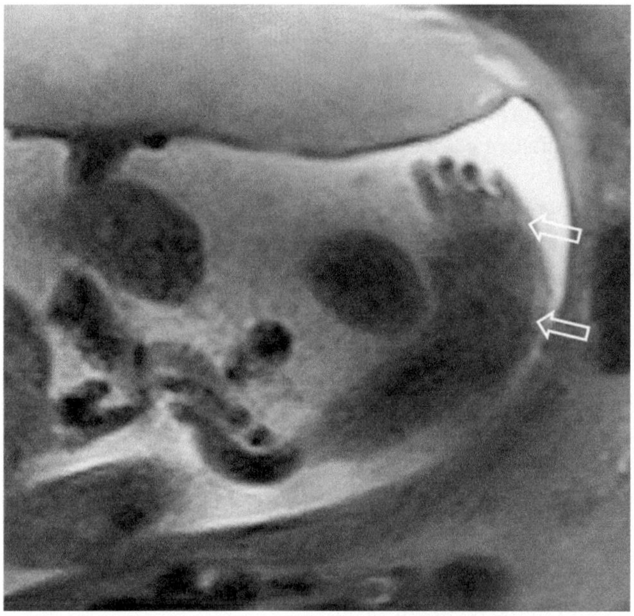

Fig. 15.14 T2W image in a 23-week fetus shows talipes of the foot (arrow). Though the leg is seen in profile (sagittal) view, the foot is seen enface

sagittal sections of the leg—the foot is seen medially deviated and is seen enface (Fig. 15.14).

15.3 Miscellaneous Fetal Conditions

15.3.1 Fetal Growth Restriction (FGR)

Synonym Intrauterine growth restriction (IUGR).

Definition and Pathology

It is defined as a condition where the estimated fetal weight (EFW) is less than the 10th percentile for the gestational age. There are two types:

1. Asymmetric FGR: The abdominal circumference is more reduced as compared to head circumference.
2. Symmetric FGR: The fetus is uniformly small and shows a reduction of all the relevant biometry values.

It is associated with several conditions—Chromosomal disorders, Several syndromes, congenital anomalies, Infection and Multiple gestations.

Imaging Features

Sonography with Doppler is the modality of choice to detect FGR. A knowledge of MRI in FGR is needed as it may be associated to a primary condition like Infection.

- MRI is very useful to calculate volumes of brain, body, lungs, and Placenta
- Placental volume/thickness may be reduced.
- Volumes of brain, body, lungs may be reduced. The usual parameters like BPD, HC, AC are also reduced.
- ADC values of some parts of the brain like Frontal white matter, centrum semiovale, thalami may be reduced [16].
- Placental perfusion is reduced [17].

15.3.2 Hydrops Fetalis

Definition and Pathology

Defined as accumulation of fluid in fluid two or more body cavities.

It is considered as a form of cardiac failure in fetuses. There are two types:

Immune hydrops fetalis—It occurs when there is feto-materal blood group/rhesus incompatibility.

Non-immune hydrops fetalis. Several causes have been identified to cause non-immune hydrops [18–20].

1. Cardiac anomalies, arrhythmia
2. Chromosomal anomalies—trisomy 13,18,21, Turner syndrome
3. Infections
4. Pulmonary anomalies
5. Certain skeletal dysplasias
6. High output flow states/AV shunts
7. Twin–twin transfusion syndrome
8. Metabolic disorders
9. Fetal masses

Imaging Features

- Fetal anasarca
- Skin/subcutaneous/Scalp edema (skin thickness > 5 mm) (Fig. 15.15)
- Ascites/Pleural effusion/Pericardial effusion
- Placentomegaly (placenta thickness > 40 mm in II trimester, >60 mm in III trimester)
- Hepatosplenomegaly
- Polyhydramnios

Prognosis

The prognosis is variable and is dependent on the causative factor.

15.3.3 Twin–Twin Transfusion Syndrome (TTTS)

Definition and Pathology

It is a prenatal condition in which monochorionic twins obtain unequal volume of placenta's blood supply. This results in the two fetuses growing at different rates.

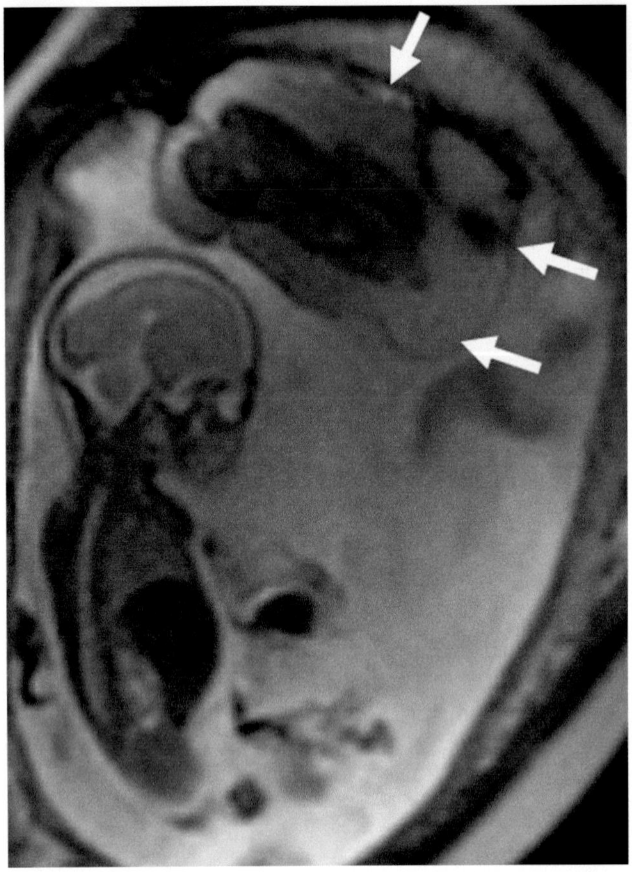

Fig. 15.15 T2W image of a twin shows diffuse subcutaneous edema (arrow) due to hydrops

In TTTS there are abnormal vascular (arteriovenous and arterioarterial) anastomoses in the placenta. Hence, the placental circulation is directed predominantly toward one twin and is supplied less to the other twin [21]. The resultant hypoperfusion in one twin leads to oliguria in the hypovolemic (donor) twin with consequent oligohydramnios. There is hypervolemia and hypertension in the other (recipient) twin with consequent polyhydramnios.

Demise of one of the fetuses in a monochorionic pregnancy is associated with a risk of hypotensive ischemic injury in the surviving twin due to the "twin embolization" syndrome. As vascular anastomoses exist between twins due to monochorionic placentation—Demise of one twin leads to sudden loss of placental bed vascular resistance. The live twin becomes acutely hypotensive resulting in ischemic lesions of brain and kidneys.

Imaging Features [22]
Recipient Twin

- Polyhydramnios
- Large urinary bladder
- Features of cardiac overload—cardiomegaly/fetal hydrops

Donor Twin

- Oligohydramnios, which may result in the twin appearing "stuck" to the side of the gestational sac.
- Small or non-visualized urinary bladder
- Though MRI is not commonly used in the initial evaluation of TTTS, it is very useful in the identification of cerebral ischemia and intraventricular hemorrhage associated with TTTS.
- There may be altered hemodynamics leading to dilated cerebral venous sinuses in donor and recipient twins which may be well demonstrated on MRI.
- There may be dilatation of the renal pelvic collecting system in the recipient twin.
- Fetal MRI is useful after laser therapy for TTTS or after death of one twin to rule out ischemic (Fig. 15.16)/hemorrhagic injury to the brain parenchyma. There can be secondary ventriculomegaly secondary to ischemic encephalomalacic changes in the brain (Fig. 15.17).

Laser coagulation is the treatment of choice for TTTS in pregnancies at <26 weeks—Selective coagulation of the anastomoses at placental vascular equator is commonly performed.

- DWI can demonstrate cerebral damage immediately after fetoscopic laser coagulation if done 1–4 days after the procedure [23].
- MRI at 4–6 weeks after the procedure is useful to see brain changes like encephalomalacia.

15.3.4 Single Umbilical Artery

It is an important marker for chromosomal anomalies. It is the result of agenesis or atrophy of one of the arteries. The umbilical cord normally has two arteries and one vein (Fig. 15.18b). Single umbilical artery should always be ruled out during a routine second-trimester scan and can be detected on cross-sectional imaging of the umbilical cord (Fig. 15.18a).

It can be associated with trisomy 18, 13 and triploidy, fetal growth retardation, abnormalities of cardiovascular, genitourinary, gastrointestinal, skeletal, and central nervous systems.

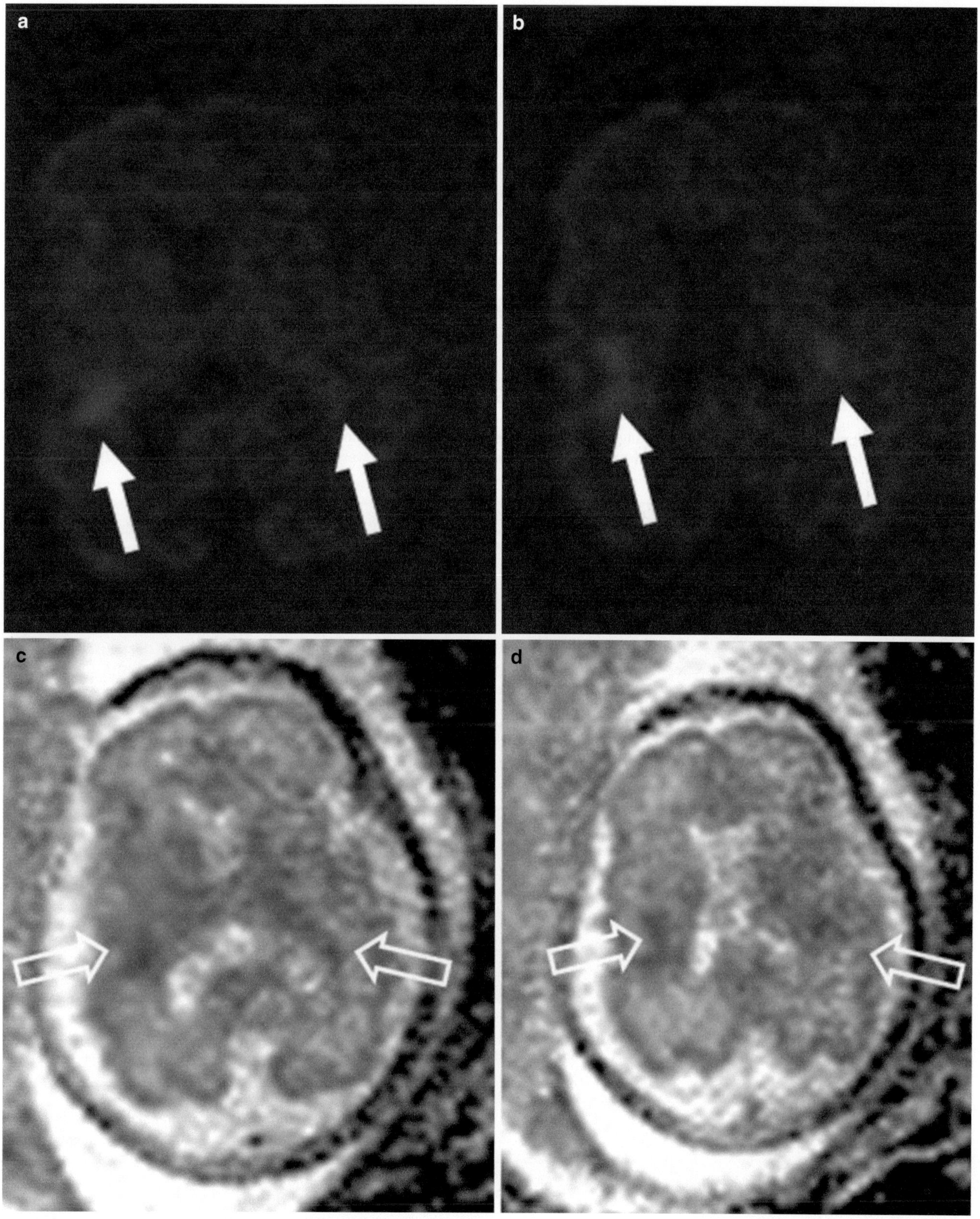

Fig. 15.16 Axial diffusion-weighted images (**a**, **b**) showing acute infarcts (arrows) in bilateral parietal region in the surviving twin following co-twin demise. ADC images (**c**, **d**) showing restricted diffusion (open arrows)

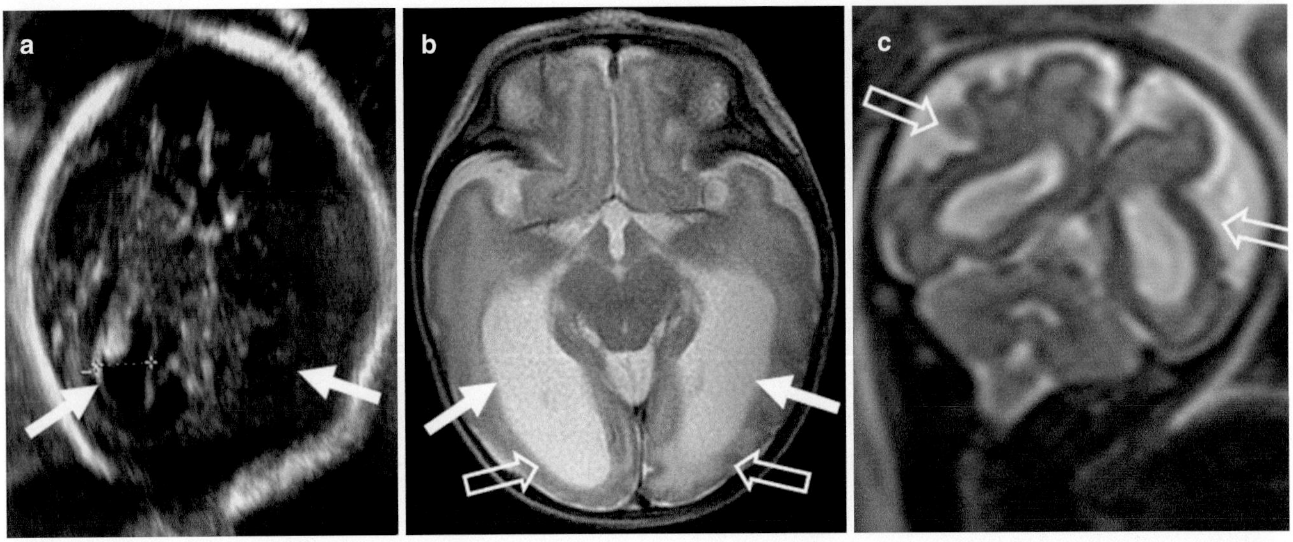

Fig. 15.17 Sonographic (**a**) and MR (**b**, **c**) T2W images show bilateral ventriculomegaly (arrows) due to encephalomalacic changes in bilateral parieto-occipital lobes (open arrows) in the surviving twin following co-twin demise at 23 weeks. The present scan was taken at 29 weeks

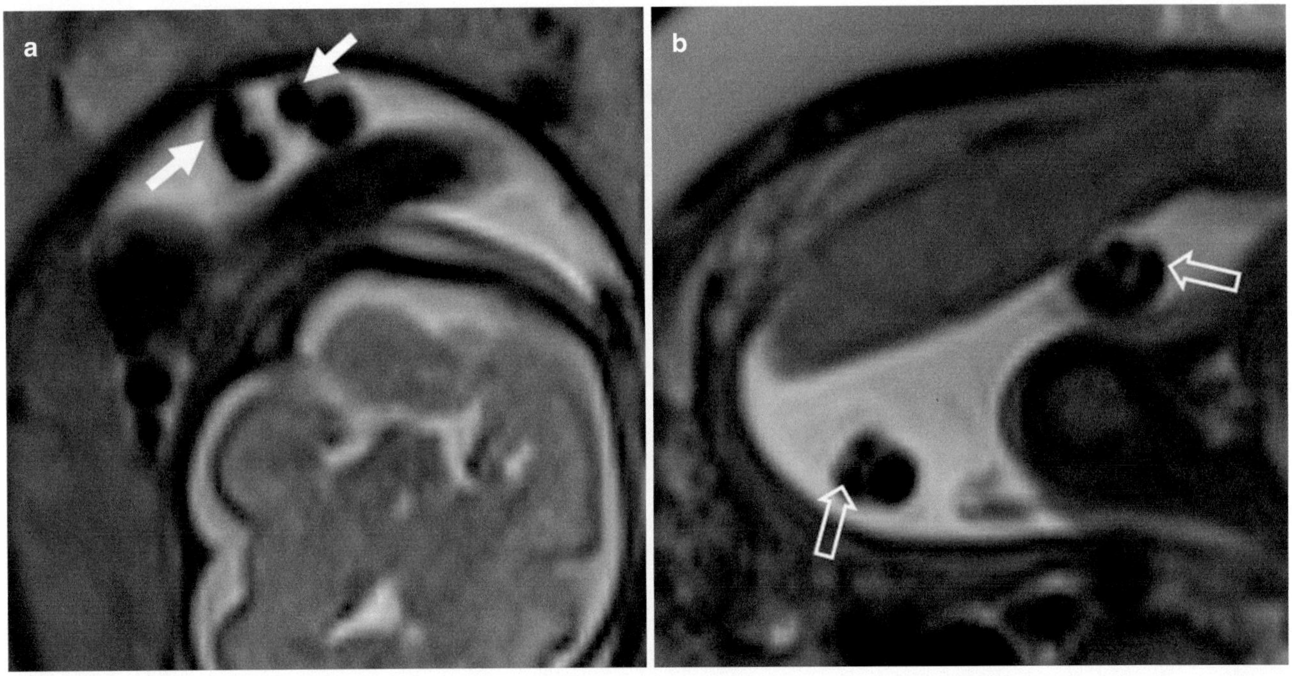

Fig. 15.18 T2W image in a 24-week fetus (**a**) shows single umbilical artery (arrow); in a 31-week fetus (**b**) 2 umbilical arteries are seen (open arrows)

References

1. Chalouhi GE, Millischer AÉ, Mahallati H, Siauve N, Melbourne A, Grevent D, et al. The use of fetal MRI for renal and urogenital tract anomalies. Prenat Diagn. 2020;40:100–9.
2. Furey EA, Bailey AA, Twickler DM. Fetal MR imaging of gastrointestinal abnormalities. Radiographics. 2016;36:904–17.
3. Gomez Huertas M, Culianez Casas M, Molina Garcia FS, Carrillo Badillo MP, Pastor PE. Complementary role of magnetic resonance imaging in the study of the fetal urinary system. Radiologia. 2016;58:101–10.
4. Gupta S, Mohi JK, Gambhir P, et al. Prenatal diagnosis of congenital anomalies of genito-urinary system on fetal magnetic resonance imaging. Egypt J Radiol Nucl Med. 2020;51:155. https://doi.org/10.1186/s43055-020-00278-z.
5. Oh KY, et al. Prenatal diagnosis of renal developmental anomalies associated with an empty renal fossa. Ultrasound Q. 2010;26(4):233–40.
6. Faghihimehr A, Gharavi M, Mancuso GSG. Fetal MR imaging in urogenital system anomalies. J Matern Fetal Neonatal Med. 2018;32:3487–94.
7. Millischer AE, Grevent D, Rousseau V, O'Gorman N, Sonigo P, Bessieres B, et al. Fetal MRI compared with ultrasound for the

diagnosis of obstructive genital malformations. Prenat Diagn. 2017;37:1138–45.
8. Irsutti M, Puget C, Baunin C, et al. Mesoblastic nephroma: prenatal ultrasonographic and MRI features. Pediatr Radiol. 2000;30:147–50. https://doi.org/10.1007/s002470050033.
9. Do AY, Kim JS, Choi SJ, Oh SY, Roh CR, Kim JH. Prenatal diagnosis of congenital mesoblastic nephroma. Obstet Gynecol Sci. 2015;58(5):405–8.
10. Grandó A, Monteggía V, Gandara C, et al. Prenatal sonographic diagnosis of adrenal neuroblastoma. J Clin Ultrasound. 2001;29(4):250–3.
11. Maki E, Oh K, Rogers S, Sohaey R. Imaging and differential diagnosis of suprarenal masses in the fetus. J Ultrasound Med. 2014;33:895–904.
12. Erol O, Süren D, Erol MB. Prenatal diagnosis of adrenal neuroblastoma: a case report with a brief review of the literature. Case Rep Obstet Gynaecol. 2013;2013:506490. https://doi.org/10.1155/2013/50649.
13. Nemec U, Nemec SF, Bettelheim D, Brugger PC, Horcher E, Schöpf V, et al. Ovarian cysts on prenatal MRI. Eur J Radiol. 2012;81:1937–44.
14. Matos APP, Duarte LB, Castro PT, Daltro P, Werner Júnior H, Araujo JE. Evaluation of the fetal abdomen by magnetic resonance imaging. Part 1: malformations of the abdominal cavity. Radiol Bras. 2018;51(2):112–8.
15. Trinh TW, Kennedy AM. Fetal ovarian cysts: review of imaging spectrum, differential diagnosis, management, and outcome. Radiographics. 2015;35:621–35.
16. Arthurs OJ, Rega A, Guimiot F, et al. Diffusion-weighted magnetic resonance imaging of the fetal brain in intrauterine growth restriction. Ultrasound Obstet Gynecol. 2017;50(1):79–87.
17. Gowland P. Placental MRI. Semin Fetal Neonatal Med. 2005;10:485–90.
18. Abrams ME, Meredith KS, Kinnard P, et al. Hydrops fetalis: a retrospective review of cases reported to a large national database and identification of risk factors associated with death. Pediatrics. 2007;120(1):84–9.
19. Jauniaux E. Diagnosis and management of early non-immune hydrops fetalis. Prenat Diagn. 1997;17(13):1261–8.
20. Holzgreve W, Curry CJ, Golbus MS, et al. Investigation of nonimmune hydrops fetalis. Am J Obstet Gynecol. 1984;150(7):805–12.
21. Sebire NJ, Talbert D, Fisk NM. Twin-to-twin transfusion syndrome results from dynamic asymmetrical reduction in placental anastomoses: a hypothesis. Placenta. 2001;22(5):383–91.
22. Khalil A, Rodgers M, Baschat A, et al. ISUOG Practice Guidelines: role of ultrasound in twin pregnancy. Ultrasound Obstet Gynecol. 2016;47(2):247.
23. Weisz B, Hoffmann C, Ben-Baruch S, Yinon Y, Gindes L, Katorza E, Shrim A, Bar Yosef O, Schiff E, Lipitz S. Early detection by diffusion-weighted sequence magnetic resonance imaging of severe brain lesions after fetoscopic laser coagulation for twin-twin transfusion syndrome. Ultrasound Obstet Gynecol. 2014;44(1):44–9.

Placental Diseases, Ectopic Pregnancy, and Other Obstetric Applications

16

Sonography is the modality of choice in imaging pregnant patients with pelvic and placental pathologies. It is inexpensive, widely available, safe, and accurate. However, US is operator-dependent and suffers from limitations like inability to image a large field of view (FOV), cannot differentiate hemorrhage from fluids, poor acoustic window in advanced pregnancy and obesity. There can be difficulty in evaluating posterior placenta and adnexal regions by US. MRI is safe in pregnancy, has advantages like high soft-tissue contrast, large FOV coverage, characterize lesions based on T1/T2 properties, and differentiate blood from fluid. Hence, MRI is being increasingly used as a complementary tool, where the USG diagnosis is ambiguous [1–4]. The other obstetric applications of MRI are summarized in Table 16.1.

Technique

While imaging the pelvis/lower abdomen, the application of Phased array torso coil is recommended to obtain better SNR. Gadolinium contrast agent is generally avoided during pregnancy. However, in select cases, dynamic contrast-enhanced images may be obtained in the evaluation of placenta morbidly adherent placenta just prior to delivery. During the 2nd and 3rd trimesters, ultra-fast sequences are employed to overcome artifacts from maternal breathing and fetal movements.

Table 16.1 The placental and other obstetric applications of MRI

• Placental pathologies – Placental adherence – Abruptio placenta – Gestational trophoblastic disease – Variants like bilobed placenta – Placental tumors • Ectopic pregnancy	• Uterine Complications—Rupture, Fibroid degeneration • Planning delivery – Placenta praevia – MR pelvimetry • Postpartum complications – Hematoma – Ovarian vein thrombosis – Uterine arteriovenous malformation Abscess

MRI protocol in early pregnancy and postpartum cases, when the Field of view to be imaged is limited to the pelvis

- High-resolution T2 Weighted Fast Spin Echo in axial, coronal, and sagittal planes. They may be obtained with respect to uterus in case of uterine pathologies.
- T1, T1 fat-suppressed Fast Spin Echo in axial plane.
- Diffusion-weighted imaging (DWI) in axial plane
- Short Tau Inversion Recovery (STIR) images in axial or coronal plane
- Gradient (GRE) images in axial plane

MRI protocol in 2nd and 3rd trimester of pregnancy, when the Field of view to be imaged is large

- T2 Weighted imaging in axial, coronal, and sagittal planes with respect to the maternal lower abdomen using Half-Fourier acquisition Single-shot Turbo Spin Echo (HASTE) or Fast Spin Echo with motion correction applied
- True Fast imaging with steady-state precession (TruFi) with fat suppression (FS) in three planes
- T1W and T1 FS axial images with Turbo FLASH or Fast Spoiled Gradient sequence (FSPGR). T1 axial images can also be obtained using Fast Spin Echo with motion correction applied.
- Diffusion-weighted images (DWI) in axial plane
- Gradient or Echo Planar imaging-gradient (EPI GRE) images in axial plane
- Imaging is preferred with respiratory triggering.

Normal Placenta

The placenta appears fairly homogeneous during 19–23 weeks (Fig. 16.1a). Subsequently, it develops faint septations that increase in number as the gestational age progresses (Fig. 16.1b). The lobules become prominent (stratification) after 36 weeks. Flow voids are seen below placenta normally. *Placental thickness* increases with gestational age at approximately 1 mm per week. The maximum thickness of a normal placenta is 4 cm.

R. Rajeswaran, *MR Imaging of the Fetus*, https://doi.org/10.1007/978-981-16-9209-3_16

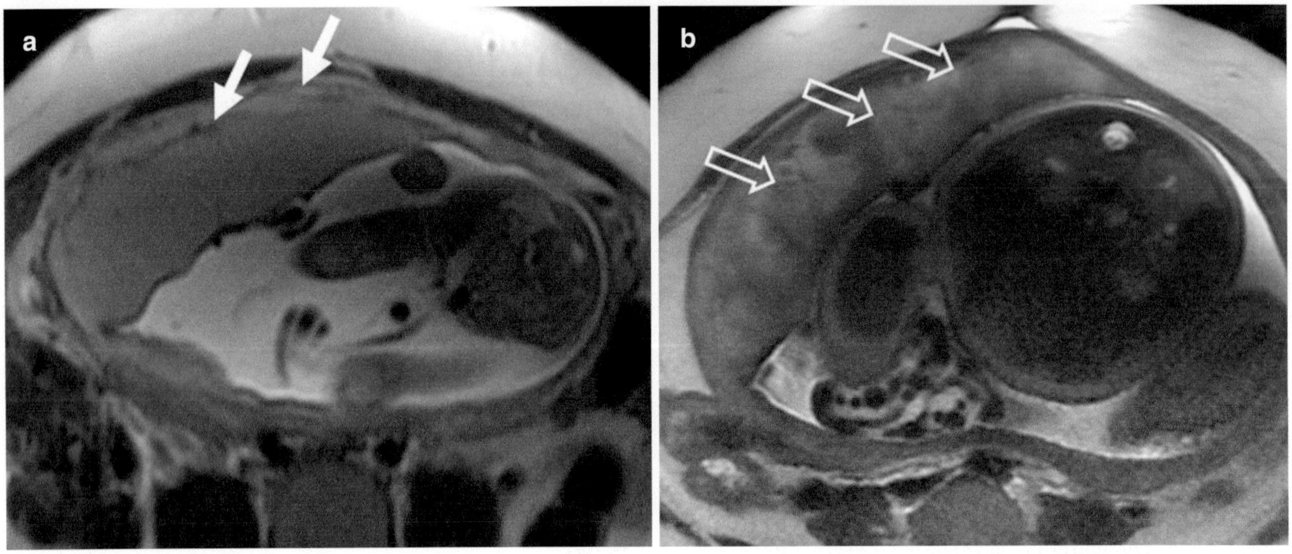

Fig. 16.1 MRI appearances of normal placentation at different gestational ages. (**a**) Axial T2 HASTE MR image shows a homogeneous placenta (arrow) at 22 weeks of gestational age. (**b**) Axial T2 HASTE MR image shows a mildly heterogeneous stratified placenta due to multiple placental septi (open arrows) at 36 weeks of gestational age

The gestational age (in weeks) = placental thickness ± 10 mm.

Morbidly Adherent Placenta (MAP)

Morbidly adherent Placenta is a condition where there is direct invasion of the placental chorionic villi into the myometrium due to defect in the decidua basalis. It can result in severe hemorrhage at the time of attempted placental separation. Common predisposing factors include previous cesarean section/uterine surgery, dilatation and curettage, placenta previa, advanced maternal age, and multiparity [3–5]. When MAP is diagnosed antenatally, these pregnant mothers are managed at adequately equipped tertiary care hospitals to reduce maternal morbidity and mortality.

Placental adherence is subclassified based on the degree of villous invasion:

- Placenta accreta (superficial myometrial invasion),
- Placenta increta (deep myometrial invasion)
- Placenta percreta (invasion through the uterine myometrium-serosa with invasion of the adjacent organs)
- Commonly imaging cannot identify these subtypes. Hence, the term Morbidly adherent Placenta is used.

MRI is complementary to USG especially in posterior placenta and to identify the depth of invasion. The following are the findings on MRI in placental adherence [1, 5]:

- Loss of retroplacental T2 dark zone/loss of placental–endometrial interface (Figs. 16.2 and 16.3). False positives due to (breathing) motion artifact can occur [6]. On DWI, myometrium appears hypointense, placenta appears hyperintense and thus the placental-myometrial interface can be defined. The invasion of placental tissue into myometrium can be seen on DWI.

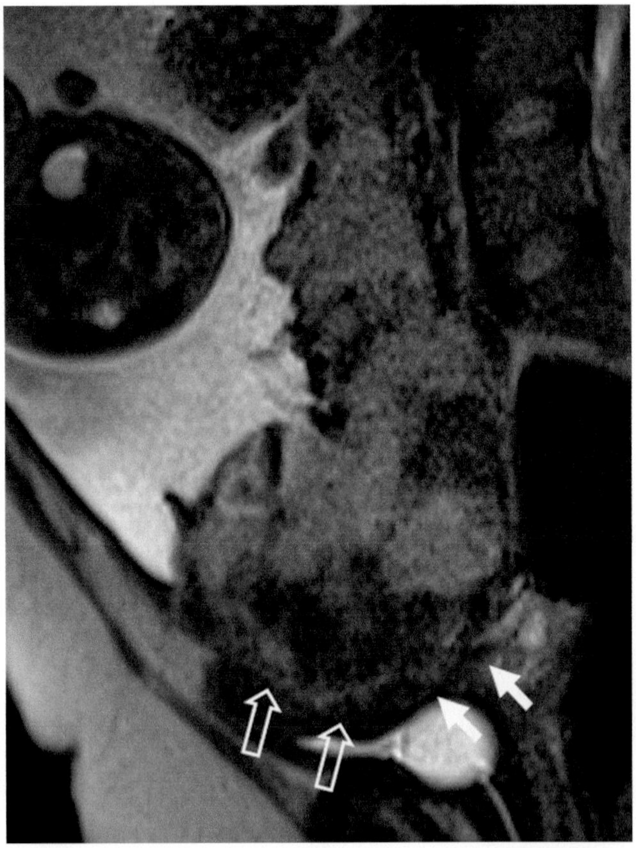

Fig. 16.2 Sagittal T2W image shows the placental edge completely covering the internal os (arrows). There is loss of interface between the placenta and decidua basalis in the anterior aspect with associated focal bulge (open arrows)—Placenta acreta

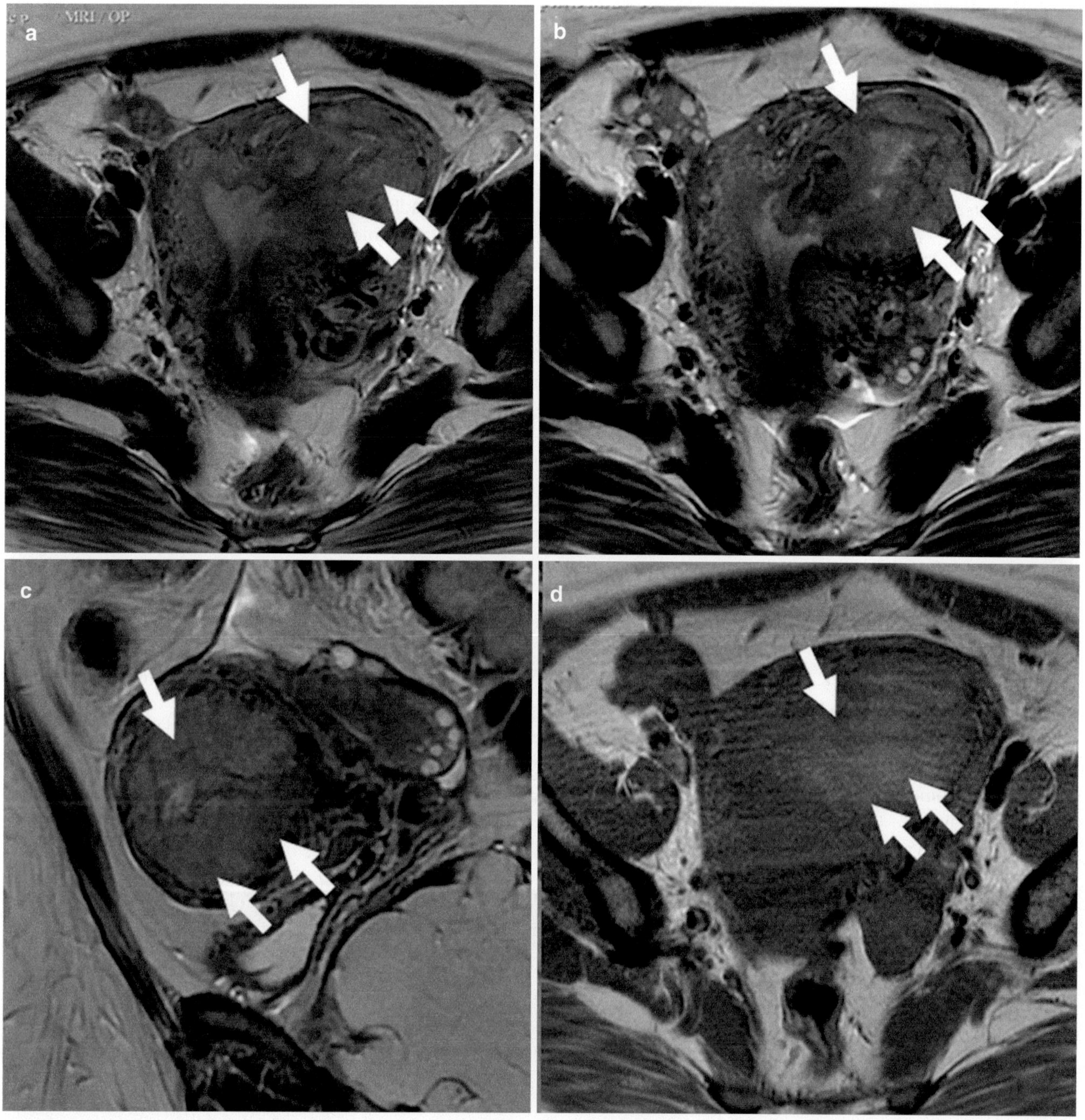

Fig. 16.3 Coronal (**a**, **b**), sagittal (**c**) and coronal (**d**) T1W images of a postpartum uterus following dilatation and curettage at 20 weeks for an anomalous fetus. Morbidly adherent placenta. Is seen in the endo-myometrium region in the left side of the uterine fundus, cornu region (arrows)

- Intraplacental dark bands on T2 WI—nodular or linear low signal intensity due to presence of fibrin.
- Focal uterine bulge (Fig. 16.2)
- Focal areas of severe myometrial thinning (<1 mm) or interruptions. False positives due to stretched uterine wall can occur in late pregnancy.
- Heterogeneous signal intensity of the placenta due to hemorrhage/lacunae within
- Presence of hypertrophied vessels and disorganized intra-placental vascularity
- Gd is used on selected patients who are elected for immediate termination of pregnancy or cesarean section [7].

Some studies have shown that MR imaging is useful in placental adherence with accuracy reaching around 70%. Sensitivity and specificity of 76.9% and 50% for MRI and

100% and 37.5% for ultrasound in the detection of morbid placental adherence has been reported in a series of 42 patients [1].

Treatment

1. Delivery by Cesarean hysterectomy at 34–35 weeks, by multidisciplinary team results in good outcomes
2. When uterine preservation is considered, prior uterine artery embolization may be done followed by delivery via Cesarean section. The placenta is left in situ or partially removed if there is separation [8, 9].

Abruptio Placenta (AP)

Placental abruption refers to premature separation of the placenta and is an important cause of vaginal bleeding during the 3rd trimester of pregnancy. It is often associated with significant perinatal mortality and morbidity, accounting for 25% of perinatal death. Masselli et al. [10] in a study on 60 patients found 100% accuracy with MRI in diagnosing AP and only 52% by USG.

Imaging Features

MRI is recommended whenever the patient is hemodynamically stable.

- Hematoma formation can be:
  - Retroplacental-hemorrhage is behind the placenta (Fig. 16.4)
  - Subchorionic—when only the margin of the placenta is separated
  - Pre-placental-hemorrhage is in the umbilical cord side of the placenta and limited by the umbilical cord (Fig. 16.5) [10].
- The stage of hemorrhage can be classified as hyperacute, acute, early subacute, late subacute, and chronic based on the age of hemorrhage.
- Underlying pathologic conditions like placenta previa, placental adherence, or vasa previa can be assessed
- Due to anechoic/isoechoic nature of the acute hemorrhage, it is sometimes difficult to diagnose on sonography. MRI is helpful to diagnose abruption and to determine the site of the blood clot.

Gestational Trophoblastic Disease

This includes hydatidiform mole and gestational trophoblastic tumors (invasive mole and choriocarcinoma).

Molar pregnancy can be further classified into partial and complete mole. USG is the modality of choice in molar pregnancy. MRI in molar pregnancy is limited to obese patients and co-existing other pathologies like leiomyoma.

Imaging features:

- Markedly hyperintense on T2WI with multiple cystic spaces distending the endometrial cavity (Fig. 16.6a, b).
- Presence of sharp border between the myometrium and the mass

Invasive Trophoblastic Tumors

- Invasion of the uterine wall is better seen on MRI than on sonography (Fig. 16.7a, b).

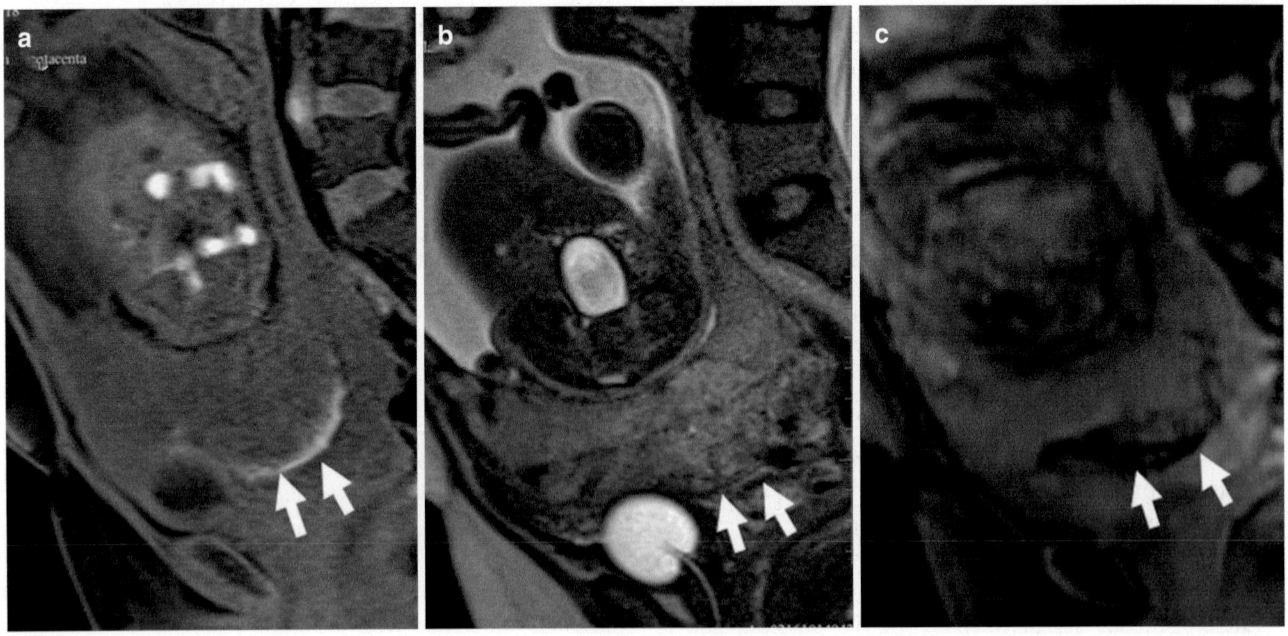

Fig. 16.4 Sagittal T1 (**a**), sagittal T2 (**b**) and sagittal GRE (**c**) images show type IV placenta praevia and retroplacental hemorrhage (arrows)

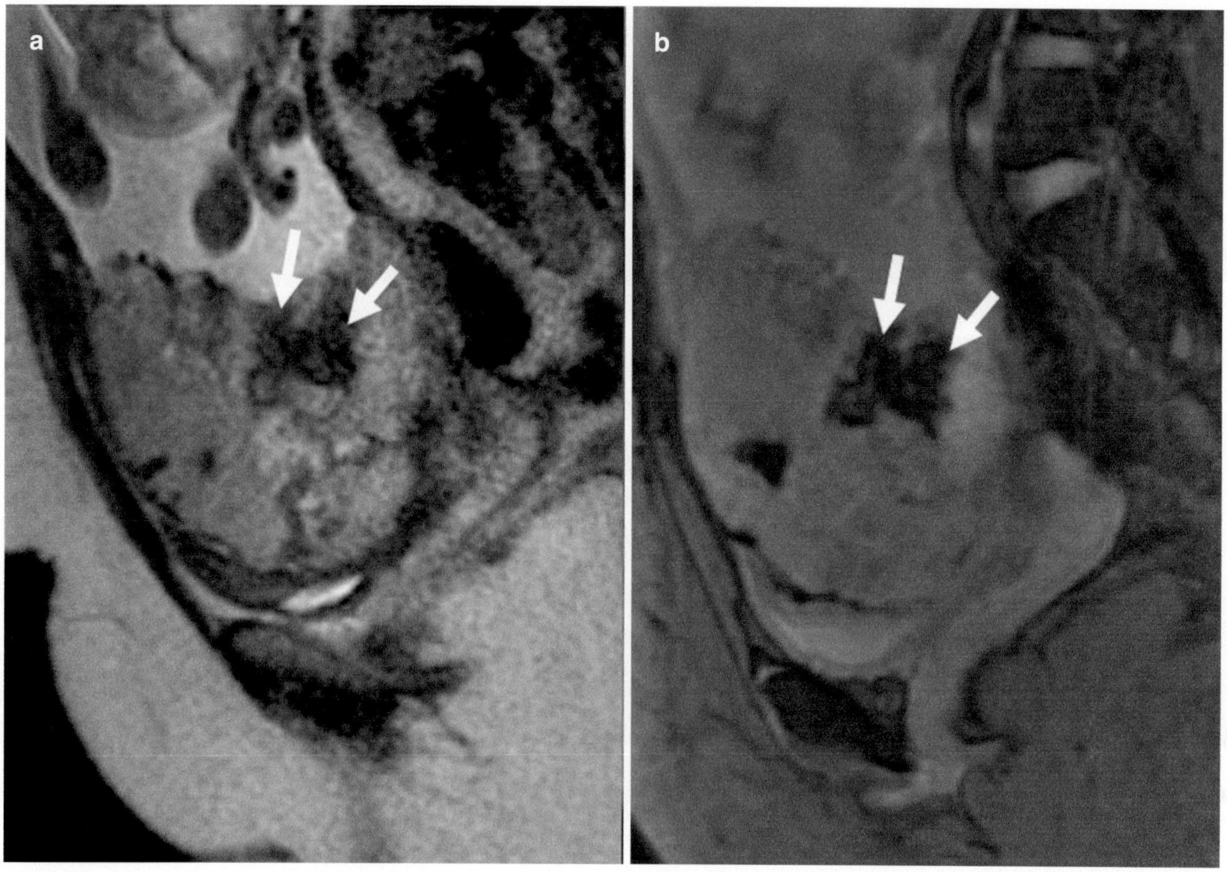

Fig. 16.5 Sagittal T2W (**a**) and GRE (**b**) sagittal images show type IV placenta praevia with Placenta acreta and preplacental hemorrhage (arrows)

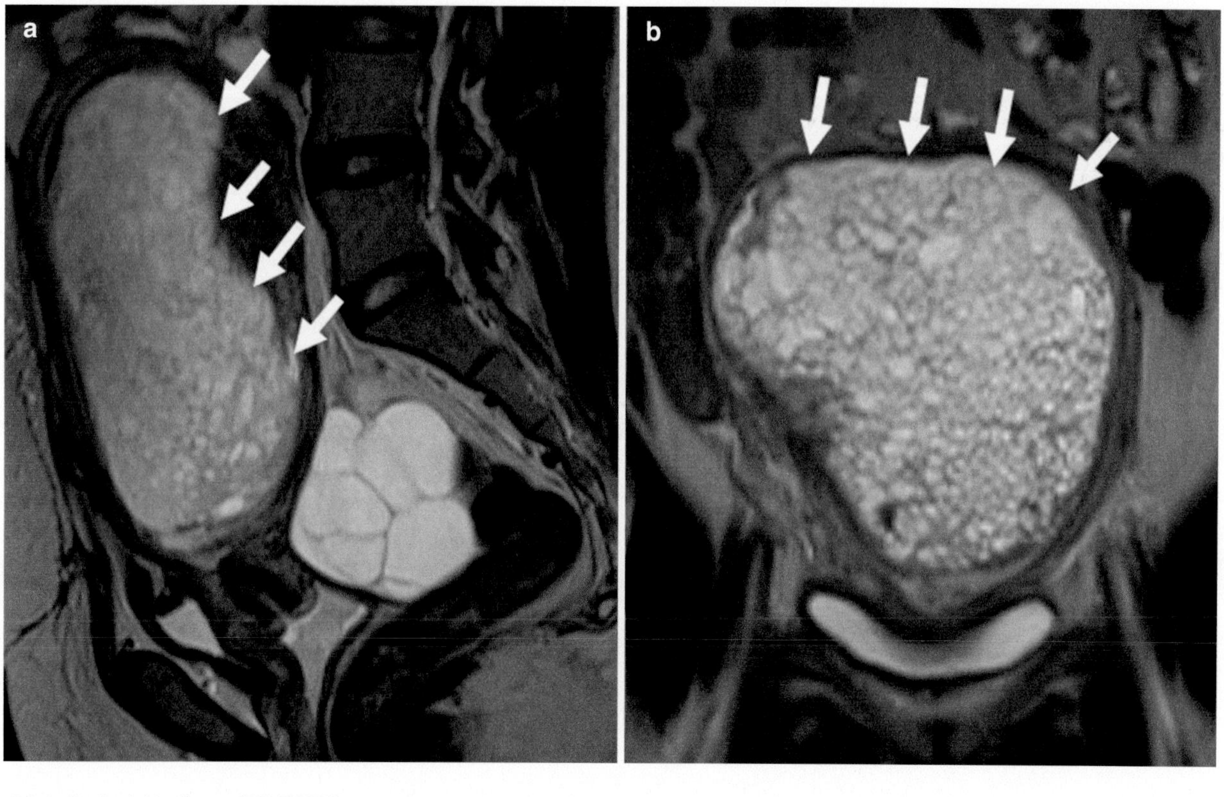

Fig. 16.6 Sagittal (**a**), Coronal (**b**) T2W images show multloculated cystic lesions (arrows) within the enlarged uterus suggesting hydatiform mole

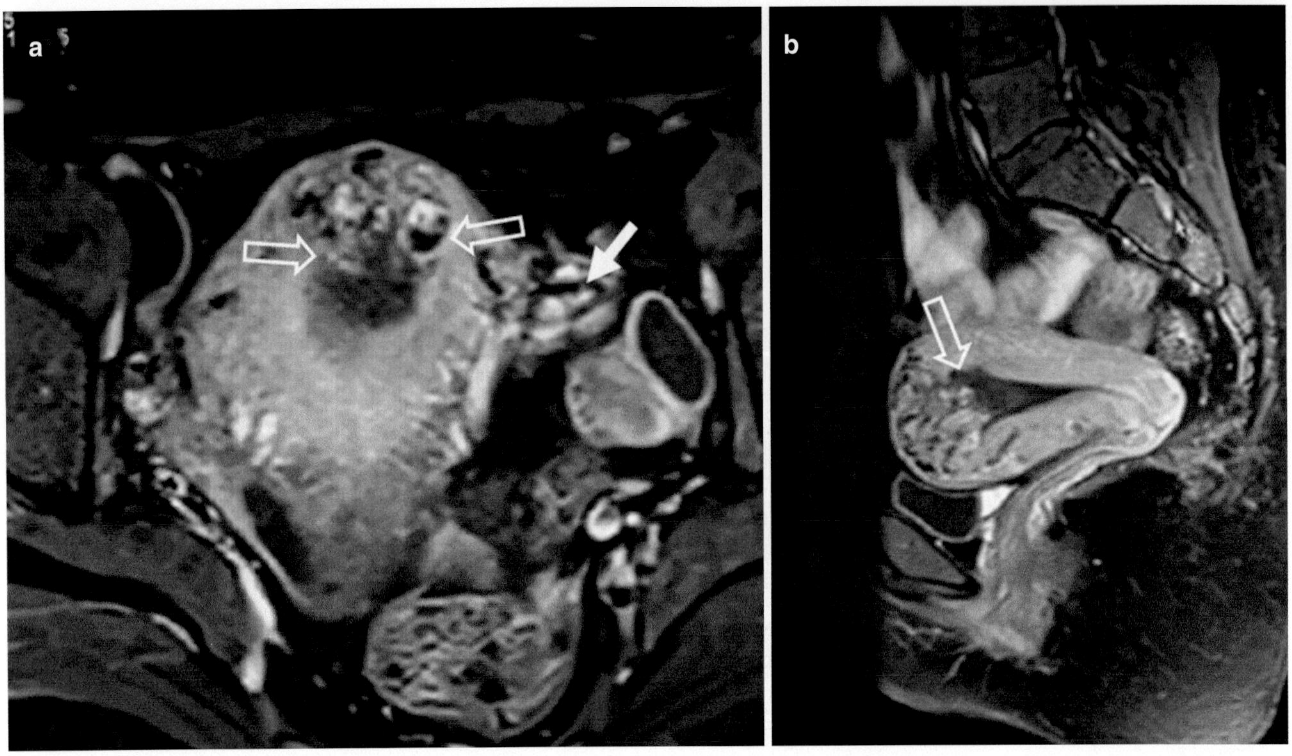

Fig. 16.7 Axial (**a**) and Sagittal (**b**), post-contrast T1 fat-suppressed images show a heterogeneously enhancing mass lesion in the endometrial cavity (open arrows) invading into the fundal myometrium suggesting Choriocarcinoma. Associated multiple flow voids are also seen (arrow)

- Extrauterine extensions when present, can be identified by MRI [11].
- These lesions show strong contrast enhancement.
- Multiple flow voids may be visualized due to hypervascularity of the lesion.

Placental Variants Include Bilobed placenta, Circumvallate placenta, succenturiate placenta, and Battledore placenta (Marginal cord insertion) [12].

MRI is rarely indicated because of poor window or sonologically "difficult" placental position.

Bilobed placenta

- Two equal-sized lobes are present separated by a membrane (Fig. 16.8).
- Umbilical cord may show insertion in either lobe or may be inserted in between the lobes.
- Can be associated with 1st trimester bleeding, abruption, and retained placenta

Succenturiate placenta

- One or more small accessory lobes are present.
- May have connecting vessels and membranes with the main placenta
- Complications—vaginal bleeding and retained placenta

Circumvallate placenta

- Annular-shaped placenta with thickened edges
- Large vessels terminate at the margin abruptly
- Complications—vaginal bleeding, placental abruption, premature rupture of the membranes (PROM) and placental insufficiency,

Battledore placenta

- Umbilical cord is inserted at or near the placental margin rather than in the center
- Complications—preterm labor, intrauterine growth restriction, and fetal distress

Placental Tumors

Placental chorioangioma—benign vascular tumor of placental origin

- *T1*: isointense to placenta, hyperintense in case of intratumoral hemorrhage
- *T2*: hyperintense similar to that of hemangioma, sometimes heterogeneous [13].
- May be multiple-chorioangiomatosis

Placental tertoma:

- Benign heterogeneous mass and may contain fat

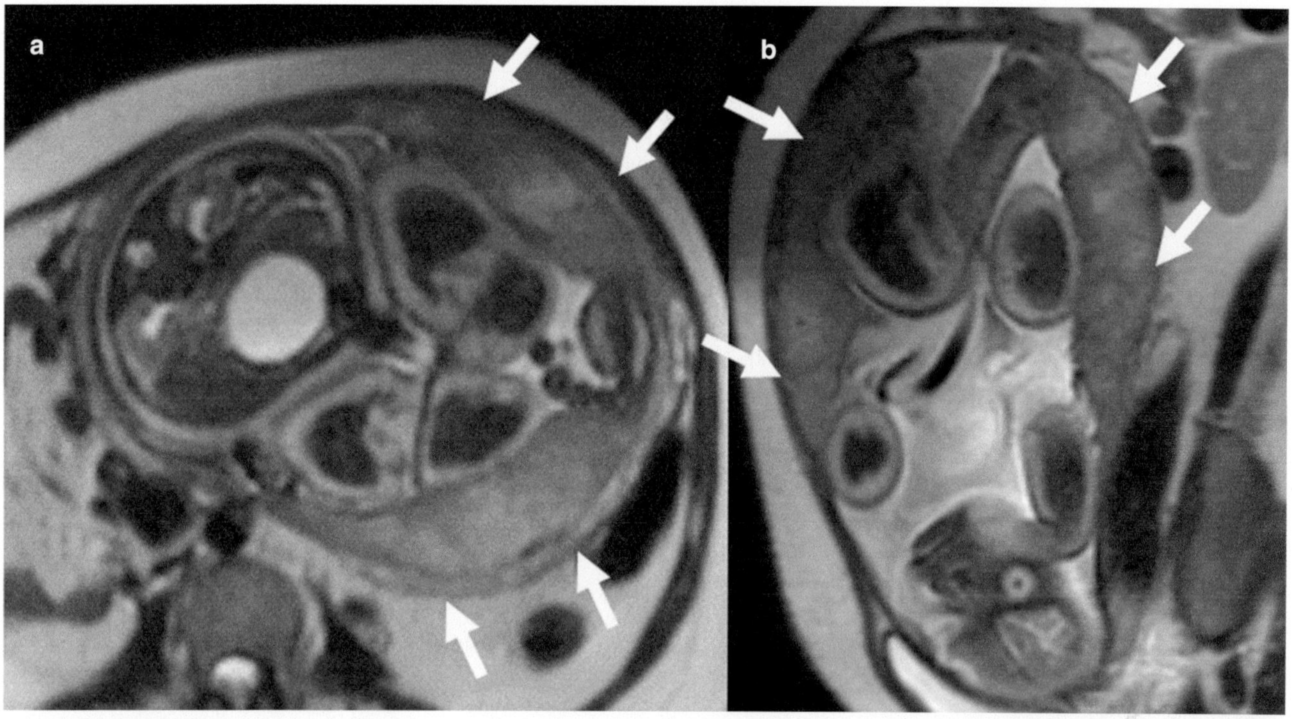

Fig. 16.8 Axial (**a**), Sagittal (**b**) T2W images showing a Bilobed placenta—along left anterolateral and posterolateral aspects of the uterus (arrow)

Placenta Praevia It is almost always diagnosed on trans abdominal/transvaginal ultrasound. Placenta is seen covering the internal os partially or completely (Fig. 16.9). In cases of posterior placenta praevia with maternal obesity or fetal cranial shadowing, MRI is preferred to obtain maximum findings. MR imaging can show the exact dimensions of the placenta that crosses the internal os.

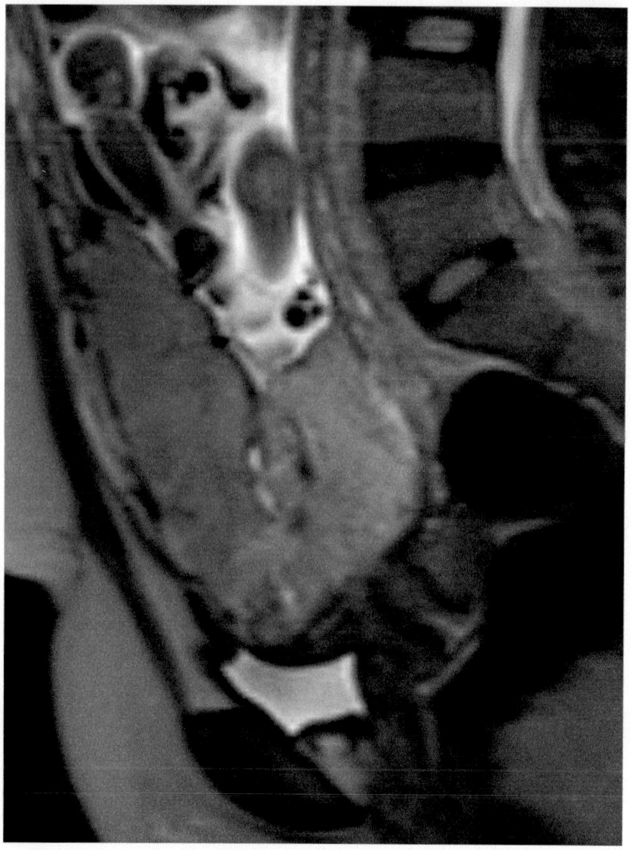

Fig. 16.9 Sagittal T2W image shows placenta completely covering the internal os suggesting placenta praevia

Ectopic Pregnancy (EP)

Ectopic pregnancy is a condition where the fertilized ovum gets implanted outside the uterine endometrium. Tubal pregnancy, occurring in the ampulla is the commonest site for ectopic pregnancy. Other sites of EP are tubal (isthmal, fimbrial), ovaries, peritoneal cavity, omentum, and intra-uterine sites like uterine interstitial, cornual, cervix, and cesarean scar [14, 15]. Transvaginal ultrasound in conjunction with clinical and laboratory data is sufficient for making an accurate diagnosis in most of the cases.

Imaging Features

- Advantage of MRI over TVS is identification of blood within the wall of GS which is diagnostic (Fig. 16.10a–d) [16].
- Empty uterine cavity with no intrauterine gestational sac (GS)
- Extra-uterine gestational sac with embryo and yolk sac within/Extra-uterine heterogenous mass with hemorrhage

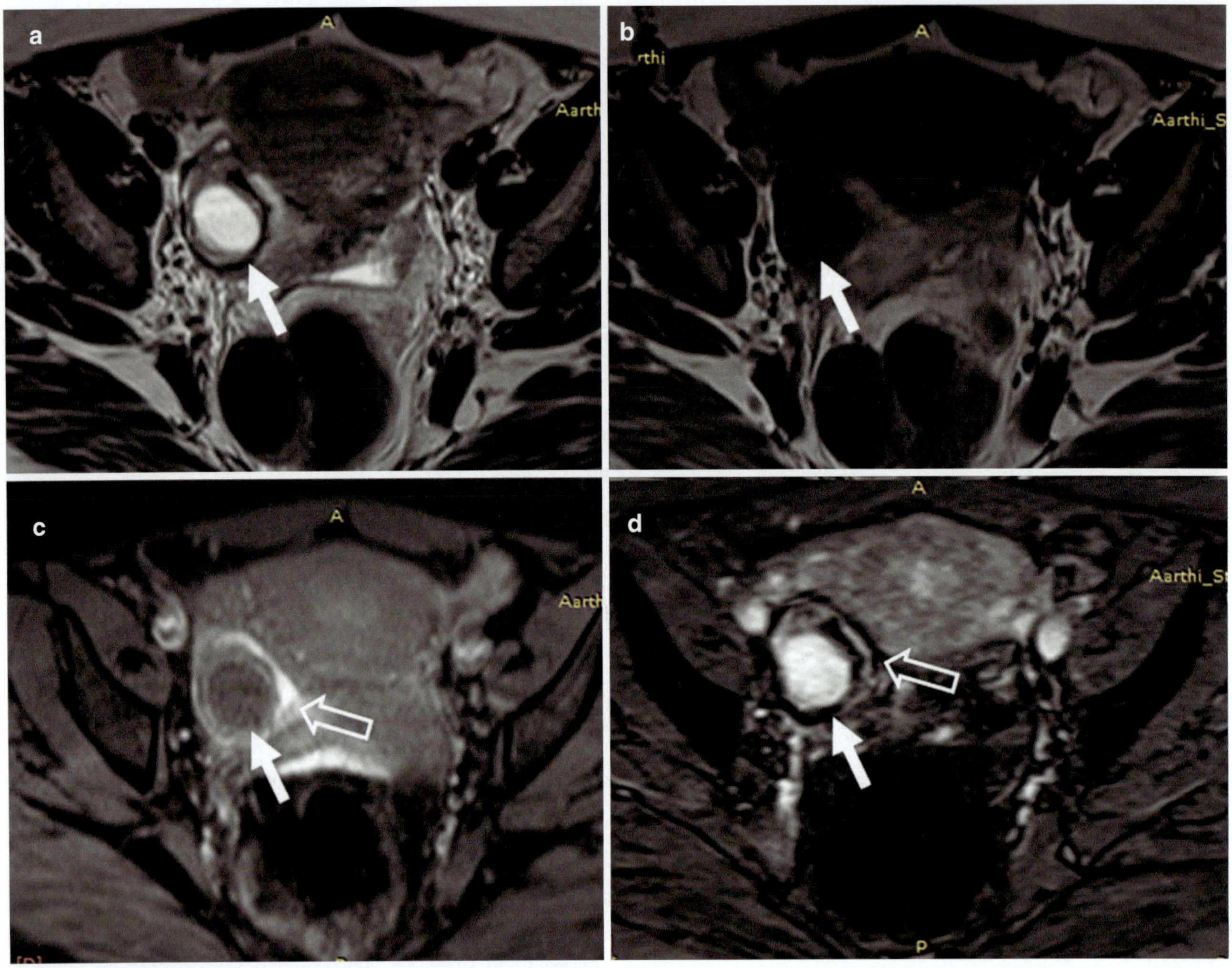

Fig. 16.10 Axial T2 (**a**), axial T1 (**b**), axial T1 FS (**c**) and axial GRE (**d**) images of a pregnancy positive patient who presented with abdominal pain show a complex right adnexal mass with cystic (gestational sac) (arrows) and hemorrhagic components (open arrows) suggesting ectopic pregnancy that was confirmed on surgery. Hemorrhage is also seen in the POD

- GS is seen as a cystic structure with low signal intensity in its wall on T2WI/GRE images [17, 18]
- Thickened endometrium
- Free fluid or hemoperitoneum in the pelvis (Fig. 16.10c, d)

Differential Diagnosis Hydrosalphinx/Corpus luteal cyst—does not show hemorrhage along the wall.

Ectopic Pregnancy in Unusual Intra-uterine Sites
MRI is complementary to TVS in confirming the diagnosis as some of these conditions may be ambiguous on TVS.

Angular pregnancy refers to implantation of fertilized ovum in the endometrium medial to the utero tubal junction (Fig. 16.11). These pregnancies can be treated conservatively as the GS may later reach the uterine cavity.

Interstitial pregnancy—GS is seen within the interstitial segment of the fallopian tube (in the lateral angle of uterine fundus) (Fig. 16.12) and is surrounded by myometrium of less than 5 mm thickness. It is more prone for uterine rupture and hemorrhage and has to be differentiated from angular pregnancy [18]. MRI is useful in demonstrating an intact junctional zone between the gestational sac and the uterine cavity (Fig. 16.12) thereby suggesting an interstitial location.

Scar pregnancy—refers to implantation of fertilized ovum over the fibrous scar of previous cesarean section or other uterine surgeries. MRI shows thinned out myometrium between GS and urinary bladder (Fig. 16.13). In addition, MRI is also useful in evaluating any bladder invasion [19].

Differential Diagnosis Cervical pregnancy, miscarriage in progress.

MR also helps in differentiating a miscarriage in progress and cervical ectopic pregnancy from a scar pregnancy. In the first two conditions, the GS is centered within the endocervical canal and the overlying anterior myometrium is of normal thickness.

Cornual Pregnancy—refers to implantation of a fertilized ovum in a rudimentary uterine horn, unicornuate uterus, cornual region of bicornuate/septate uterus/uterus didelphis.

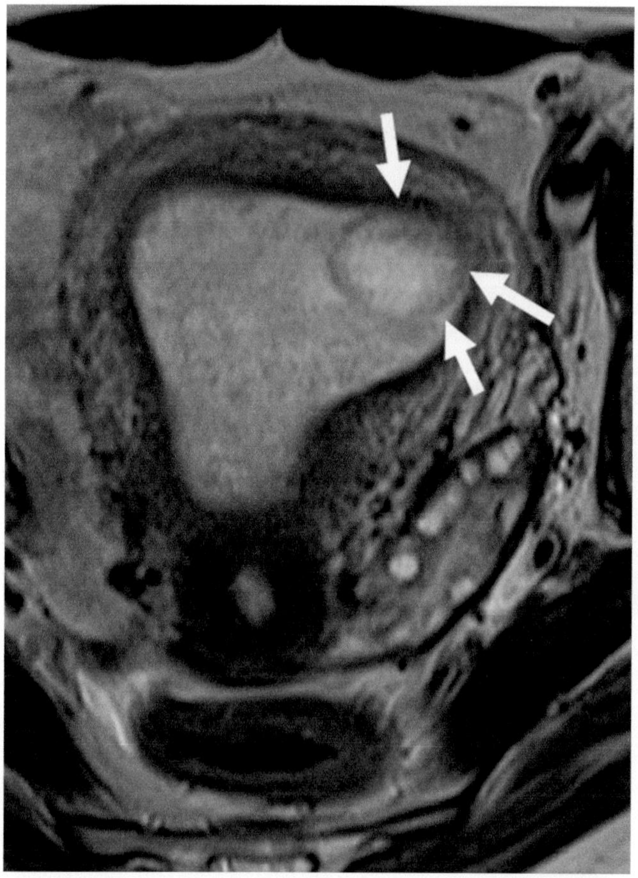

Fig. 16.11 Coronal T2W image showing gestational sac on the left superolateral aspect of the uterus (arrows)

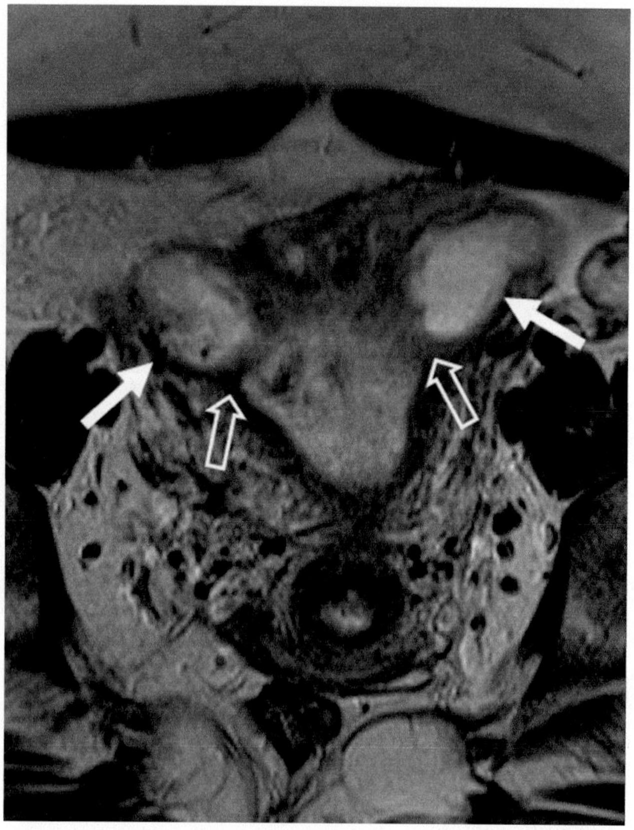

Fig. 16.12 Coronal T2 weighted image showing two gestational sacs, one in each cornu (arrows) and lateral to the uterotubal junctions (open arrows)—bilateral interstitial pregnancy

Sonographically cornual pregnancy may be misinterpreted as tubal ectopic pregnancy or a normal intrauterine pregnancy. On MRI, cornual pregnancy appears as a GS surrounded by a wall which is isointense to normal myometrium in all pulse sequences.

MRI is also useful in distinguishing a bicornuate uterus from septate uterus and in evaluating the nature of the septum, whether fibrous/muscular.

Abdominal pregnancy—MRI shows an extrauterine fetus and placenta. The uterus is seen separately. Severe bleeding is a dreadful complication and accurate diagnosis is possible with MRI.

Uterine Pathologies

Red degeneration in uterine fibroid

It is the most common degeneration occurring during pregnancy in a fibroid and patient may present with acute abdominal pain.

Draining vein of fibroid is obstructed leading to hemorrhagic infarction and may be demonstrated by MRI [20, 21].

- Peripheral (rim) or diffuse of hyperintensity within the fibroid may be visualized on T1 weighted images.
- Presence of hemorrhagic products in the fibroid (Fig. 16.14) is pathognomonic of red degeneration.

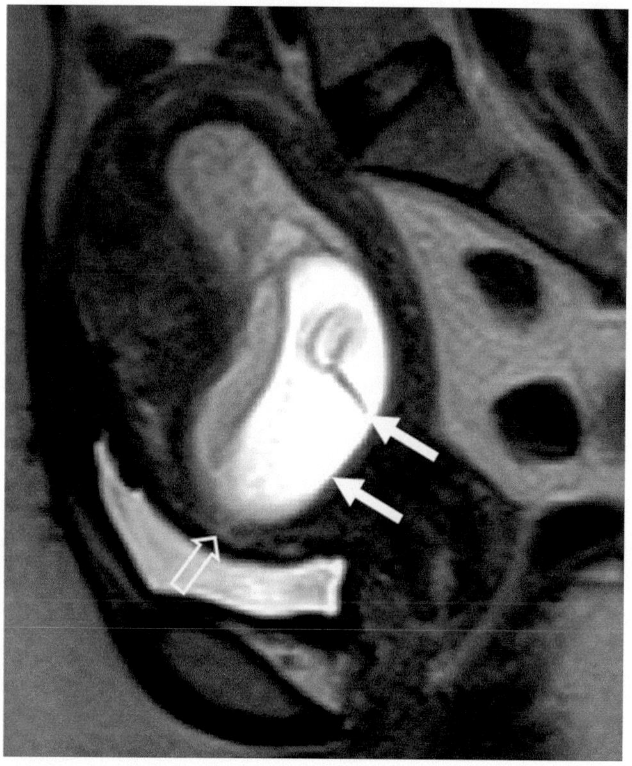

Fig. 16.13 Sagittal T2W image showing gestational sac along the lower uterine segment scar (arrows). The overlying myometrium shows thinning

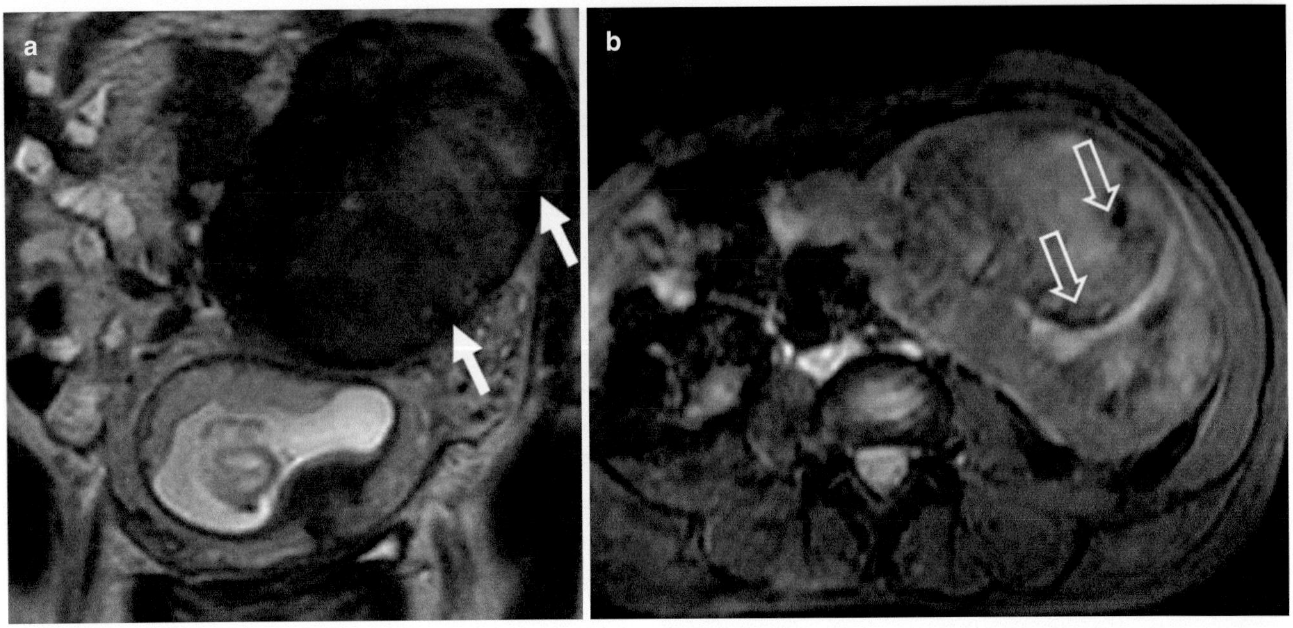

Fig. 16.14 Coronal (**a**) T2W image of a pregnant woman who presented with abdominal pain shows a large sub-serosal fibroid in the fundus (arrows) Axial gradient image (**b**) shows areas of hemorrhage within (open arrows) suggesting red degeneration. The patient was treated conservatively and myomectomy was performed after delivery

Uterine rupture

Uterine rupture is defined as a full-thickness tear of uterus and its covering visceral peritoneum [17].

- MRI is useful to show the exact site of uterine disruption (Fig. 16.15) when it is not properly demonstrated on USG.
- Hemoperitoneum
- MRI is recommended only when the patient is hemodynamically stable.

Ovarian Pathologies

MRI is useful in the assessment of ovarian masses, ovarian torsion, and hemorrhagic cysts.

Ovarian torsion

- Enlarged ovaries with hemorrhage/stromal edema (Fig. 16.16)
- Twisting and thickening of the pedicle (>10 mm) [17]
- Free fluid in the pelvis
- Absence of post-Gd enhancement

Obstetric MR Pelvimety MRI data such as obstetric conjugate, interspinous distance, intertuberous distance, transverse diameter, and sagittal outlet diameter are useful in cases of suspected cephalo pelvic disproportion and to decide the mode of fetal delivery [22].

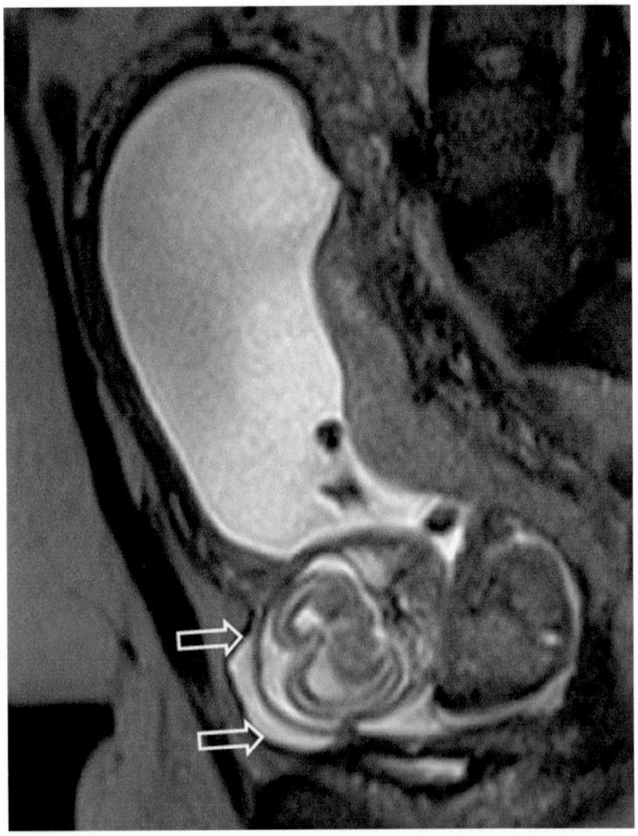

Fig. 16.15 Sagittal T2W image shows myometrial thinning with focal bulge in the anteroinferior aspect of the uterus, in the region of the previous cesarean scar suggesting incomplete uterine rupture (open arrows)

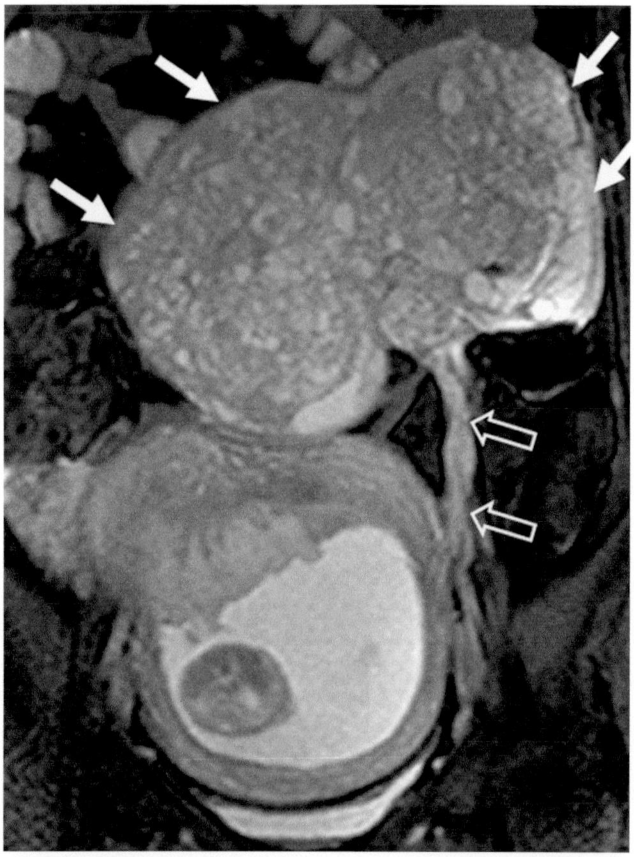

Fig. 16.16 22-year-old pregnant woman presenting with abdominal pain. Coronal TRUFI FS image shows a left ovarian mass (arrows) with twisted pedicle (open arrows) suggesting torsion. The mass was excised and HPE revealed ovarian immature teratoma with changes secondary to torsion

Postpartum Complications

Abscess/hematoma: MR is useful in demonstrating *abscess/ hematoma* formation in the various layers of the anterior abdominal wall, peritoneum, uterus following Cesarean section/uterine surgeries. Abscess appears hypointense on T1, hyperintense on T2 (Fig. 16.17) and shows diffusion restriction. Hematoma shows variable appearance on T1 and T2 WI depending on the stage; however, blooming may be seen on gradient images.

Puerperal ovarian vein thrombosis is rare and the patient presents with lower abdominal pain [23]. One of the serious complications is septic pulmonary embolism. MRI especially Contrast-enhanced dynamic MR venography is useful to demonstrate the thrombosed ovarian.

Uterine arteriovenous malformation may be of the congenital or acquired types [23]. The acquired type is often associated with obstetric disorders or procedures such as multiple pregnancies, abortions, cesarean section, and dilation and curettage. Multiple serpiginous flow-voids are visualized in the uterine wall, parametrium, and endometrial cavity on T1 and T2 weighted images (Fig. 16.18a–c) Contrast-enhanced dynamic MR angiography is useful in depicting the feeding vessel, nidus, complex tuft of vessels, and draining vein (Fig. 16.18d). This information can be used to plan transcatheter embolization.

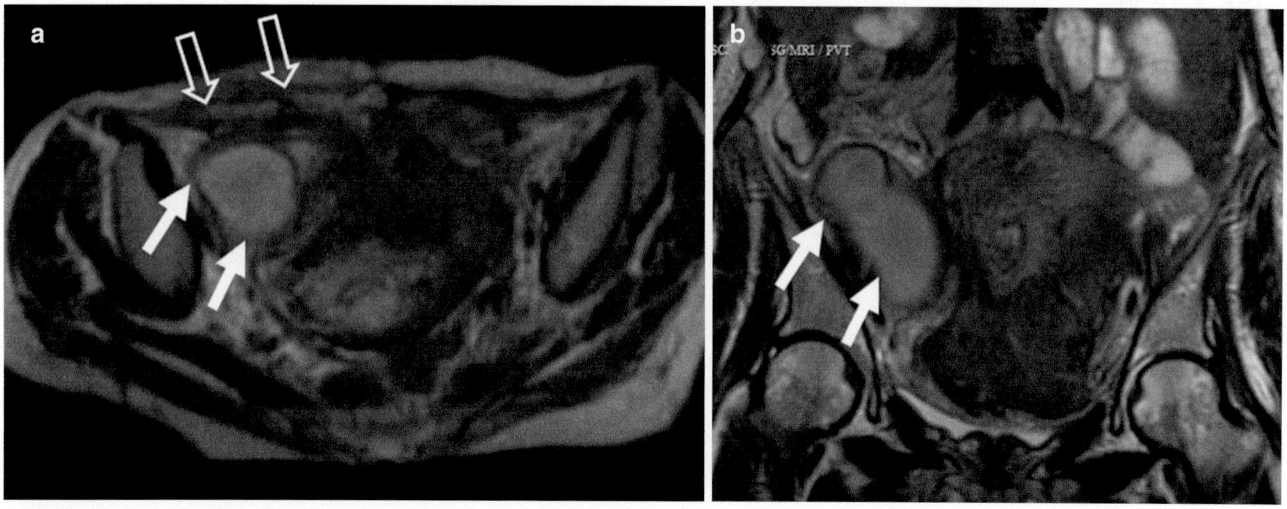

Fig. 16.17 Axial (**a**) and Coronal (**b**) T2W images, Post-LSCS shows an abscess in the right iliac region (arrow), draining through a tract along the right side of the Pfannenstiel incision (open arrows)

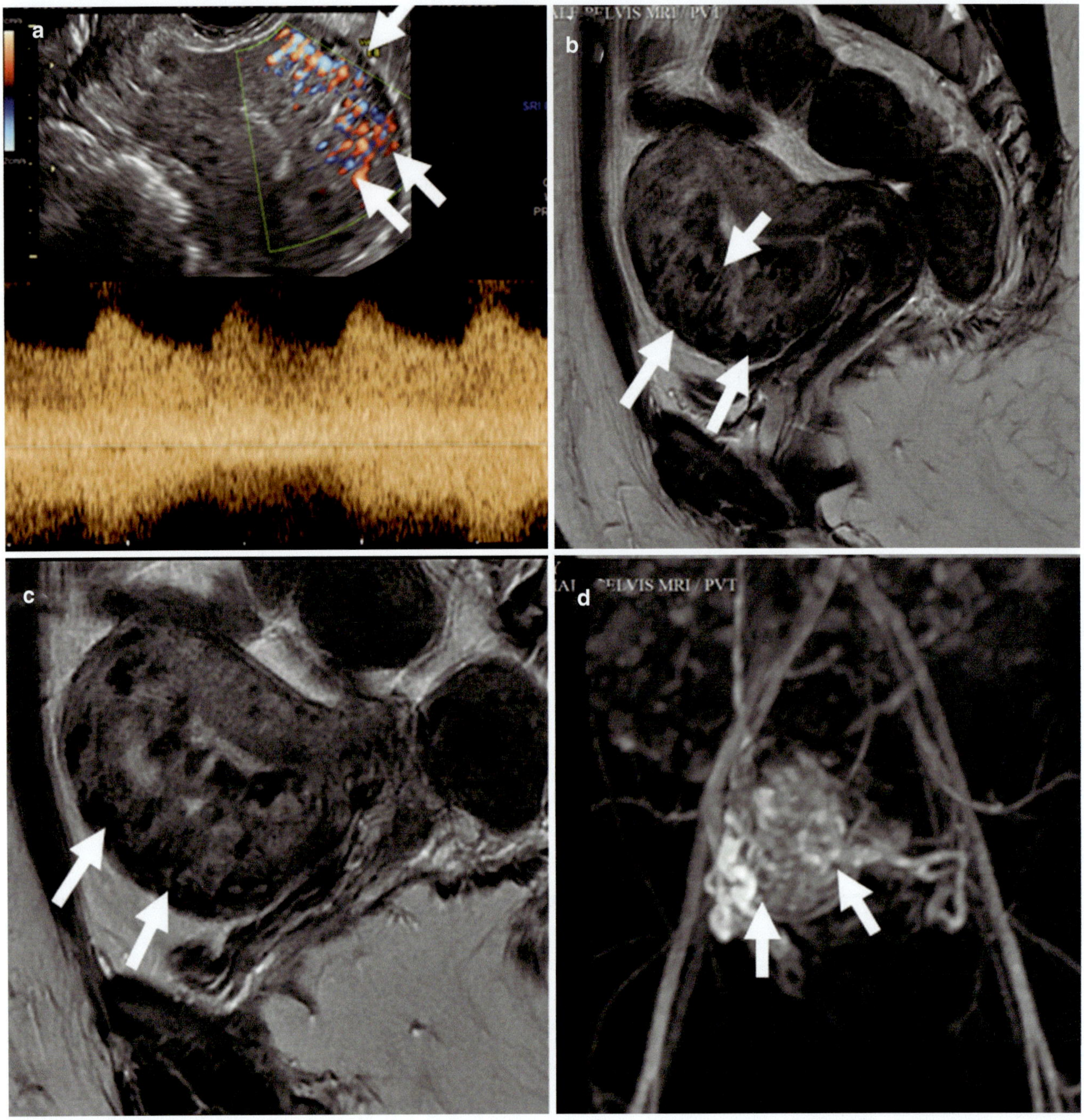

Fig. 16.18 Color Doppler (**a**) for history of bleeding following Medical Termination of Pregnancy reveals increased vascularity in the anterior myometrium. Sagittal T2W (**b**, **c**) images show multiple serpentine T2 flow voids within the anterior myometrium. MR angiography (**d**) confirms uterine Arteriovenous malformation (arrow) predominantly involving the anterior myometrium with feeders arising from bilateral uterine arteries ($R > L$)

References

1. Riteau A, Tassin M, Chambon G, et al. Accuracy of ultrasonography and magnetic resonance imaging in the diagnosis of placenta accreta. PLoS One. 2014;9:e94866.
2. Yoshigi J, Yashiro N, Kinoshita T. Diagnosis of ectopic pregnancy with MRI: efficacy of T2 weighted imaging. Magn Reson Med Sci. 2006;5:25–32.
3. Christopher Baughman W, Corteville JE, Shah RR. Placenta accreta: spectrum of US and MR imaging findings. Radiographics. 2008;28:1905–16.
4. Varghese B, Singh N, George RAN, et al. Magnetic resonance imaging of placenta accreta. Indian J Radiol Imag. 2013;23:379–85.
5. Mahalingam HV, Rangasami R, Premkumar J, et al. Placenta accreta scoring system (PASS)—assessment of a simplified clinico-radiological scoring system for antenatal diagnosis of placenta accreta. Egypt J Radiol Nucl Med. 2021;52:42. https://doi.org/10.1186/s43055-021-00427-y.
6. Nagenthran G, Rangasami R, Chandrasekharan A, et al. Role of magnetic resonance imaging in pregnancy-associated obstetric and gynecological complications. Egypt J Radiol Nucl Med. 2019;50:98. https://doi.org/10.1186/s43055-019-0112-x.
7. Millischer AE, Deloison B, Silvera S, Ville Y, Boddaert N, Balvay D, et al. Dynamic contrast enhanced MRI of the placenta: A tool for prenatal diagnosis of placenta accreta? Placenta. 2017;53:40–7.
8. Bailit JL, Grobman WA, Rice MM, et al. Eunice Kennedy Shriver National Institute of Child Health and Human Development (NICHD) Maternal-Fetal Medicine Units (MFMU) Network. Morbidly adherent placenta treatments and outcomes. Obstet Gynecol. 2015;125(3):683–9.
9. Silver RM, Fox KA, Barton JR, et al. Center of excellence for placenta accreta. Am J Obstet Gynecol. 2015;212(5):561–8.
10. Masselli G, Brunelli R, Di Tola M, et al. MR imaging in the evaluation of placental abruption: correlation with sonographic findings. Radiology. 2011;259:222–30.
11. Shaaban AM, Rezvani M, Haroun RR, et al. Gestational trophoblastic disease: clinical and imaging features. Radiographics. 2017;37:681–700.
12. Rathbun KM, Hildebrand JP. Placenta abnormalities. In: StatPearls. Treasure Island, FL: StatPearls Publishing; 2018.
13. Kirkpatrick AD, Podberesky DJ, Gray AE, et al. Best cases from the AFIP: placental chorioangioma. Radiographics. 27(4):1187–90.
14. Priya M, Rajeswaran R, Anupama C, Chitra A. Role of MRI in the localisation of uncommon forms of ectopic pregnancies. Int J Contemp Med Res. 2017;4:1898–901.
15. Tamai K, Koyama T, Togashi K. MR features of ectopic pregnancy. Eur Radiol. 2007;17:3236–46.
16. Parker RA, Yano M, Tai AW, Friedman M, Narra VR, Menias CO. MR imaging findings of ectopic pregnancy: a pictorial review. Radiographics. 2012;32:12–5.
17. Gupta R, Bajaj SK, Kumar N, et al. Magnetic resonance imaging—a troubleshooter in obstetric emergencies: a pictorial review. Indian J Radiol Imaging. 2016;26:44–51.
18. Smith F, Adam A, Phillips W. NMR imaging in pregnancy. Lancet. 1983;1:61–2.
19. Ash A, Smith A, Maxwell D. Caesarean scar pregnancy. BJOG. 2007;114:253–63.
20. Radhika BH, Naik K, Shreelatha S, Vana H. Case series: pregnancy outcome in patients with uterine fibroids. J Clin Diagn Res. 2015;9:QR01–4.
21. Wilde S, Scott-Barrett S. Radiological appearances of uterine fibroids. Indian J Radiol Imaging. 2009;19:222–31.
22. Keller TM, Rake A, Michel SCA, Selfert B, Efe C, Treiber K, et al. Obstetric MR pelvimetry: reference values and evaluation of inter- and intraobserver error and intraindividual variability. Radiology. 2003;227:37–43.
23. Nagayama M, Watanabe Y, Okumura A, Amoh Y, Nakashita S, Dodo Y. Fast MR imaging in obstetrics. Radiographics. 2002;22:563–82.

MIX
Papier aus verantwortungsvollen Quellen
Paper from responsible sources
FSC® C105338

If you have any concerns about our products,
you can contact us on
ProductSafety@springernature.com

In case Publisher is established outside the EU,
the EU authorized representative is:
Springer Nature Customer Service Center GmbH
Europaplatz 3, 69115 Heidelberg, Germany

Printed by Libri Plureos GmbH
in Hamburg, Germany